THE

S/NVQ Level 3
Health Award
For Health Care Assistants

Julia Watling   Alexandra Boyle
Julie Boyd   Jane Fraser   Wendy Flynn
Nicki Pritchatt   Yvonne Nolan

www.heinemann.co.uk

ort
nks
ing

0

Heinemann

Heinemann is an imprint of Pearson Education Limited, a company incorporated in England and Wales, having its registered office at Edinburgh Gate, Harlow, Essex, CM20 2JE. Registered company number: 872828

www.heinemann.co.uk

Heinemann is a registered trademark of Pearson Education Limited

First published 2008

12 11 10 09 08
10 9 8 7 6 5 4 3 2 1

British Library Cataloguing in Publication Data is available from the British Library on request.

ISBN: 978 0 435 402 41 9

Edited by Sarah Christopher
Designed by Tony Richardson
Typeset by 𝗧\ Tek-Art, Crawley Down, West Sussex
Illustrated by 𝗧\ Tek-Art
Original illustrations © Pearson Education Limited, 2008
Picture research by Caitlin Swain
Cover design by Pearson
Cover photo/illustration © Digital Stock; © Getty Images/PhotoDisc; © Image Source; © iStockphoto/Christine Balderas; © iStockphoto/Maciej Bogacz; © iStockphoto/Michael Riccio; © Pearson Education/Jules Selmes; © Pearson Education/MM Studios; © Pearson Education/Tudor Photography; © PhotoDisc; © PhotoDisc/Arthur S. Aubrey; © PhotoDisc/Steve Cole; © PhotoDisc/Lawrence Lawry; © PhotoDisc/Jim Wehtje
Printed in China (CTPS/01)

Acknowledgements

Every effort has been made to contact copyright holders of material reproduced in this book. Any omissions will be rectified in subsequent printings if notice is given to the publishers.

Norfolk and Norwich University Hospital NHS Trust
Jenny Chen and colleagues of Bath Royal United Hospitals Trust
Hilary Whyatt of South Manchester Universities Hospital Trust

Photo acknowledgements

The authors and publisher would like to thank the following for permission to reproduce photographs:
© Alamy Images/Mediscan page 301; © ConvaTec page 278; © Digital Vision/Rob van Petten page 226; © ERRG Photography/Alamy page 312; © Eyewire page 226; © Getty Images/Chris Baker page 75; © Getty Images UK/Thinkstock page 226; © Harcourt Education/Jules Selmes page 76; © Helen King/CORBIS page 58; © iStockPhoto/Daniel Fascia page 309; © iStockPhoto/Maartje van Caspel page 138; © iStockPhoto/Michael Riccio, © iStockphoto/Christine Balderas, © iStockphoto/Maciej Bogacz, front cover; © KPT Power Photos page 226; © Louise Murray/Science Photo Library page 272; © Dr P. Marazzi/Science Photo Library pages 138, 258, 259, 273, 276, 278, 279; © MedicBeds page 249; © Pearson Education Ltd page 19; © Pearson Education Ltd/Gareth Boden page 226; © Pearson Education/Jules Selmes pages 25, 33, 57, 60, 61, 144; ©Pearson Education Ltd/ Lord & Leverett pages 2, 12, 83, 101, 104, 129, 229; © Pearson Education Ltd/Mind Studio pages, 6, 44, 86, 88, 94, 144, 146, 147, 142, 152, 154, 162, 163, 173, 237, 283, 287, 289, 320, 324, 325, 330, 334, 336; © Pearson Education Ltd/Richard Smith pages 46, 55; © Pearson Education Ltd/Studio 8 pages 77, 160; © Pearson Education Ltd/Tudor Photography page 11; © PhotoDisc page 231; © PhotoDisc, ©Pearson Education Ltd/ Jules Selmes, © Pearson Education Ltd/Jules Selmes , front cover; © Photofusion page 118; © rcsed.ac.uk pages 273, 278; © Richard Smith pages 245, 298, 300; © Richard Smith/Pearson Education Ltd page 64; © R. P. R. Groenedijk/Surgical-Tutor.org.uk page 276; © Sinclair Stammers/ Science Photo Library page 139; © St. Mary's Hospital Medical School/Science Photo Library page 139; © Volker Steger/Science Photo Library page 280; © Westholme page 250

Contents

Introduction

The health sector is undergoing some of the biggest and most far reaching changes since it was created in 1948. The changing role of the nurse, and more recently, the healthcare assistant are central to these changes. The requirement placed upon employers to ensure that their healthcare assistants are trained to at least National Vocational Qualification (NVQ) level 2, alongside calls to establish a central register of all trained healthcare assistants with a Code of Practice, is indicative of the growing role of healthcare assistant in the healthcare sector alongside nurses.

Since the creation of the health sector in 1948 we have seen numerous advances in medical sciences each ushering in advances in the diagnosis and treatment of a range of illnesses. Arising from these changes we have witnessed the growth of 'specialism's' in health care amongst all professions in the healthcare sector. In his report *Health Care for London* (July 2007) and the later report *Our NHS Our future: Next Stage Review* (Department of Health, October 2007) Professor Lord Darzi presents the case to continue this process of change and the increased use of specialisms to provide healthcare.

This book is a response to these changes taking place across the healthcare sector. The revised NVQ award with its different health pathways reflects some of these changes and the advancing roles not only of the healthcare assistant but also those supporting midwives, physiotherapists and occupational therapists, radiographers and those working within operating theatres.

Healthcare assistants have always been key members of the nursing team, but in recent years their role has begun to evolve and extend. In addition to the more traditional tasks such as personal care and assisting with meals, healthcare assistants now undertake some procedures previously undertaken by qualified nurses. Trained healthcare assistants now take and record observations; they undertake blood glucose and venous sampling procedures, perform wound care and carry out electrocardiograms.

In addition, some trusts are creating the band 4 'assistant practitioner' for those healthcare assistants in more advanced roles and as a result, healthcare assistants are required to provide evidence of undertaking further training, usually in the form of a National Vocational Qualification. Such a qualification provides an opportunity for the care worker to demonstrate they not only have the practical skills required, but also the knowledge and understanding which underpins their practice. The Health Award provides flexible pathways of achievement which can be tailored to meet individual need as well as the needs of employing organisations to provide competency based accreditation which can be used for continuous professional development, acquisition of an S/NVQ qualification and career progression.

Not everyone reading this book will be undertaking a qualification: some will use it for reference or to keep up to date with current practice. We hope that the reflections aspect will help you to think about, reflect upon and help you to develop your practice.

Following the revised NVQ in Health and Social Care award in 2005 the new Health Pathways came into place in 2006. The revised NVQ Level 3 health qualification consists of a combination of both core, optional, and pathway specific units. A total of ten units must be completed. This book will introduce you to the knowledge base needed to complete the core units and some of the more popular clinical units needed for your award.

Each NVQ unit is incorporates the following features:

Introduction – an introduction to the unit and how it links to the NHS Knowledge and Skills Framework.

How to generate evidence – different methods to demonstrate competence, for example direct observation by your assessor, question and answer and reflective accounts of your actions in the workplace – what you did and why you did it this way.

Evidence in action – by answering these questions you will be able to provide the knowledge evidence for the numbered questions and generate some of the evidence for your portfolio.

Reflections – if you consider the reflections, think about your practice and how you might do things differently on another occasion. This may generate evidence for the core unit HSC 33: Reflect on and develop your practice.

Memory joggers – are a feature that will remind you to look at NVQ units you have already covered to see if you might have already generated evidence in a previous unit. This feature will also help you to take a holistic approach to your NVQ and perhaps avoid you having to repeatedly provide the same evidence.

You will find that this book closely follows the structure of the NVQ. As an adult learner your time is precious so all of the activities are designed to generate evidence for your portfolio.

We wish you good luck in your studies and the development of your practice. Working within the health sector can be challenging but very rewarding. We hope you enjoy the book and put it to good use as you continue to develop your professional skills, knowledge and competence within an ever changing profession.

How to use this book

How to use this book

The book covers core underpinning knowledge for the level 3 award, accompanied by a range of popular option units. A particular feature of the book is the emphasis on assessment: portfolio activities and underpinning knowledge are referenced to the qualification to make planning your assessment simple and holistic. Look out for the following special features as you work through the book.

Knowledge specifications

The main headings in each unit link to the knowledge specifications of the S/NVQ elements, helping you develop the knowledge and understanding required for the qualification.

(KS 1, 2, 3, 4, 5, 8, 9, 10, 15)

Performance criteria

Highlighted against the evidence you need to collect and show to help identify the skills you need for the qualification.

HSC 31 Identify ways to communicate effectively

Reflect

Reflection is a core tool for health care assistants. This feature will enable you to carefully assess your practice and its implications for service users, colleagues and your working environment.

Activity

These practical activities test your understanding and give you opportunities to apply your knowledge and skills.

Case study

Realistic and diverse stories that you can relate to and learn from, with thought-provoking questions at the end.

Evidence through reflection / Evidence in action / Evidence with a case study

These features show what you can do to collect evidence for your portfolio, in the form of 'Reflect' 'Case study' or 'Activity' features like those above.

Evidence through reflection

Evidence in action

Evidence with a case study

Memory jogger

This will remind you if you already have plenty of evidence or prior learning from other units.

Key terms

Clear definitions of words and phrases you need to know.

Test yourself

Questions to test your knowledge.

Remember

Reminders of important information.

Best practice

Summary lists and reminders to ensure best practice.

Did you know?

Additional information to illustrate points covered in the unit.

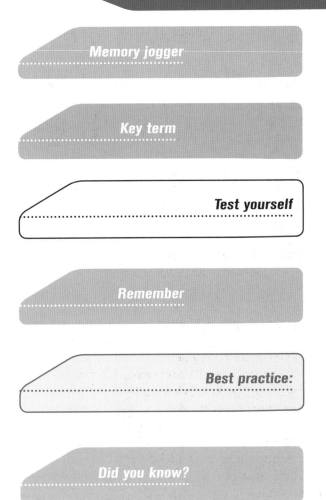

Checklist

Reminder lists or step-by-step instructions to help you cover every point during procedures.

References and further reading

Recommended books, journals and websites to develop your knowledge on subjects covered in the unit.

Legislation grid

The legislation grid on page 000 will help you to ensure you are learning all that you need for the level 3 award.

Knowledge Specification Framework grid

You will find a grid detailing coverage of the knowledge specification points on page 000.

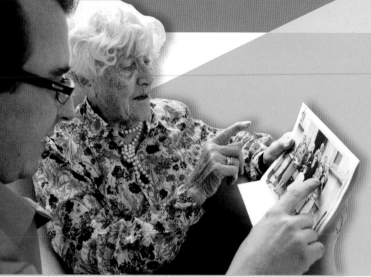

Promote effective communication for and about individuals

Introduction

Communication is all about the way people reach out to one another. It is an essential part of all relationships, and the ability to communicate well with patients, colleagues and others is a basic requirement for doing your job.

Communication is not just talking – we use touch, facial expressions and body movements when we are communicating with people personally, and there are many means of written and electronic communication in today's society.

It is important that you learn to communicate well even where there are differences in individuals' abilities and methods of communication; you will need to be able to communicate effectively on complex and sensitive issues within the hospital environment.

It is also important that you develop skills in effective listening. This is an important part of communicating; in fact, listening and communicating go hand in hand. Listening effectively to our patients enables us to meet their needs.

Recording information serves many valuable purposes. You need to understand the significance of what you record and how it is recorded, in order to be sure that you are doing the best you possibly can for the individuals you work with.

This unit will help you to understand how all of these aspects of communication can be used in order to build and develop relationships, and to improve your practice as a health care assistant.

What you need to learn

- Ways in which people communicate
- Listening effectively
- Communicating about difficult and sensitive issues
- Undertaking difficult, complex and sensitive communications
- Communication differences
- Sensory impairment
- Cultural differences
- How to find out about likely communication problems
- Ways of receiving and passing on information
- Confidentiality
- Protecting patients' personal information
- How to record information

What evidence you need to generate for your portfolio

For your award you will mainly be required to produce observations of you carrying out tasks in your workplace. Your assessor will observe you undertaking real-life activities to cover the performance criteria and scope. This can be supported by witness testimonies from colleagues who have seen you working.

In addition, you will need to demonstrate your knowledge and understanding. You can do this by providing written accounts that identify how you integrate theory with practice, and answering verbal or written questions. Communication is a core skill that will be used when carrying out most tasks so evidence can be derived in all work situations.

The knowledge specifications identified under the headers of each section are intended as a guide.

HSC 31 Identify ways to communicate effectively

Ways in which people communicate

(KS 1, 2, 3, 4, 5, 8, 9, 10, 15)

This section is about supporting people to communicate with each other. Communication is much more than talking – it is about how people respond to each other in many different ways: facial expression, body movements, dress, written communication, telephone or electronic messages.

More than talking

In order to be an effective health care assistant, you must learn to be a good communicator. You will have to know how to recognise what is being communicated to you, and be able to communicate with others without always having to use words.

Signs and signals

When we meet and talk to people, we will usually do so in two different ways: the first is spoken language and the second is **non-verbal communication** or **body language**. You may be surprised to learn that over 80 per cent of what you communicate to others is understood without you speaking a word.

> ### Key term
>
> **Non-verbal communication** or **body language** Ways of communicating without words, through positioning and posture, gestures, facial expression and eye contact.

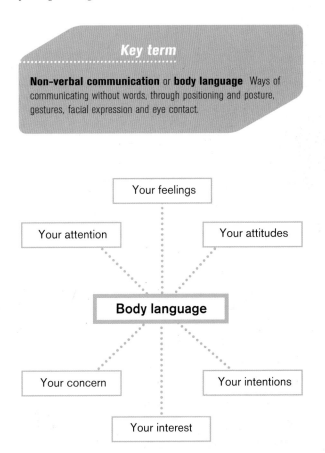

The way in which you use your body can convey messages about many things, without you even realising it.

Effective communication in care work requires the ability to analyse your own and other people's non-verbal behaviour. Some of the most important parts of the body that 'send messages' are shown above.

Research shows that people pay far more attention to facial expressions and tone of voice than they do to spoken words. For example, in one study, words contributed only 7 per cent towards the impression of whether or not someone was liked, tone of voice contributed 38 per cent and facial expression 55 per cent. The study also found that, if there was a contradiction between facial expression and words, people believed the facial expression.

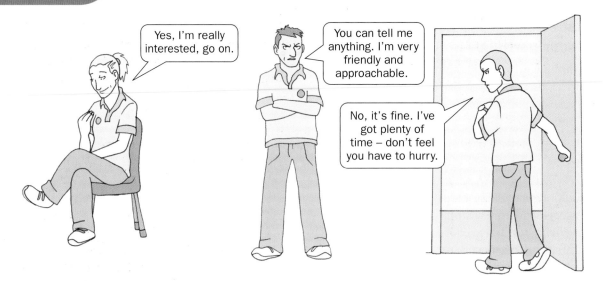

Our bodies send messages to other people – often without us meaning to send those messages.

The eyes

We can often anticipate the feelings or thoughts that another person has by looking at their eyes. We can sometimes understand the thoughts and feelings of another person by eye-to-eye contact. Our eyes get wider when we are excited, or when we are attracted to or interested in someone. A fixed stare may send the message that the person is angry. Looking away is often interpreted as showing boredom in European cultures.

The face

Faces can send very complex messages and we can read them easily – even in diagram form.

Our faces often indicate our emotional state. When a person is sad, he or she may look down, there may be tension in the face, and the mouth will be closed. The muscles in the person's shoulders are likely to be relaxed, but his or her face and neck may show tension. A happy person will have wide-open eyes that make contact with you, and will smile. When people are excited, they may move their arms and hands quickly or expansively.

Voice tone

If we talk quickly in a loud voice with a fixed tone, people may see us as angry. A calm, slow voice with varying tone may send a message of being friendly.

Body movement

The way we walk, move our heads, sit, cross our legs and so on send messages about whether we are tired, happy, sad or bored.

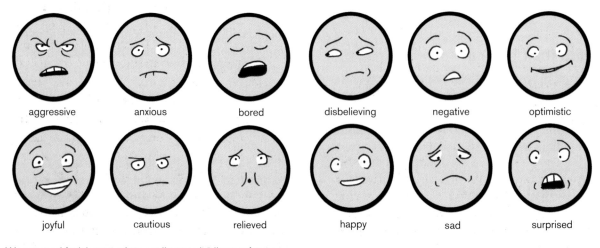

We can read facial expressions easily, even in diagram form.

Posture

Sitting with crossed arms can mean 'I'm not taking any notice'. Leaning back or to one side can send the message that you are relaxed or bored. Leaning forward can show interest.

Muscle tension

The tension in our feet, hands and fingers can tell others how relaxed or how tense we are. If people are very tense, their shoulders might stiffen, their face muscles might tighten and they might sit or stand rigidly. A tense face might have a firmly closed mouth with lips and jaws clenched tight. A tense person might breathe quickly and become hot.

Gestures

Gestures are hand and arm movements that can help us to understand what a person is saying. Some gestures carry a generally agreed meaning of their own within a culture.

Contact

Touching another person can send various messages, such as affection, power, sexual interest or sympathy. Health care assistants should not make **assumptions** about touch, and consent should always be gained before touching a patient. See page 283 for more information on consent.

Key term

Assumptions Something believed to be true without proof.

Proximity and personal space

The space between people can sometimes show how friendly or intimate the conversation is. Different cultures have different assumptions about how close people should be when they are talking.

In Britain, when talking to strangers, we may keep an arm's length apart. The ritual of shaking hands indicates that you have been introduced. When you are friendly with someone, you may accept the person coming even closer to you. Relatives and partners may not be restricted in how close they can come.

Face-to-face positions

Standing or sitting face to face can send a message of being formal or being angry. A slight angle can create a more relaxed and friendly feeling.

Responding to others

Looking at a patient's body language and non-verbal communication may tell you a lot about how that patient is feeling.

- Notice whether someone is looking at you, or at the floor, or at a point over your shoulder. Lack of eye contact should give a first indication that all may not be well. It may be that the individual is not feeling confident. He or she may be unhappy, or feel uneasy about talking to you. You will need to follow this up.

- Look at how a person sits. Is he or she relaxed and comfortable, sitting well back in the chair, or tense and perched on the edge of the seat? Is he or she slumped in the chair with the head down? People who are feeling well and cheerful tend to hold their heads up, and sit in a relaxed and comfortable way. An individual who is tense and nervous, who feels unsure and worried, or is in pain is likely to reflect that in the way he or she sits or stands.

- Observe hands and gestures carefully. Someone twisting his or her hands, or fiddling with hair or clothes, is signalling tension and worry. Frequent little shrugs of the shoulders or spreading of the hands may indicate a feeling of helplessness or hopelessness.

Communication through actions

For many people, it is easier to communicate by actions than by words. You will need to make sure that you recognise the significance of a touch or a sudden movement from someone who is ill and bedridden, or a gesture from someone who speaks a different language. A gesture can indicate what his or her needs are and what sort of response the person is looking for from you. You may be faced with a young person with challenging behaviour who throws something at you – this is a means of communication. It may not be a very pleasant one, but nonetheless, it expresses much of the person's hurt, anger and distress. It is important that you recognise this for what it is and respond

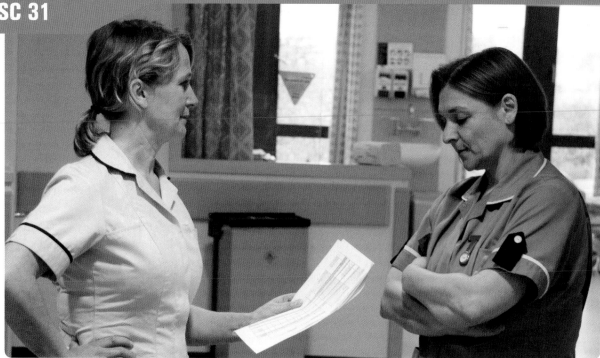

Be aware of your own body language.

in the same way you would if that patient had been able to express his or her feelings in words.

Giving out the signals

Being aware of your own body language is just as important as understanding the person you are talking to.

Best practice: Communication skills

✔ Make sure that you maintain eye contact with the person you are talking to (having made sure this is appropriate as some cultures find eye contact threatening). Remember to avoid staring. Looking away occasionally is normal, but if you find yourself looking around the room, or watching others, then you are failing to give people the attention they deserve.

✔ Be aware of what you are doing and, if you are losing attention, try to think why.

✔ Sit where you can be comfortably seen. Don't sit where someone has to turn in order to look at you.

✔ Sit a comfortable distance away – not so far that any sense of closeness is lost, but not so close that you 'invade their space'.

✔ Make sure you are showing by your gestures that you are listening and interested in what people are saying – sitting half turned away gives the message that you are not fully committed to what is being said.

✔ Folded arms or crossed legs can indicate that you are 'closed' rather than 'open' to what someone is expressing.

✔ Nodding your head will indicate that you are receptive and interested – but be careful not to overdo it and look like a nodding dog!

✔ Lean towards someone to show that you are interested in what they are saying. You can use leaning forwards quite effectively at times when you want to emphasise your interest or support. Then move backwards a little at times when the content is a little lighter.

✔ Using touch to communicate your caring and concern is often useful, but not always appropriate. Many individuals find it comforting to have their hand held or stroked, or to have an arm around their shoulders, but others do not, so ensure you have asked if they would like this before doing so.

✔ Be aware of a person's body language, which should tell you if he or she finds touch acceptable.

✔ Always err on the side of caution if you are unsure about what is acceptable in another culture, for example with regard to touching. Always gain consent.

✔ Think about age and gender in relation to touch. An older woman may be happy to have her hand held by a female health care assistant, but may be uncomfortable with such a response from a man.

✔ Ensure that you are touching someone because you think it will comfort him or her, and not because you feel helpless and can't think of anything to say.

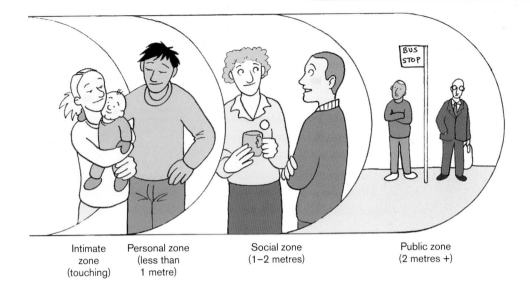

Intimate zone (touching) Personal zone (less than 1 metre) Social zone (1–2 metres) Public zone (2 metres +)

Listening effectively

(KS 1, 2, 3, 4, 5, 8.4, 9, 10, 12, 15)

Communication is a two-way process. A great deal of communication is wasted because only one of the parties is communicating.

As a health care assistant, if you are not listening effectively and receiving the information a patient is trying to communicate, the conversation is a waste of time.

Health care assistants are often busy with many patients to care for and sometimes may not listen carefully enough when patients communicate with them. This shows a lack of respect and may result in mistakes being made.

Learning how to listen effectively is a key task for anyone working in health care. You may think that you know how to listen and that it is something you do constantly. After all, you are hearing all sorts of noises all day long – but simply hearing sounds is not the same thing as actively listening.

For most people, feeling that someone is really listening makes a huge difference to how confident they feel about talking. You will need to learn how you can show people you are listening to what they are saying.

You should practise your listening skills in just the same way you would practise any other skill – you can learn to listen well.

Evidence through reflection (KS 2)

1 Think about a time you have talked to someone you felt was really interested in what you were saying and listening carefully to you. Try to note down what it was that made you so sure he or she was really listening. Did the fact you thought the person was really listening to you make it easier to talk?

2 Think about the last time you were talking to someone and you knew that they were not listening to what you were saying. How did this make you feel? Try to note down what made you think they were not listening to you.

Write notes for your portfolio.

'Listening' using body language

The way in which you use your body can convey messages about many things. Your body language can let people know that you are really listening to what they are saying.

You should always:

1 look at the person who is talking to you

2 maintain eye contact when appropriate, but without staring

3 nod your head to encourage the person to talk and show that you understand

4 use 'aha', 'mm' and similar expressions which indicate that you are still listening

5 lean slightly towards the person who is speaking – this indicates interest and concern

6 have an open and interested facial expression, which should reflect the tone of the conversation – happy, serious, etc.

Making the right noises

Body language is one key to effective listening, but what you say in reply is also important. You can back up the message that you are interested and listening by checking that you have understood what has been said to you.

Using sentences beginning 'So ...' to check that you have got it right can be helpful. 'So ... it's only since you had the fall that you are feeling worried about going home alone.' You can also use expressions such as 'So what you mean is ...' or 'So what you are saying is ...'

Short, encouraging phrases used while people are talking can show concern, understanding or empathy. Phrases such as 'I see', 'Oh dear', 'Yes', or 'Go on' all give the speaker a clear indication that you are listening and want him or her to continue.

Using questions to 'listen' better

Sometimes questions can be helpful to prompt a patient who is talking, or to try to move a conversation forward. There are two different kinds of questions. Questions that can be answered with just 'yes' or 'no' are closed questions. 'Would you like to get out of bed today?' is a closed question.

An open question needs more than 'yes' or 'no' to answer it. 'What is your favourite kind of outing?' is an open question. Open questions usually begin with:

1 'What ...'
2 'How ...'
3 'Why ...'
4 'When ...'
5 'Where ...'

Depending on the conversation and the circumstances, either type of question – open or closed – may be appropriate. For example, if you are encouraging a patient to talk because he or she has always been quiet, but has suddenly begun to open up, you are more likely to use open questions to encourage him or her to carry on talking. On the other hand, if you need factual information or you just want to confirm that you have understood what has been said to you, then you may need to ask closed questions.

One of the main points to remember when listening is to keep what you say to a minimum.

Evidence in action (KS 2, 9, 10, 15)

Over the next few days, listen to the interactions that are taking place between patients and the practitioners working with them and identify the style of questioning used (open or closed). Identify and make notes for your portfolio about whether you thought the style of questioning used influenced patient's choice. Was the questioning style effective? Discuss your thoughts with your assessor.

Best practice: Good listening

Good listening includes:

✔ Not interrupting – always let people finish what they are saying, and wait for a gap in the conversation.

✔ Not giving advice – even when asked. Do not respond to questions by saying 'If I were you . . .'. You should try to encourage patients to take responsibility for their own decisions.

✔ Not telling patients about your own experiences, unless you are doing this in order to encourage them to talk. Any conversation about yourself should support your role as a listener, not make people listen while you talk about yourself.

✔ Not dismissing fears, worries or concerns by saying 'That's silly' or 'You shouldn't worry about that'. Patients' fears are real and should not be made to sound trivial.

✔ Ensuring that you feedback to the practitioner in charge any concerns the patient may have.

Evidence in action (KS 10, 12, 16)

Write a brief description for your portfolio about two particular occasions when you have been involved in communicating with patients, one where sensitive communication was involved. Include the following points.

- How did you show patients you were listening to what they said?
- Why was body language important?
- What factors affected the way patients responded to you?
- Were there any barriers to communication? How did you deal with each of them?
- What environmental factors did you need to consider when planning sensitive communication?
- What open questions and closed questions did you use?
- If you were in the situation again, would you do things differently?

Communicating about difficult and sensitive issues

(KS 1, 2, 3, 4, 8, 9, 10, 13, 14, 15, 18)

The patient's needs should be at the centre of the care process. Your role is to make sure that the patient has every opportunity to state exactly how they wish their needs to be met – and this is especially important when the issues are difficult, sensitive or complex. Some patients will be able to give this information personally; others will need an advocate who will support them in expressing their views.

Developing relationships

Communication is the basis of all relationships, regardless of whether the relationships are personal or professional. As individuals communicate, a relationship is formed. This is usually a two-way process, as each individual involved gets to know the other through a process of communicating and sharing information.

When you provide care for someone, you will get to know and talk to him or her, and a relationship will grow. This is not easy with all patients you care for. When there appears to be little communication, you may have to find alternatives – but you should persist. Developing strong relationships with your patients is a crucial part of your role as a health care assistant, and can be one of the most rewarding aspects of your work.

Stages of an interaction

Communication between individuals is called an 'interaction'. As you spend time in communication with someone, the nature of the interaction will go through changes.

- Stage 1: Introduction, light and general. At first, the content of the communication may be of little significance. This is the stage at which both parties decide whether they want to continue the discussion, and how comfortable they feel. Body language and non-verbal communication are very important at this stage.

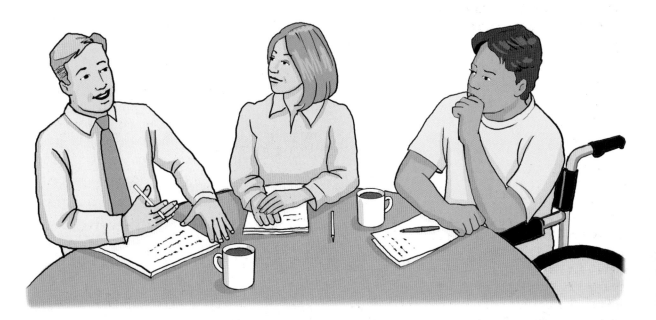

Patient takes an advocate when visiting the doctor.

- Stage 2: Main contact, significant information. The middle of any interaction is likely to contain the 'meat', and this is where you will need to use active listening skills to ensure that the interaction is beneficial.
- Stage 3: Reflect, wind up, end positively. People often have the greatest difficulty in knowing how to end an interaction. Ending in a positive way where all participants are left feeling that they have benefited from the interaction is very important. You may find that you have to end an interaction because of time restrictions, or you may feel that enough has been covered – the other person may need a rest, or you may need a break.

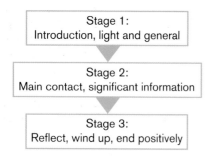

At the end of an interaction you should always try to reflect on the areas you have covered, and offer a positive and encouraging ending – 'So we'll do this now, and hopefully that will mean you feel more comfortable.'

Even if the content of an interaction has been fairly negative, you should encourage the individual to see the fact that the interaction has taken place as being positive in itself.

If you are called away before you have had a chance to properly 'wind up' an interaction with an individual, make a point of returning to end things in a positive way. If you say 'I'll be back in a minute', make sure that you do go back.

Life stages and development

One of the most significant influences on communication and the way people deal with difficult or stressful issues is the life stage they are at. The chart on the next page will help you to understand the life stages patients are either at, or have experienced.

Communicating with children

It will be important to communicate with children in a different way from adults. Children will have different emotional, social, intellectual and language needs. They may not understand some of the long words that adults might use. Children will also think differently from adults; conversation may not work in the same way. If you ask children to tell you about their past life, they might only be able to tell you about very practical, concrete experiences such as a birthday party or where they went on holiday. Adults, on the other hand, might be able to organise their life story into themes about jobs, relationships and aspirations.

Communicating with older adults

Older adults may also have quite different emotional, social, intellectual and conversational needs to young adults.

Characteristics of different life stages

	Intellectual/cognitive	Social/emotional	Language	Physical
Infant birth–1 year	Learns about new things by feeling with hands and mouth objects encountered in immediate environment	Attaches to parent(s), begins to recognise faces and smile; at about 6 months begins to recognise parent(s) and expresses fear of strangers, plays simple interactive games like peekaboo	Vocalises, squeals, and imitates sounds, says 'dada' and 'mama'	Lifts head first then chest, rolls over, pulls to sit, crawls and stands alone. Reaches for objects and rakes up small items, grasps rattle
Toddler 1-2 years	Extends knowledge by learning words for objects in environment	Learns that self and parent(s) are different or separate from each other, imitates and performs tasks, indicates needs or wants without crying	Says some words other than 'dada' and 'mama', follows simple instructions	Walks well, kicks, stoops and jumps in place, throws balls. Unbuttons clothes, builds tower of 4 cubes, scribbles, uses spoon, picks up very small objects
Pre-school 2-5 years	Understands concepts such as tired, hungry and other bodily states, recognises colours, becomes aware of numbers and letters	Begins to separate easily from parent(s), dresses with assistance, washes and dries hands, plays interactive games like tag	Names pictures, follows directions, can make simple sentences of two or three words, vocabulary increases	Runs well, hops, pedals tricycle, balances on one foot. Buttons clothes, builds tower of 8 cubes, copies simple figures or letters, for example O, begins to use scissors
School age 5-12 years	Develops understanding of numeracy and literacy concepts, learns relationship between objects and feelings, acquires knowledge and understanding	Acts independently, but is emotionally close to parent(s), dresses without assistance, joins same-sex play groups and clubs	Defines words, knows and describes what things are made of, vocabulary increases	Skips, balances on one foot for 10 seconds, overestimates physical abilities. Draws person with 6 parts, copies detailed figures and objects
Adolescent 12-18 years	Understands abstract concepts like illness and death, develops understanding of complex concepts	Experiences rapidly changing moods and behaviour, interested in peer group almost exclusively, distances from parent(s) emotionally, concerned with body image, experiences falling in and out of love	Uses increased vocabulary, understands more abstract concepts such as grief	May appear awkward and clumsy while learning to deal with rapid increases in size due to growth spurts
Young adult 18-40 years	Continues to develop the ability to make good decisions and to understand the complexity of human relationships – sometimes called wisdom	Becomes independent from parent(s), develops own lifestyle, selects a career, copes with career, social and economic changes and social expectations, chooses a partner, learns to live co-operatively with partner, becomes a parent	Continues to develop vocabulary and knowledge of different styles of language use	Fully developed
Middle age 40-65 years	Continues to develop a deeper understanding of life – sometimes called wisdom	Builds social and economic status, is fulfilled by work or family, copes with physical changes of ageing, children grow and leave nest, deals with ageing parents, copes with the death of parents	Vocabulary may continue to develop	Begins to experience physical changes of ageing
Older adult 65+ years	Ability may be influenced by health factors; some individuals will continue to develop 'wisdom'	Adjusts to retirement, adjusts to loss of friends and relatives, copes with loss of spouse, adjusts to new role in family, copes with dying	Ability may be influenced by health factors; some individuals may continue to develop language skills	Experiences more significant physical changes associated with ageing

Imagine you are talking with Mrs Hemshore (see photograph opposite). She is 85 years old and has been telling you her life story. She then says: 'Now you won't understand this – you're too young to understand this – but I've had my life, and it's been a good life. I've done everything I wanted to do, and now I'm ready to die. It's not that I want to be dead, it's just that I'm very tired and it's right and proper that my life should end now. I'm not depressed and I'm not ill. What I really appreciate is just having you here to listen to me. There isn't anything for you to say – I just want someone to listen to me while I make sense of things. At your age, I guess you can't understand just how important this is for me.'

If a 25-year-old said something like this it might suggest an underlying depression, but the needs of people in later life may be quite different from the needs of young adults. The ability to listen and provide a 'caring presence' may be central to meeting the needs and preserving the self-esteem of people in later life.

Key term

Distress Suffering resulting from anxiety, grief or unhappiness.

Difficult and strong emotions

In growing and developing, most of us learn to control our powerful emotions. The sight of a two-year-old lying on the floor in a supermarket kicking and screaming is not uncommon, but it is socially unacceptable for an adult to do the same thing.

Most of the time people behave within the accepted norms of society. However, on occasion, the emotions may become too powerful or the normal control which people exercise over their emotions may relax, resulting in a display of emotion that is recognised as **distress**.

People can become distressed because of a wide range of causes, but some common causes of distress can be identified and it is helpful for you to be aware of situations and circumstances that can act as triggers.

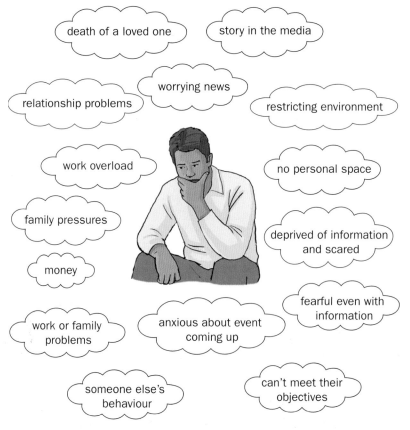

death of a loved one

story in the media

worrying news

relationship problems

restricting environment

work overload

no personal space

family pressures

deprived of information and scared

money

fearful even with information

work or family problems

anxious about event coming up

someone else's behaviour

can't meet their objectives

Common reasons for people becoming depressed.

The illustration on the previous page shows some of the more common triggers for distress. Clearly there are many others which you may come across depending on the setting in which you work.

How to identify when someone is becoming distressed

When you have a close working knowledge of a patient's behaviour over a period of time, it becomes easy to identify when he or she is becoming distressed. You will find that you have become 'tuned-in' to the patient's behaviour and can recognise the signs that indicate a change in mood.

For example, someone who is normally talkative may become quiet and someone who is normally quiet may start to shout or talk very quickly. Even if the signs are far less extreme than these examples, if you know a patient well, you may still notice something out of character, and be able to use your skills to help reduce the effects of the their distress.

However, you will not always know your patient so well as they are often not with you long enough to do this. Also, you may have to deal with the distress not only of the patient, but of the relatives or carer.

There are some general indications that a patient is becoming distressed, which you can use in order to take immediate action. You are most likely to notice:

1   changes in voice – it may be raised or at a higher pitch than usual

2   changes in facial expression – this could be scowling, frowning, snarling

3   changes in eyes – pupils could be dilated and eyes open wider

4   agitated body language – an aggressive stance, leaning forwards with fists clenched

5   reddening of the face and neck

6   excessive sweating

7   changes in breathing patterns – the person may breathe faster than normal.

Undertaking difficult, complex and sensitive communications

(KS 2, 3, 4, 9, 10, 12, 13, 15, 16)

If patients are upset as the result of an outside event, such as the death of a close friend or relative, or because they have received some bad news, there is probably little you can do to prevent the distress, but the way you communicate with them on the topic and the way you handle the situation can often reduce it.

This is where effective listening skills are important. Patients may need to discuss with you what the doctor said about their condition and you may need to ask the practitioner in charge to talk to the patient about difficult, complex or sensitive issues.

Your acknowledgement and recognition of their distress may be sufficient for some people, and they may be able to resolve their distress themselves if they know that they can obtain additional support from you if necessary.

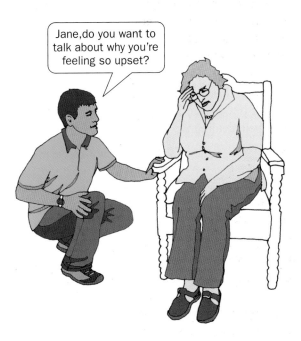

Jane, do you want to talk about why you're feeling so upset?

Health care workers need to give patients the chance to decide whether they want to talk about the causes of distress.

Interacting with someone who is distressed

You need to be aware of the ways in which you are using your own communication skills to interact with a patient who is distressed. While you are taking into account the patient's body language and the clues of non-verbal communication, you will need to be conscious of the messages your own non-verbal communication is sending. You need to demonstrate openness with an open welcoming position, but you should not encroach on a patient's personal space, as this often heightens tension. Make eye contact in a way that demonstrates you are willing to listen, but only if this is appropriate – some patients may find this threatening.

It is important you approach any patient who is distressed or displaying anger or excitement in a calm and non-threatening way. This will minimise the risks to the patient, to any other people in the immediate area and to yourself. If at any point you feel your personal safety is at risk, you should immediately summon help.

Don't feel you have to cope alone

No one is able to deal with every situation with which they are faced, and you may feel that a particular situation is beyond your capability. This is nothing to be ashamed of. Knowing your own limitations is important and demonstrates a higher degree of maturity and self-awareness. Contact other members of your team or other professionals with the experience to deal with the situation – never hesitate to summon help when you feel unsure in dealing with an individual in distress.

A distressed patient can become aggressive in some circumstances. If you observe a patient becoming aggressive and potentially violent, as in the case of someone changing from crying or expressing anger to shouting or throwing things, then you should immediately summon help.

Anger is not always directed at others; it can be turned inwards, directed against patients themselves. You may be faced with a distressed, hurt and angry patient who makes it clear that they intend to self-harm. In this case, you have a responsibility to take immediate action to protect the patient. You must also advise the patient that you will have to take these steps to protect them and attempt to stop them from harming themselves.

Deciding the level of support

When communicating with someone who is distressed, one of the first things to do is decide on the support and assistance you need to offer. People in distress can benefit from a wide range of different forms of support.

Evidence through reflection (KS 2, 4, 6, 7, 10, 15)

Think back to an occasion when you have supported a distressed patient. Make notes for your portfolio on the support you gave, what made you decide that was the correct level of support and what, if anything, would you have done differently.

Memory jogger

What are reflection skills? Refresh your understanding by looking at Unit HSC 33 on page 76.

You should establish with the distressed individual the extent of the help needed and what you can usefully provide. Providing unwanted support can sometimes be as damaging and as unhelpful as too little or none. The risks of providing unwanted support are that:

1 patients may feel they are disempowered and are no longer able to help or support themselves – this is not good for their self-esteem or self-confidence;

2 patients may feel you have interfered and they have been forced to reveal more about themselves and their personal life than they would have wished to;

3 patients may become over-dependent on you for help and support, which may reduce their ability to manage for themselves.

Offering too little or no help may mean that:

1 patients feel they are isolated and there is nobody who cares for them or is interested in their problems;

2 patients may feel they are unworthy and not liked as individuals;

3 patients may get very angry and frustrated at the apparent lack of care or interest from the rest of the world.

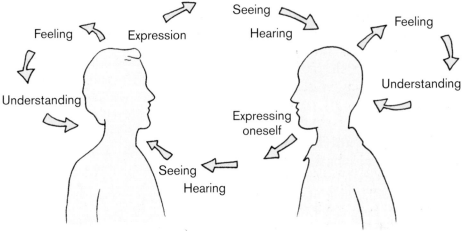

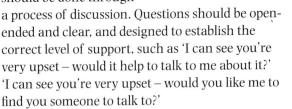

The level of help and support you should offer is always best decided along with the patient themselves. Wherever possible, this should be done through a process of discussion. Questions should be open-ended and clear, and designed to establish the correct level of support, such as 'I can see you're very upset – would it help to talk to me about it?' 'I can see you're very upset – would you like me to find you someone to talk to?'

There may be circumstances in which it is not possible to discuss this with patients, perhaps because they are extremely agitated, angry or distressed and are unable to hold a calm conversation. It may even be that they are threatening to harm themselves or others. In these circumstances, you will need to judge how best to intervene or refer for help.

Broadly, the necessary support you are likely to identify will fall into one of three categories.

Practical support	Giving information, making a telephone call, providing transport or other practical assistance, contacting someone on behalf of the distressed person, or meeting an appropriate professional
Emotional support	Using listening skills
Immediate emergency assistance	Summoning immediate help from a colleague, a senior member of staff, or an appropriate professional

How to offer support

Do not underestimate the support you will be able to provide by using good communication skills and a

Developing a sense of empathy may involve a communication cycle of active listening.

genuine **empathy** and care for your patients – you can encourage them to express how they feel about what is causing them worry, anxiety or distress.

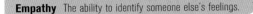

Key term

Empathy The ability to identify someone else's feelings.

Empathising with another person is a skill that develops from good active listening, and involves developing an accurate understanding of the feelings and thoughts of another person. It is a characteristic of a caring attitude, where an individual can see beyond his or her own assumptions about the world and can imagine the thoughts and feelings of someone who is quite different.

You will need to ensure that you have access to the appropriate information and resources for the circumstances. Within a hospital, there are specialist organisations that will offer particular support for those who are bereaved, for those who are experiencing relationship difficulties or for those who are feeling depressed and may harm themselves.

Again, however, if you feel the situation calls for more support than you can offer, it is important that you recognise this and make an appropriate referral.

How distress can affect you

It can be very upsetting to deal with someone who is displaying powerful emotions. Patients' stories or experiences can be so moving and troubling that you may feel grateful, or perhaps even guilty, for your own happier circumstances. On the other hand, if you are having difficulties yourself, you could find these echoed or brought to the surface by dealing with an individual in distress. In this case, it is important to talk to your manager as soon as possible and arrange for someone else to continue to offer support to the patient.

Feeling concerned, upset or even angry after a particularly emotional experience with a patient is normal. You should not feel that such a response is in any way a reflection on the quality of your work or your ability as a health care assistant.

After such an experience most people are likely to continue to think about it for some time. One of the best ways to deal with this is to discuss it with your manager or the professional in charge. It is often useful to have the opportunity to **debrief** following a situation that has occurred and to reflect on the experience with other members of the working team. This does not necessarily need to take long – even a short discussion or conversation can be valuable. The chaplaincy can often offer support to both yourself or the patient concerned following stressful situations. This forms the basis of reflective practice, something we will examine further in Unit HSC 33 page 76.

The distress of others, whether in the form of anger, sadness or anxiety, will always be upsetting for the person who works with them. However, if you are able to develop your skills and knowledge so that you can identify distress, work towards reducing it and offer effective help and support to those who are experiencing it, then you are making a useful and meaningful contribution to the provision of quality care.

The principles of good communication are an important part of making sure that the patient is fully involved in dealing with any issues or difficult situations. The impact of dealing with situations in a way that makes patients feel valued is enormous. Often the steps are small and do not take a great deal of effort or demand major changes – but the results are so effective that any effort you have made will be repaid many times over by the positive benefits for the patients you care for.

Best practice: Skilled communication

Skilled communication involves:

✔ watching other people

✔ remembering what they do

✔ identifying what words and actions mean and then checking your guesses with the person

✔ never relying on your own impressions, because these might turn into assumptions

✔ do not make assumptions as this can lead to **discrimination** – see Unit HSC 35 (page 101)

✔ ensuring all interactions have a communication cycle, i.e. a beginning, middle and end.

Key term

Discrimination Unfair treatment of a person or a group of people.

Evidence through reflection (KS 22, 23)

Research the communication cycle and write about your understanding of this cycle for your portfolio. Give an example of how you put this into practice during a situation of conflict, identifying the different ways of communicating patient's choice while ensuring their well-being and protection. Make notes for your portfolio.

Communication differences

(KS 1, 2, 3, 4, 5, 6, 7, 8.2, 8.3, 8.4, 9, 10, 11, 12, 16, 19)

There are many factors that can get in the way of good communication. You will need to understand how to recognise these and to learn what you can do to overcome them yourself, and to support individuals in overcoming them. Until you do this, your communication will always be less effective than it could be.

It is easy to assume that everyone can communicate, and that any failure to respond to you is because of someone's unwillingness rather than inability. There are as many reasons why people find communication difficult as there are ways to make it easier.

The most common effect of communication differences is for the patient receiving care to feel frustrated and isolated. It is an important part of your job to do everything in your power to reduce the effect of communication differences and to try to lessen the feelings of isolation and frustration that people experience.

You must also be alert to the fact that a patient's needs may change, and that a method of communication which was effective in the past may not continue to be appropriate. Be prepared to change your approach and to seek additional help if necessary.

Evidence through reflection (KS 10)

Identify two different ways in which you communicate with people, for example talking, writing, or speaking on the telephone. Consider the most important element in each one. For example, for talking it could be language, for the telephone it could be hearing, and so on. Now think about how you would manage that communication without that important element. List the problems you would have and the ways you could try to overcome them. Include these notes in your portfolio.

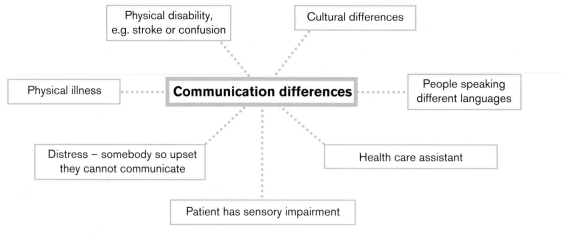

Communication differences.

Removing the physical barriers first

Communication can be hindered by physical and environmental factors. This may seem obvious, but they need to be considered when planning communication. Always provide a private situation if you have personal matters to discuss – it is rarely the case that the best that can be arranged is to pull the curtains around a bed. You need to think about the surroundings. People find it difficult to talk in noisy, crowded places. A communal lounge with a television on is not a good place for effective communication.

Remember the temperature – make sure it is comfortable. Think about lighting, ensuring it is not too dark or too bright, ensuring the sun is not shining in someone's eyes. It is very disconcerting not to be able to see someone's face when talking to him or her – remember what you have learned about non-verbal communication.

Styles of speaking

Register

Speaking is about much more than just passing information between people. For example, many people can speak with different degrees of formality or informality. This is called the **register** of language.

If you went to a hospital reception, you might expect the person on duty to greet you with a formal phrase, such as: 'Good morning, how can I help you?' An informal greeting might be: 'Hello mate, what's up then?' or 'How's it going?'

> **Key term**
>
> **Register** Degree of formality or informality in language.

But in some situations, the informal greeting might make people feel that they are not being respected.

The degree of formality or informality establishes a context. At a hospital reception, you are unlikely to want to spend time making friends and chatting things over with the receptionist. You may be seeking urgent help; your expectations of the situation might be that you want to be taken seriously and put in touch with professional services as soon as possible. You might see the situation as a very formal encounter. If you were treated informally, you might interpret this as not being taken seriously, or not respected.

Speech communities

People from different localities, different ethnic groups, different professions and work cultures all have their own particular jargon, phrases and speech patterns. Where communities or groups of people have particular ways of speaking we call this a **speech community**: for example, people who are deaf often refer to themselves as being part of the 'deaf community' where sign language is the first or preferred method of communication.

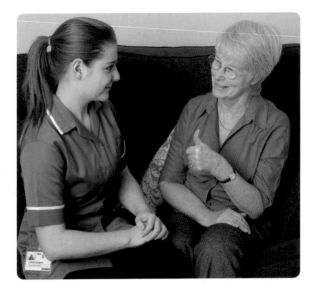

The particular jargon that may be used by health care assistants could also be referred to as a speech community. This can create barriers for patients who may not understand what is being said and are therefore excluded from communicating effectively.

Making sure you have been understood

You should never talk down to people, but equally there is no point in you using so much jargon and medical terminology no one understands what you are talking about. Instead of saying 'The doctor thinks you have a UTI so you need to increase your fluids', you could say 'The doctor thinks you may have a water infection so can you drink a glass of water regularly?' This is much easier for a patient to understand. You must be sure that your communication is being understood. The most straightforward way to do this is to ask someone to recap what you have discussed. You could say something like: 'Can we just go over this so that we are both sure about what is happening – you tell me what is happening tomorrow'. Alternatively you can rephrase what you have just said and check with the patient has understood.

and they are not in a position to ask or to have any questions answered. The patient may feel excluded from the health care setting, and could find making relationships with health care workers difficult. Misunderstanding could occur due to lack of effective listening and communication skills on the part of the health care assistant.

Different languages

Where a patient speaks a different language from those who are providing care, it can be an isolating and frustrating experience. The patient may become distressed and frightened as they may not understand exactly what is happening

Dealing with language differences

Make sure that you know what language an individual is comfortable with – don't assume it is the same as yours without making certain. Find out if you need to provide any translation facilities, or written information in another language. If translation is needed, your team leader or manager should be able to help you to arrange it. Language preferences should be recorded on a patient's care plan so all staff can have access to this information.

You should always use professional interpreters wherever possible. It may be very tempting to use other members of the family – very often children have excellent language skills – but it is inappropriate in most care settings. This is because:

- their English and their ability to interpret may not be at the same standard as a professional interpreter, and misunderstandings can easily occur
- you may wish to discuss matters which are not appropriate to be discussed with children, or the patient may not want members of his or her family involved in very personal discussions about health or care issues.

It is unlikely that you would be able to have a full-time interpreter available throughout a patient's period of care, so it is necessary to consider alternatives for encouraging everyday communication.

There are other simple techniques that you may wish to try which can help basic levels of communication. For example, you could use flashcards and signals, similar to those you would use for a patient who has suffered a stroke. This gives the patient the opportunity to show a flashcard to indicate his or her needs. You can also use them to find out what kind of assistance may be needed.

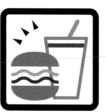
Food

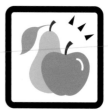
Fruit

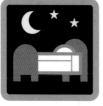
Bed

Drink

Evidence with a case study (KS 2, 6, 11, 13)

A lady who speaks no English is admitted to your ward. She has a teenage daughter who can speak English and is spending a great deal of time on the ward.

1 What conflicts and dilemmas do you as a health care assistant face when communicating with this patient?

2 Find out how to access an interpreter and which languages they support.

Make notes for your portfolio.

Evidence in action (KS 10, 11)

Try to arrange some time to shadow the Speech and Language Therapist in your workplace. Make notes for your portfolio on the patients you see, the aids the therapist uses and the support they offer. Try to go back to visit to the patients you have encountered and identify if the aids have helped with communication. Make notes for your portfolio.

Do not forget that an effective way of communicating with a patient who speaks a different language is through non-verbal communication (see page 3). A smile and a friendly face are understood in all languages, as are a concerned facial expression and a warm and welcoming body position.

Sensory impairment

(KS 1, 2, 3, 4, 5, 6, 7, 8, 9, 10, 11, 12, 15)

Hearing impairment

A loss or reduction of ability to hear clearly can cause major differences in the ability to communicate.

Communication is a two-way process, and it can be difficult for somebody who does not hear sounds at all, or hears them in a blurred and indistinct way, to be able to respond and to join in. As with speaking different languages, the result can be that patients become withdrawn and feel isolated from others around them. This can lead to frustration and anger, sometimes resulting in patients resorting to challenging behaviour.

Profound deafness is not as common as partial hearing loss. People are most likely to suffer from the loss of hearing of certain sounds at particular volumes or pitches, such as high sounds or low sounds. It is also very common for people to find it difficult to hear if there is background noise – many sounds may jumble together, making it difficult to pick out the voice of one person. You should remember that wards and clinics are often very noisy places. Hearing loss can also have an effect on speech, particularly for those who are profoundly deaf and are unable to hear their own voices as they speak. This can make communication doubly difficult.

Supporting patients with hearing difficulties

1 Ensure that any means of improving hearing that a patient uses, for example a hearing aid, is working properly and is fitted correctly, that the batteries are working, that it is clean and that it is doing its job properly in terms of improving the patient's hearing.

2 Ensure that you are sitting in a good light, not too far away and that you speak clearly, but do not shout. Shouting simply distorts your face and makes it more difficult for a patient with hearing loss to be able to read what you are saying.

3 Be prepared to write things down if the patient prefers you to do this in order to communicate clearly.

Some patients may be able to lip read, while many will use a form of sign language for understanding. This may be British Sign Language (BSL).

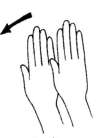
wait

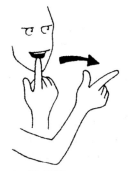
Tell/Say

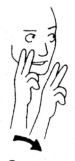
Go to see

BSL signs are the ones you'll see interpreters use on TV programmes.

Some deaf people may use Makaton, a system that uses speech, signs and symbols to help people with learning difficulties to communicate and to develop their language skills. It may involve speaking a word and performing a sign using hands and body language. There is a large range of symbols that may help people with a learning difficulty to recognise an idea or to communicate with others.

Other services which are extremely helpful to people who have hearing difficulties include telecommunication services, such as using a minicom or typetalk service. These allow a spoken conversation to be translated in written form using a form of typewriter, and the responses can be passed in the same way by an operator who will relay them to the hearing person. These services have provided a major advance in enabling people who are hard of hearing or profoundly deaf to use telephone equipment. For people who are less severely affected by hearing impairment, there are facilities such as raising the volume on telephone receivers to allow them to hear conversations more clearly.

Did you know?

The British Deaf Association says that BSL is a first or preferred language for nearly 70,000 people in the UK.

When communicating with people with hearing impairments:

✔ make sure the person can see you clearly – check whether they wear glasses

✔ face both the light and the person at all times

✔ include the person in your conversation

✔ do not obscure your mouth

✔ speak clearly and slowly – repeat if necessary, or rephrase your words

✔ do not shout into a person's ear or hearing aid

✔ minimise background noise

✔ use your eyes, facial expressions and hand gestures, where appropriate.

Act as the patient's advocate by providing active support when the patient is communicating with other members of the health care team.

Evidence through reflection (KS 3, 6, 8, 11)

As a health care assistant, how can you ensure someone from the deaf community is able to communicate effectively with health care professionals? Write notes for your portfolio.

Visual impairment

Visual impairment causes many communication difficulties. A patient may not be able to pick up the visual signals given out by someone who is speaking – and, being unaware of these signals, he or she may also fail to give appropriate signals in return. This could lead to you misinterpreting communication, or thinking that the patient is behaving in an inappropriate way.

When caring for people with limited vision, it may be important for you to use language to describe things that a sighted person may take for granted, such as non-verbal communication or the context of certain comments.

Touch can be an important aspect of communication for the patient. For example, some registered blind people can work out what you look like if they can touch your face, to build an understanding of your features. However, health care assistants must not take this for granted, and **consent** must be obtained before doing so.

Key term

Consent Freely given, specific and informed indication of wishes.

Supporting patients with visual difficulties

One of the most common ways of assisting patients who have visual impairment is to ensure they have access to their glasses or contact lenses. You need to be sure that these are clean and that they are the correct prescription. Has the patient's eyesight or requirements for glasses changed recently? If so, he or she will obviously have difficulty picking up many of the non-verbal signals you will be giving out when you are communicating.

For patients with more serious loss or impairment, you will need to take other steps to ensure that you minimise the differences that will exist in your styles of communication.

Best practice: Communicating with patients who have visual impairment

✔ Make sure that you introduce yourself when you come into a room. It is easy to forget that a patient may not be able to see. A simple 'Hello Mr Smith, it's Sue' is all that is needed so that you don't 'arrive' unexpectedly.

✔ Do not suddenly begin to speak to a patient without first letting him or her know that you are there. One way to do this is to touch him or her, but check that the patient is comfortable with this approach.

✔ You may need to use touch more than you would in speaking to a sighted person, because the concerns that you will be expressing through your face and your general body movements will not be seen. So, if you are expressing concern or sympathy, it may be appropriate to touch the patient's hand or arm, while saying you are concerned and sympathetic. Make sure this is appropriate and you have asked the patient's permission.

✔ Ask the patient what system of communication they require – do not impose your idea of appropriate systems on the person. Most people who are visually impaired know very well what they can and cannot do and, if you ask, they will tell you exactly what they need you to do.

✔ Do not decide that you know the best way to help. Never take the arm of someone who is visually impaired to help him or her to move around. Allow the patient to take your arm or shoulder, to ask for guidance and tell you where he or she wishes to go.

Evidence in action (KS 7)

Make notes in your portfolio about where in your organisation you can find information about translation support services for those registered with a sight or hearing impairment.

Physical disabilities

Depending on the disability, there can be different problems with communication.

Patients who have suffered strokes will often have communication difficulties, and not only in forming words and speaking. They often also suffer from **aphasia**, which is the inability to understand and to express meaning through words. This condition is very distressing, both for the patient and for those who are trying to communicate. Aphasia is often coupled with a loss of movement and a difficulty in using facial muscles to form words.

Key term

Aphasia A condition where someone has difficulty understanding and expressing meaning through words.

In some cases, the communication difficulty is a symptom of a disability. For example, many people with cerebral palsy and motor neurone disease have difficulty controlling the muscles that affect voice production, and find it hard to speak in a way that can be readily understood.

Other disabilities may have no effect at all on voice production or the thought processes that produce spoken words, but the lack of other body movements may mean that non-verbal communication may be difficult or not what you would expect.

Supporting patients with physical disabilities
Again, the way you can help depends on the type of physical disability or illness; communication will depend on what sort it is. For example, if you were communicating with a patient who has had a stroke, you could deal with his or her aphasia by:

- using very simple, short sentences, speaking slowly and being prepared to wait while the patient processes what you have said and composes a reply

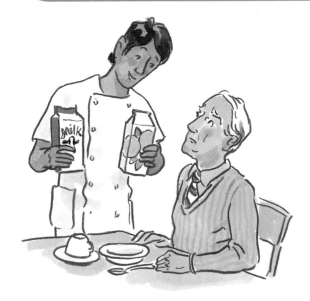

You have a responsibility to respect all service users' choices.

- using gestures – they make it easier for people to understand the ideas you are trying to get across
- using drawing, writing or flashcards to help understanding
- using closed questions which only need a 'yes' or 'no' answer. Avoid long, complicated sentences containing lots of ideas. For example, do not say: 'It's getting near teatime now, isn't it? How about some tea? Have you thought about what you would like?' Instead, say: 'Are you hungry? Would you like fish? Would you like chicken?' and so on, until you have established what sort of meal the patient would prefer.

However, you need to make sure that you do not talk down to any patient, but treat them appropriately, as an individual you respect. One of the commonest complaints from people with physical disabilities is that people will talk to their carers about them rather than talk to them directly – this is known as the 'does he take sugar' approach.

With a condition such as motor neurone disease the patient may have difficulties in making speech, although not in understanding it. The patient will understand perfectly what you are saying to him or her but the difficulty will be in communicating with you.

In this instance, there is no need for you to speak slowly, although you will have to be prepared to allow time for a response owing to the difficulties that the patient will have in producing words.

It can be hard to understand people who have illnesses that affect their facial, throat or larynx muscles. You will have to become familiar with the sound of the patient's voice and the way in which he or she communicates. You should give patients time to express their needs and not rush them, as this may cause frustration and anxiety. Be careful not to make assumptions about a patient's **cognitive** capability based on their ability to speak.

Key term

Cognitive Intellectual ability.

Evidence through reflection (KS 8, 9)

Write a short report identifying which patients may have problems communicating within your work setting. Identify the reasons why this may be the case. If you were the patient within that setting how would this make you feel?

Learning difficulties

Depending on the severity, a learning difficulty can create differences in communication, in terms of how well the patient can understand any form of communication, and in terms of their ability to respond appropriately to it.

Learning difficulties may affect the ability of a patient to understand and process information. Patients may have a short attention span, so that communications have to be repeated several times, or perhaps paraphrased in a different form.

Supporting patients with learning difficulties

Where people have a learning difficulty, you will need to adjust your methods of communicating to take account of the level of difficulty that they experience. You should have gathered sufficient information about the patient to know the level of understanding that he or she has – how simply and how often you need to explain things and the kinds of communication which are likely to be the most effective. You should use words and phrases that the patient is familiar with. Many people with a learning difficulty respond well to physical contact and are able to relate and communicate on a physical level more easily than on a verbal level. If you do not yet know the patient well, you may be able find out

more by talking to the patient's relatives or carer. The relative or carer can supply a wealth of information on the patient's needs and choices. The views of relatives and carers of patients with learning difficulties should be valued by the caring profession. There may be opportunity to visit a patient in their own environment prior to a planned admission, and this can give the health care assistant invaluable insight into the patient's daily routine and abilities.

Evidence through reflection (KS 15)

If you are planning communication with a patient who has a sensory impairment or who has a learning disability, you will need to take account of this and adjust your communication so it can be understood and made sense of by your patient. Write notes for your portfolio on how you might do this.

Dementia/confusion

This condition is most often found in older people, the most common type being caused by Alzheimer's disease. People with Alzheimer's can ultimately lose the ability to communicate, but in the early stages will have short-term memory loss: they may be unable to remember the essential parts of a conversation or a recent exchange.

Supporting patients with dementia or confusion
People with memory disorders often substitute inappropriate words. A 90-year-old patient may say: 'My mother visited me yesterday'. On the surface, such a statement appears to be irrational – but you might know that the visitor was in fact, a daughter, and the patient has simply used an incorrect word. From a care perspective, it is very important not to challenge the rationality of what is being said; the most important thing is to make the older person feel valued and respected.

Sometimes a patient may be disorientated and make statements about needing to go to work or to go home to look after the children. Again, it is important not to argue, but rather to try to divert the conversation in a way that interests and values the person.

Evidence in action (KS 1, 2, 3, 8, 9, 10, 11)

Over the next few days, talk to patients you are caring for about the work they used to do, their family, their hobbies, etc. Remember: memories of the past are often clear and accurate. Write notes for your portfolio about this experience, for both yourself and the patients.

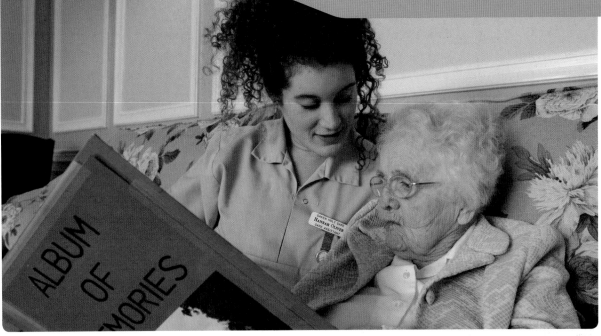

A book of memories can help patients communicate about their past.

Cultural differences

(KS 1, 2, 3, 4, 5, 6, 7, 8, 9, 10, 11)

You will also need to be aware of cultural differences between you and the person you are talking to.

Culture is about more than language – it is about the way that people live, think and relate to each other. In some cultures, for example, children are not allowed to speak in the presence of certain adults. Other cultures do not allow women to speak to men they do not know, and this must be respected when undertaking any aspect of care. In some cultures it is acceptable to stand very close to someone, whereas in others people feel extremely uncomfortable if others stand too close.

Different cultures interpret body language differently too. An almost infinite variety of meanings can be given to any type of eye contact, facial expression, posture or gesture. Every culture develops its own special system of meanings. For example, in Britain the hand gesture with palm up and facing forwards means: 'Stop, don't do that.' In Greece it can mean 'You are dirt' and is a very rude gesture. All health care assistants need to show respect for all the different styles of non-verbal communication and guard against making assumptions based on their own upbringing and culture.

Evidence with a case study
(HSC 31: KS 1, 2, 13, 14; HSC 35: KS 13)

A patient's beliefs

Hafsah is from Somalia in Africa and is a devout Muslim. She had her first baby in hospital in the UK.

Following the delivery, Hafsah refused to get out of bed, and would press the buzzer every time she wanted anything, including asking staff to take her baby from the cot and give him to her to feed. This was in accordance with her own culture in which a new mother remains in bed for ten days after giving birth. During that time, everything is done for her and her baby, and all she does is feed the baby. It is usually her mother-in-law or another female relative who takes control during this time.

The ward staff became resentful of the demands that Hafsah was making. They were not always as pleasant as they might have been when they were called into her room. Hafsah became very distressed and was agitated and nervous each time she needed assistance. She began to have problems feeding the baby. There was a great deal of concern about this and about her refusal to get out of bed, and she was encouraged to do so. The midwives explained to her that she ran the risk of thrombosis or other circulatory problems if she continued to lie in bed.

A solution was eventually found by allowing her mother-in-law to remain with her in a side room to provide the care needed. But Hafsah still couldn't be persuaded to get out of bed. As she had been provided with all the information about possible consequences, and she had made an informed choice consistent with her own beliefs, her decision to stay in bed had to be respected.

1 What were the issues presented by Hafsah's beliefs?

2 Do you think the situation was handled correctly?

3 What would you have done?

4 How could you tell Hafsah was distressed?

Write notes for your portfolio.

Time can be just as important as place in shaping someone's culture. Many older men and women consider it disrespectful to address people by their first names. You will often find older people with neighbours they have known for 50 years, who still call each other 'Mrs Baker' or 'Mr Wood'.

In some eras, challenging authority by asking questions was not seen as acceptable. Some patients may find it hard to ask questions of doctors or other health professionals, and are unlikely to feel able to raise any queries about how their care or treatment should be carried out.

Evidence in action (KS 1, 2, 3, 4, 5, 6, 8, 9, 13, 14)

Discuss with your supervisor the appropriate way to approach other health professionals when wanting to discuss a difference of opinion on a patient's treatment. Make notes for your portfolio.

Supporting patients with cultural differences

You need to find out about a patient's background when you are thinking about how you can make communication work for him or her. For example, you may want to find out whether you can use someone's first name, or touch someone without seeming disrespectful.

To find out the information you need, ask the patient if possible, and/or:

- look in the patient's records
- speak to a member of the family or a friend, if this is possible
- ask someone else from the same culture, such as a colleague
- use reference books, if necessary.

It is important that you identify the different interpretations that words and body language can have for patients. This is not a straightforward issue; words and signs can mean different things depending on their context.

Be aware that the words you use can mean different things to different people and generations – words like 'web', 'chip' or 'gay'. Be aware of particular local words used in your part of the country, which may not mean the same to someone from another area.

Think carefully about the subject under discussion. Some people from particular cultures, or people of particular generations, may find some subjects very sensitive and difficult to discuss.

It is also important that you communicate with your patient at the correct intellectual level. Make sure that you communicate with them at a language level they are likely to understand, but not find patronising. Everyone has the right to be spoken to as adults and not patronised or talked down to.

Evidence in action (KS 6, 7)

Find out if there is a policy in your workplace for identifying a patient's cultural preferences. Ask who establishes the information about the cultural background of people who use your service, and what policies there are to ensure individual needs are met. If there is no policy, make notes for your portfolio on the information that you feel should be contained in one.

Evidence through reflection (KS 7)

Write notes for your portfolio on the following.

- Find out what sort of support you could access to assist any of your patients with communication difficulties.

Identify whether there is a policy in your workplace relating to patients with communication difficulties. If there is not, write down what you feel such a policy should include.

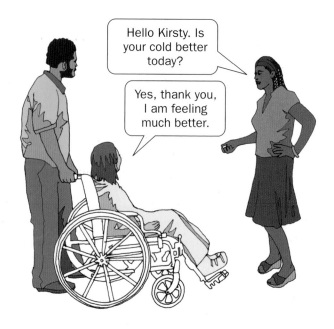

Hello Kirsty. Is your cold better today?

Yes, thank you, I am feeling much better.

Thinking about the obstacles

Never assume that you can be heard and understood, and that you can be responded to, without first thinking about the individual and his or her situation. Check first to ensure you are giving the communication the best possible chance of success by dealing with as many barriers as possible.

Practical difficulties

If you need to communicate with someone who has a known disability, such as hearing loss, impaired vision, mobility problems or speech impairment, you must consider the implications for your communication.

If someone is profoundly deaf, you will need to establish what sort of assistance he or she needs. If he or she communicates by signing, you will need to have a sign language interpreter available. Do not assume that you can do this yourself – it is highly skilled and people train for a long time to do this. If someone uses a hearing aid, consider that it may not be operating efficiently if you seem to be having communication problems.

Consider the level of someone's hearing. Many people are hard of hearing, but this may not be a profound hearing loss. It can mean that they have difficulty hearing where there is background noise and other people talking. In these situations, try to ensure background noise is kept to a minimum (this might mean taking the patient to a quiet room).

If someone has a physical disability, you will need to consider whether this is likely to affect his or her non-verbal communication. Also, his or her body language may not be what you would expect.

Individuals who have visual impairment to any significant degree will need to be addressed with thought and care. Do not rely on your facial expressions to communicate your interest and concern – use words and touch where appropriate. Remember to obtain any information they may need in a format they can use. Think about large print books, braille or audio tapes. If you need any further information, the Royal National Institute for the Blind (RNIB) will be able to advise you about local sources of supplies.

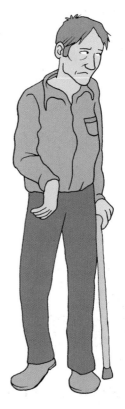

The non-verbal communication of someone with a physical disability may be different from what you expect.

Evidence with a case study (KS 8, 9,11)

Solving communication problems

Mr Talan lives alone. For many years he has been well known in the neighbourhood. He was never particularly chatty, but always said a polite 'Good morning' on his way to the shops, and had a smile and a kind word for the children. His wife died about 15 years ago. They only had one son, a soldier killed in action many years previously.

Recently, Mr Talan's health has begun to deteriorate. He had a bad winter with a chest infection and a nasty fall in the snow. This seemed to shake his confidence, and he accepted the offer of a home care assistant twice a week. Neighbours began to notice that Mr Talan no longer spoke to them, and he failed to acknowledge the children. His outings to the shops became less frequent. Jean, his home care assistant, was worried that he hardly responded to her cheerful chat as she worked. She realised that Mr Talan's hearing was deteriorating.

After medical investigations, Mr Talan was provided with a hearing aid. He began to be much more like his old self – he spoke to people again, smiled at the children and enjoyed his visits to the shops.

1 How do you think Mr Talan felt when he began to have problems hearing people?

2 Why do you think he reacted in the way he did?

3 What other factors might Jean have thought were causing Mr Talan's deterioration?

4 How are people likely to have reacted to Mr Talan?

Make notes for your portfolio.

The way you address people who have an impairment needs to be thought through carefully.

How to find out about likely communication problems

(KS 1, 2, 3, 4, 5, 6, 7, 17, 19)

You can discover likely communication problems by simply observing an individual during a care episode. You can find out a great deal about how a patient communicates and what the differences are between their way of communicating and your own.

Through observation, you should be able to establish:

- which language is being used
- if the patient experiences any hearing difficulties or visual impairment
- if there is any physical illness or disability
- if there is a learning difficulty.

Any of these factors could have a bearing on how well a patient will be able to communicate with you, and what steps you may need to take to make things easier. Observation is a useful tool, but you should work with the patient to establish exactly what is needed to assist with communication.

Best practice: Finding out about likely communication problems

As a health care assistant, you can find out about and anticipate possible problems with communication by:

✔ discussing with colleagues who have worked with the patient before – they are likely to have some background information and advice

✔ consulting other professionals who have worked with the patient – they may know means of communication that have been effective for them

✔ reading previous case notes or case histories

✔ finding out as much as you can about a patient's particular illness or disability, where you have been able to establish this – the most useful sources are likely to be the specialist agencies for the particular condition

✔ talking to family or friends – they are likely to have a great deal of information about what the differences in communication are for the patient. They will have developed ways of dealing with communication, possibly over a long period of time, and are likely to be a very useful source of advice and help.

Evidence with a case study
(HSC 31: KS 6; HSC 35: KS 9)

A patient is admitted to the ward having experienced a cerebral vascular accident (CVA) with resulting aphasia. Write notes for your portfolio about how you could gain information about this patient's communication needs, wishes and preferences.

Recording the information

There would be little point in finding out about effective means of communication with someone and then not making an accurate record so that other people can also communicate with that person.

Evidence in action (KS 19)

Discuss with your practitioner in charge where information on a patient's communication difficulties is recorded. Make notes for your portfolio.

When making notes regarding a patient's communication difficulties make sure you note:

- the nature of the communication differences
- how they show themselves
- ways which you have found to be effective in overcoming the differences.

(See page 41 for an example of poor recording.)

Information recorded in notes may look like this:

Best practice: Communicating effectively

✔ Check what the differences in communication are – remember they can be cultural as well as physical.

✔ Work with the patient to understand their preferred methods of communication and language.

✔ Use all possible sources to obtain information and advice.

Encouraging communication

The best way to ensure that someone is able to communicate to the best of his or her ability is to make the patient feel as comfortable and as relaxed as possible. There are several factors to consider when thinking about how to make people feel confident enough to communicate.

> Mr Parkins has communication difficulties following his stroke. He has speech problems with left side hemiplegia. Speech is slurred but possible to understand with care. Most effective approaches:
>
> a) allow maximum time for communication responses
> b) modify delivery if necessary in order to allow understanding
> c) speak slowly, with short sentences
> d) give only one piece of information at a time
> e) physical reassurance (holding hand) seems to help while waiting for a response
> f) can use flashcards on bad days (ensure they are placed on the right-hand side)
> g) check Mr Parkins has understood the conversation.

Communication differences	Encouraging actions
Different language	• Smile • Have a friendly facial expression • Use appropriate gestures • Use pictures • Show warmth and encouragement – repeat their words with a smile to check understanding
Hearing impairment	• Speak clearly, listen carefully, respond to what is said to you • Remove any distractions and other noises • Make sure any aids to hearing are working • Use written communication where appropriate • Use signing where appropriate • Use properly trained interpreter if high level of skill is required
Visual impairment	• Use contact, if appropriate, to communicate concern, sympathy and interest • Use tone of voice rather than facial expressions to communicate mood and response • Do not rely on non-verbal communication, e.g. facial expression or nodding head • Ensure that all visual communication is transferred into something which can be heard, either a tape or somebody reading
Confusion or dementia	• Try to make sense of communication by interpreting non-verbal behaviour • Focus on showing respect and maintaining the dignity of the other person • Do not challenge confused statements with logic • Re-orientate the conversation if you need to • Remain patient • Be very clear and keep conversation short and simple • Use simple written communication or pictures where they seem to help
Physical disability	• Ensure that surroundings are appropriate and accessible • Allow for difficulties with voice production if necessary • Do not patronise • Some patients' body language may not be appropriate because of their disability
Learning difficulty	• Judge appropriate level of understanding • Make sure that you respond at the right level • Remain patient and be prepared to keep covering the same ground • Be prepared to wait and listen carefully to responses

The risk of stereotyping

It can be very hard to really understand people's needs. Sometimes it can be tempting to make life easier by relying on fixed ideas to explain 'what people are like'. When a person has fixed ideas and regards certain types of people as all being the same, this is called stereotyping. Skilled caring starts from being interested in people's individual differences.

Stereotypes of people with disabilities are common. Disabled people are often understood as damaged versions of 'normal' people. When disabled people are negatively stereotyped in this way, they may be pitied or ignored.

Key term

Stereotype Oversimplified opinion of a person.

Older people are often negatively stereotyped. Old age is sometimes thought of as a time of decline and decay. The individual potential of a person is ignored and he or she becomes just another 'problem'.

A negative stereotypical view of an older person might include concepts such as those shown in the diagram on the following page.

This concept is developed further in Unit HSC 35 on page 118.

Stereotypical thinking might result in a health care assistant ignoring a patient's rights. For example, a health care assistant might think 'I won't offer this patient a choice because she's old – old people don't remember, so it doesn't matter what I do'.

When working in a health care setting with patients, you will need to be aware of the potential views of others and be ready to counteract any stereotyping or **labelling** which may be taking

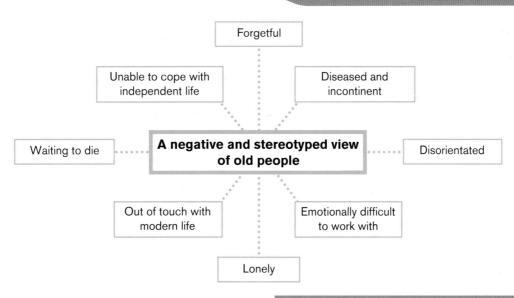

place. Be aware of the fact that assumptions may be made about the abilities of the patient. For example, it is not uncommon to underestimate what people with learning difficulties can achieve. There is also a commonly held belief that people with Alzheimer's disease need round-the-clock protection. This is not always the case: many people who have Alzheimer's are capable of achieving a great deal of independence, provided that the environment in which they live is suitably adapted. You will need to be aware of the assumptions that may be made, and the ways in which stereotyping and labelling can affect individuals.

Key term

Labelling Describing someone in a way that treats them as one of a category, rather than as an individual.

Best practice: Supporting patients to communicate

✔ Support patients to express how they want to communicate and to use their preferred methods of communication.

✔ Ensure that any aids to communication, such as hearing aids, are set up and working properly and glasses are clean.

✔ Support others who are communicating with patients to understand them and use appropriate methods of communication.

✔ Encourage patients to respond, to express their feelings and emotions appropriately, and to overcome barriers to communication.

✔ Enable patients to maintain contact with relatives and friends.

HSC 31 Update and maintain records and reports

Updating and maintaining the accuracy of records and reports is vitally important for any care setting. The information in records or reports could be about a patient who is being cared for in your workplace, a relative or friend, or it could be about the organisation itself, or about someone who works there, or for administrative purposes.

The information could come to you in a range of ways:

1 verbally, for example in a conversation either face to face or on the telephone

2 on paper, for example in a letter, a patient's health record or instructions from a health professional

3 electronically, or by fax.

Whatever the purpose of the information, it is a legal requirement that you record it accurately.

Evidence through reflection (KS 1)

Which law relates to the accurate recording of information within your workplace? Research information governance in your hospital and any related Code of Practice. Write notes for your portfolio.

It is also important that you pass on any information correctly, in the right form and to the right person. Recording information is essential in health care services, because the services that are provided are about people rather than objects. It is vital that information is accurate, accessible and readable and not your own thoughts and assumptions. Information about the communication and language needs of patients is of daily importance, and something that is recorded in the patient's care plan. It is always worth remembering that all records could be required as evidence in a court of law.

Ways of receiving and passing on information

(KS 1, 2, 3, 4, 5, 17, 18, 19)

Today, within health care, there are many ways in which information is circulated between agencies, colleagues, other multi-disciplinary team members, patients, relatives, carers, volunteers and so on. The growth of electronic communication has meant a considerable change in the way that people receive and send information, in comparison to only a few years ago when information sharing was limited to face-to-face meetings, telephone calls or posted letters.

Telephone

One of the commonest means of communication is the telephone; it has advantages because it is instant. However, there are some disadvantages to using the telephone to communicate. You can never be entirely sure who you may be talking to, and it can often be difficult to ensure that you have clearly understood what has been said. There can be problems with telephone lines, which cause crackling and technical difficulties. It is also possible to misinterpret someone's meaning when you cannot pick up other signals, such as facial expression and body language. If you regularly take or place messages on the telephone, there are some very simple steps that you can take to ensure that you cut down the risk of getting a message wrong.

Make sure that you check the name of the person who is calling. If necessary, ask the person to spell his or her name and repeat it to make sure you have it right. It is easy to mix up Thomas and Thompson, Williams and Wilkins, and so on. You may also need to take the person's address, and again it is worthwhile asking him or her to spell the details to ensure that you have written them correctly.

Always ask for a return telephone number so that the person who receives the message can phone back if necessary. You should read back the message itself to the person who is leaving it, to check that you have the correct information and that you have understood his or her meaning. Remember – **confidentiality** must be maintained at all times.

Key term

Confidentiality Treating patient's information with discretion according to the law.

Evidence in action (KS 1, 17)

Within your workplace, do you have access to a code of conduct, policy or guideline relating to the use of information technology? Write notes for your portfolio about the contents of this code and how it impacts on your practice.

Research the Caldicott Report and identify the principles and their application to practice. Identify the role of the Caldicott Guardian. Make notes for your portfolio.

Incoming post

If it is part of your role to open and check any incoming post, you must make sure that you:

- open it as soon as it arrives
- follow your own workplace procedures for dealing with incoming mail – this is likely to involve stamping it with the date it is received
- pass it on to the appropriate person for it to be dealt with or filed. See page 33 for advice on how to deal with confidential information.

Faxed information

The steps for dealing with an incoming fax message are as follows.

- Read the cover sheet – this will tell you who the fax is for, who it is from (it should include telephone and fax numbers) and how many pages there should be.
- Check that the correct number of pages have been received. If a fax has misprinted or has pages missing, contact the telephone number identified on the cover sheet and ask for the information to be sent again. If there is no

telephone number, send a fax immediately to the sending fax number, asking for the fax to be resent.

- Follow your organisation's procedure for dealing with incoming and outgoing faxes. Make sure the fax is handed to the appropriate person as soon as possible.

Email

Email is a frequently used means of communication within and between workplaces. It is fast, convenient and easy to use for many people. Large reports and complex information that would be cumbersome to post or fax can be transmitted as an attachment to an email in seconds. However, not everyone in all workplaces has access to email, and not all electronic transmission is secure. Be aware of this if you are sending highly sensitive and confidential material. If you do send and receive information by email you should:

1 follow the guidelines in your workplace for using email and the transmission of confidential material

2 open all your emails and respond to them promptly

3 save any confidential messages or attachments in an appropriate, password-protected file or folder, and delete them from your inbox (unless that is also protected)

4 return promptly any emails you have received in error

5 never share your password with anyone.

Outgoing post

If you have to write information to send to another organisation, whether by letter, fax or email, you should be sure that the contents are clear, cannot be misunderstood and are to the point. Remember that anything you write down in the course of your work becomes a legal document.

Within many organisations, you will need to show any faxes or letters to your manager before they are sent. This safeguard is in place in many workplaces for the good reason that information being sent on behalf of your employer must be accurate and appropriate. As your employer is the person ultimately responsible for any information sent out, he or she will want to have procedures in place to check this.

Confidentiality

(KS 1, 2, 3, 4, 5, 19)

Confidentiality involves keeping information safe and only passing it on where there is a clear right to it and a clear need to do so. Confidentiality is an important right because:

- patients will not trust a health care assistant who does not keep information confidential
- patients will not feel valued or able to keep their self-esteem if their private details are shared with others
- patients' safety may be put at risk if details of their property and habits are shared publicly.

A professional service that maintains respect for individuals must keep private information confidential. Patients have a right to confidentiality under the terms of the Data Protection Act (1998) – see the table on page 37. Confidentiality has to be kept within boundaries, and the rights of others have to be balanced with the patient's rights. It is also essential that personal information in relation to staff is kept confidential.

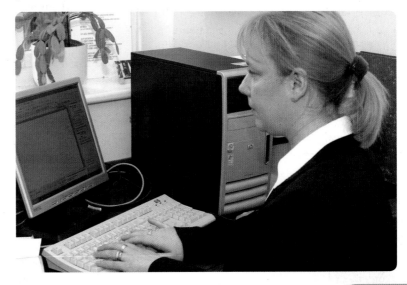

Passing on information

In many cases, the passing of information is routine and related to the care of the patient. For example, medical information may be passed to another hospital, to a residential home or to a private care agency. However, it must be made clear to the patient that this information will be passed on in order to ensure that they receive the best possible care.

A health care assistant may have to tell his or her manager something learned in confidence. Again, the patient has a right to know that you mean to pass on their confidence to someone else. The information is not made public, so it is still partly confidential.

Consent

Best practice involves asking patients if we can let other people know things. For example, it would be wrong to pass on even the date of a person's birthday without asking him or her first. Some people might not want others to celebrate their birthday – for example, Jehovah's Witnesses believe that it is wrong to do so. Whatever we know about a patient should be kept private, unless the person tells us that it is acceptable to share the information. However information on aspects of care can be passed on when others have a right and a need to know it.

Right to know, need to know or want to know?

There are always some people who do *need* to know information about a patient, either because they are directly involved in providing care for the individual or because they are involved in some other support role. However, it is essential that you only pass on the information that is required for the purpose. For example, you don't need to tell the hearing aid clinic that Mr Sampson's son is currently serving a prison sentence. However, if Mr Sampson became seriously ill and the hospital wanted to contact his next of kin, you would need to pass that information on. In other words, people should be told what is necessary for them to carry out their role.

Some examples of people who have a need to know about work with patients are:

- managers – they may need to help make decisions which affect the patient
- colleagues – they may be working with the same person
- other professionals – they may also be working with the patient and need to be kept up to date
- Mental Capacity Act (2007).

When information is passed to other professionals, it should be on the understanding that they keep it confidential.

Be sure who you are talking to

It is important to check that people asking for information are who they say they are. If you answer the telephone and the caller says he or she is a social worker or other professional, you should explain that you must call back before giving any information. Phoning back enables you to be sure that you are talking to someone at a particular number or within a particular organisation. If you meet a person you don't know, you should ask for proof of identity before passing on any information. Information should be passed on only on a 'need to know' basis and should be agreed with the practitioner in charge before doing so.

Supporting relatives

Relatives will often claim that they have a 'right to know'. The most famous example of this was Victoria Gillick, who went to court to try to gain access to her daughter's medical records. She claimed that she had the right to know whether her daughter had been given the contraceptive pill. Her GP had refused to tell her and she took the case all the way to the House of Lords, but the ruling was not changed and she was not given access to her daughter's records. The rules remain the same. Even for close relatives, the information is not available unless the patient agrees.

Sometimes it is possible to ask relatives to discuss issues directly with the patient rather than giving information yourself, as shown in the illustration on the following page.

Even if you are faced with angry or distressed relatives who believe that you have information they are entitled to, you must not disclose any information that is confidential.

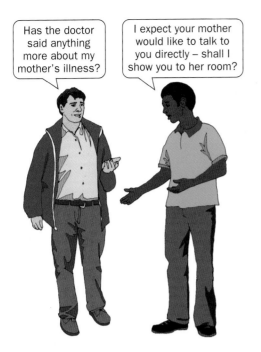

Has the doctor said anything more about my mother's illness?

I expect your mother would like to talk to you directly – shall I show you to her room?

The patient's rights

The Data Protection Act (1998) gives people a right to see the information recorded about them. This means that people can see their medical records, or social services files. Providing the consultant in charge of the patient agrees there may be potential damaging information that needs delicate handling, such as adopted children, etc. Since January 2005, the Freedom of Information Act (2000) has provided people with a right to access general information held by public authorities, including local authorities and the National Health Service. Examples include how much the Chief Executive earns, how many patients survive surgery with a specific consultant, etc. Personal information about other people cannot be accessed and is protected by the Data Protection Act (1998).

Patients also have a right to expect that information about them is accurately recorded. This and the right to confidentiality are backed by the Data Protection Act (1998). Other important legislation includes the Mental Capacity Act (2007), the Human Rights Act (1999), etc. All services now have to have policies and procedures on the confidentiality of recorded information. For more details, see the table on page 37.

How you can maintain confidentiality

The most common way in which workers breach confidentiality is by chatting about work with friends or family. It is very tempting to discuss the day's events with your family or with friends over a drink or a meal. It is often therapeutic to discuss a stressful day, and helps get things into perspective. But you must make sure that you talk about issues at work in a way that keeps patients' details confidential and anonymous.

For example, you can talk about how an encounter made you feel without giving any details of the other people involved. For example, you can say: 'Today this patient accused me of not drying between his toes properly – at first I was so angry I didn't know what to say! What would you have done?' The issue can be discussed without making reference to gender, ethnicity, age, physical description, location or any other personal information that might even remotely identify the person concerned.

It might be considered a breach of the Data Protection Act (1998) to discuss patients' details with people who do not have a need to know. The essential issue is trust; even if no one can identify the name of the person involved, others might perceive you as displaying a lack of respect if you talk about the people you work with in places where you might be overheard.

You also need to be sure that you do not discuss one patient you care for with another, at any time.

you never know who's listening!

CARELESS TALK COSTS LIVES

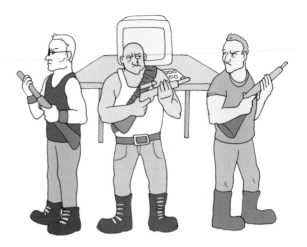

Computer records must be surrounded by proper security.

The basic rule is that all information a patient gives, or that is given on his or her behalf, to an organisation is confidential and cannot be disclosed to anyone without the consent of the patient. You will need to support patients in contributing to and understanding records and reports concerning them, and ensure they understand how the rules of confidentiality affect them.

Best practice: Respecting confidentiality

✔ Generally you should only give information with consent.

✔ Only give people the information they need to know to do their job.

✔ Information should be relevant to the purpose for which it is required.

✔ Check the identity of the person to whom you give information.

✔ Make sure that you do not give information carelessly.

Protecting patients' personal information

(KS 1, 2, 3, 4, 5, 18, 19)

Once something is written down or entered on a computer, it becomes a permanent record. For this reason, you must be very careful what you do with any files, charts, notes or other written records.

Written records must always be stored somewhere locked and safe, and records kept on computers must also be kept safe and protected. Your workplace will have policies relating to records on computers, which will include access being restricted by a password, and the computer system being protected against the possibility of people 'hacking' into it.

The information that you write in files should be clear and useful. Do not include irrelevant information, and write only about the patient concerned. Anything you write should be true and able to be justified, and not your personal opinion. Any mistakes made while writing on documentation should be crossed out with a single line and then rewritten. Under no circumstance should corrective fluid be used.

Best practice: ACES

The purpose of a file is to reflect an accurate and up-to-date picture of a patient's situation, and to provide a historical record, which can be referred to at some point in the future. Some of it may be required to be disclosed to other organisations.

Always think about what you write. Make sure it is **ACES**:

✔ **A**ccurate

✔ **C**lear

✔ **E**asy to read

✔ **S**hareable.

All information, however it is stored, is subject to the rules laid down in the Data Protection Act (1998), which covers medical records, social service records, credit information, local authority information – in fact, anything which is personal data.

Anyone processing personal data must comply with the eight enforceable principles of good practice. These say that data must be:

1 fairly and lawfully processed

2 processed for limited purposes

3 adequate, relevant and not excessive

4 accurate

5 not kept longer than necessary

6 processed in accordance with the data subject's rights

7 kept secure

8 not transferred to countries without adequate protection.

Written records

The confidentiality of written records is extremely important. You will need to make sure that, when you receive information in a written form (perhaps intended for someone's file or a letter concerning someone you are caring for), the information is not left where it could be easily read by others.

Do not leave confidential letters or notes lying in a reception area, or on a desk where visitors or other staff members might see them. You should ensure that the information is filed, or handed to the

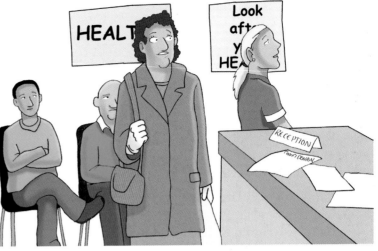

Leaving confidential material lying around in public may be more than just embarrassing – it could be against the law.

person it is intended for, or that you follow your organisation's procedure for handling confidential information as it comes into the organisation.

You may need to stamp such information with a 'confidential' stamp so that people handle it correctly.

The dos and don'ts of dealing with information

Type of information	Do	Don't
Telephone calls, incoming	Check the identity of the caller	Give out any information unless you are sure who the caller is
Telephone calls, outgoing	Make sure that you are passing on information to which the caller is entitled	Give out details that the individual has not agreed to disclose
Written information	Check that it goes immediately to the person it is intended for	Leave written information lying around where it can be read by anyone
Receiving faxed material	Check your organisation's procedure for dealing with faxed material. Collect it as soon as possible from any central fax point	Leave it in a fax tray where it could be read by unauthorised people
Sending faxed material	Ensure that it is clearly marked 'Confidential' and has the name on it of the person to whom it should be given Ensure that you are sending the fax to the correct address	Fax confidential material without clearly stating that it is confidential and it is only to be given to a named person If in doubt, do not use a fax to send confidential information
Receiving emailed information	Save any confidential attachments or messages promptly into a password-protected file Acknowledge safe receipt of confidential information	Leave an email open on your screen
Sending emailed information	Ensure that you have the right email address for the person who is receiving the information Clearly mark the email 'Confidential' if it contains personal information Ask for the recipient to acknowledge receipt	Leave an email open on your screen Send confidential information to an address without a named mailbox, e.g. info@ . . . Share your password

Choosing the best way to pass on information

There are different ways of passing on information, some quicker than others. For example, the situation may require an immediate response in which case you could telephone the person you need to speak to, or send an email. These methods are fast, almost instant, and relatively reliable for getting information accurately from one place to another.

There may be other occasions when, on the grounds of confidentiality, something is sent through the post marked 'Strictly confidential' and only to be opened by the person whose name is on the envelope. This method may be entirely appropriate for information that is too confidential to be sent by fax and would be inappropriate in a telephone conversation or to be sent by email.

You will have to take a number of factors into account when deciding which method to use, as the diagram shows.

The purpose of keeping records

In any organisation, records are kept for a variety of different purposes. The type of record that you keep is likely to be dictated by the purpose for which it is required. It could be:

- information that is needed for making decisions
- information to provide background knowledge and understanding for another health care worker
- information about family and contacts of people who are important to a patient
- information to be passed to another health professional who is also involved in providing patient care
- information to be passed from yourself to a colleague over a short space of time to ensure that the care you provide offers an element of continuity
- information to help in planning and developing services.

The kind of record you keep within your own organisation may well be different from the type you would keep if you were going to send that information to another agency, or if it was going into someone else's filing system.

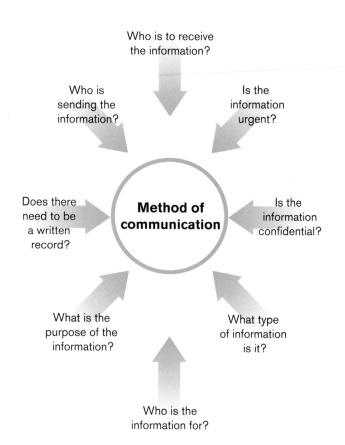

Factors to consider when choosing a method of communication.

Sally:

Mary Johnson

Please could you make sure that you check on Mrs Johnson several times during the next shift. Nothing I can put my finger on, nothing that could go on the handover record, but she just doesn't seem herself. Please keep an eye on her.

See you tomorrow

Sue

An informal note like this is often used to pass on information that is not appropriate for a formal file or record sheet, but it is still important for a colleague to take note of. This is different from information that has to go outside the organisation – that would need to be formally written, and word-processed using a more structured format.

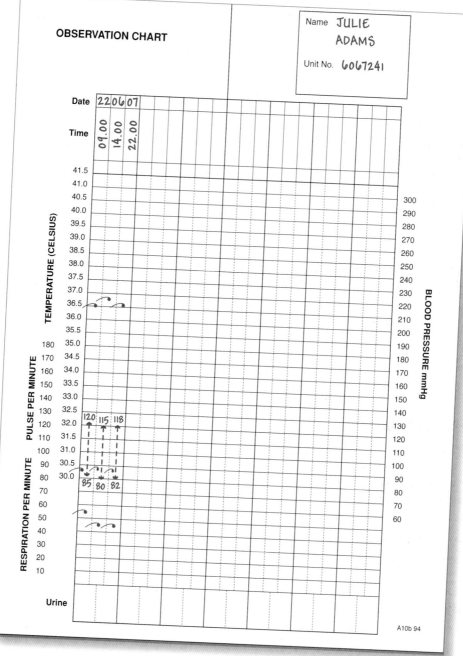

An observation chart.

Types of record

Medical records

One of the common means of transmitting information and keeping records in health care is an observation chart recording temperature and blood pressure.

This is done in a very simple form on a graph, so it is easy to see at a glance if there are any problems. The purpose of this record is simply to monitor a patient's physical condition so that everybody who is caring for them can check on the patient's well-being.

Other types of record

Information that is likely to be used in making decisions about a patient is very important. Where such records are being kept, it is important that reports are not written in such a way that people have to read through vast amounts of material before finding the key points. It may be necessary

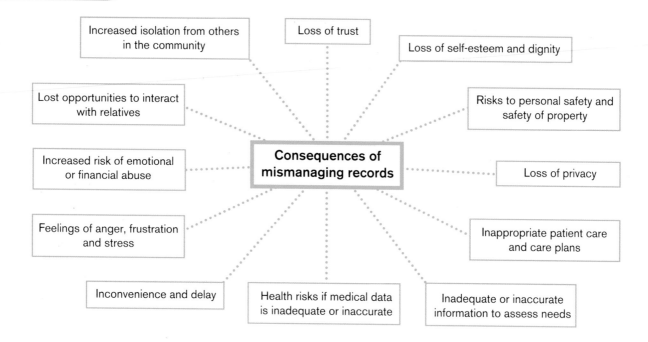

Increased isolation from others in the community

Loss of trust

Loss of self-esteem and dignity

Lost opportunities to interact with relatives

Risks to personal safety and safety of property

Consequences of mismanaging records

Increased risk of emotional or financial abuse

Loss of privacy

Feelings of anger, frustration and stress

Inappropriate patient care and care plans

Inconvenience and delay

Health risks if medical data is inadequate or inaccurate

Inadequate or inaccurate information to assess needs

to include a significant amount of information to make sure that all of the background is there, but a summary at the beginning or the end covering the main points is always useful.

Evidence in action (KS 5)

Find out how many different types of record are kept in your workplace. There may be reports, charts, notes or index cards. Note what each is used for. Identify which records are about a patient's communication abilities. Make notes for your portfolio.

Why keeping good records is so important

If patient's records are not managed in accordance with the Data Protection Act (1998) and hospital policies, patients might suffer a range of damaging consequences (see diagram top).

How to record information

(KS 1, 2, 3, 4, 5, 18, 19)

If you think about the purpose for which the information is to be used, this should help you to decide on the best way to record it. There is little point in going to the trouble of typing out a piece

of information that you were simply going to pass over to a colleague on the next shift. Alternatively, if you were writing something which was to go into a patient's case notes or case file and be permanently recorded, you would need to make sure that the information is of use to colleagues, or others who may need to have access to the file.

You may need to record and report:

- signs and symptoms indicating a change in the condition of a patient
- signs of a change in the care needs of a patient
- actions you have taken relating to a patient's needs or condition following discussion with the professional in charge
- difficulties or conflicts that have arisen, and actions taken to resolve them in discussion with the professional in charge.

It is good practice to have any reports or records that you have written about a patient's care countersigned by the professional in charge.

Evidence in action (KS 17, HSC 35, KS 9)

Find out your organisation's policy about record-keeping, and where different types of information should be recorded and kept. Check whether there are clear guidelines on what should be handwritten and information that needs to be word-processed. Make notes for your portfolio.

You must make sure that you follow the guidelines and provide information in the format that your organisation needs. If you are unsure about how you should produce particular kinds of records, ask your manager.

Key term

Objective Not influenced by emotions or personal prejudices.

Methods of storing and retrieving records

Imagine going into a music shop which has thousands of CDs stored in racks but in no recognisable order; they are not filed by the name of the artist, nor by the title of the album. Imagine how much time it would take to trace the particular CD that you are looking for. This is exactly what it is like with a filing system – unless there is a system that is easily recognisable and allows people to trace files quickly and accurately, it is impossible to use.

Records are stored in filing systems. These may be manual or computerised. All organisations will have a filing system, and one of the first jobs you must undertake is to understand how it works and learn how to use it.

Some organisations have people who deal specifically with filing, and they do not allow untrained people to access the files. This is likely to be the case if you work for a large organisation, such as an NHS trust.

Evidence with a case study (KS 18)

Maintaining records and reports

Look at the following report on K by CS, K's named health care assistant.

Write notes for your portfolio covering the following questions.

1 What is your opinion of this report? Consider the factual detail, the attitude shown towards K by his health care assistant and the practical suggestions made.

2 List the improvements that you would make to this report.

3 What problems could be caused by poor report writing like this?

4 If you were CS's manager, how would you respond to receiving a report like this?

K has been bad this week. He said he felt ill but he didn't have a temperature or anything. I think he wanted to stay in hospital rather than go home on his own.

Tuesday 12 noon. After I had just fed him he vomited all over me. I know he can't help throwing up, but he could give me some warning so I didn't have to change all my clothes. I cleaned him up in the usual way.

Thursday the physio came and asked us to get K to mobilise using his zimmer frame. So I told him he had to get out of bed and walk with the frame. He got really stroppy and refused to get up in the end. I think we ought to fix set times for him to get out of bed and walk each day. Then we won't have these fights about him getting about. What do you think?

If you learn to appreciate the importance of records and the different systems that can be used for their storage, you can assist rather than hinder the process of keeping records up to date, in the right place and readily accessible when people need them.

Manual systems

In a manual filing system, the types of file used can vary. The most usual type of file is a brown manila folder with a series of documents fastened inside. Other types include ring binders, lever arch files and bound copies of computer printouts.

All of the files have to be organised (indexed) and stored in a way that makes them easily accessible whenever they are required.

Alphabetical system

If there are not too many files, they can be kept in an alphabetical system in a simple filing cabinet or cupboard. In this sort of system, files are simply placed according to the surname of the person they are about. They are put in the same order as you would see names in a telephone directory, starting with A and working through to the end of the alphabet, with names beginning *Mc* being filed as *Mac* and *St* being filed as *Saint*. When working in the ward environment, patient records are usually kept using an alphabetical system within a locked notes trolley.

Numerical systems

Where there are large numbers of files, an alphabetical system would not work. In that situation an alphabetical filing system would become impossible to manage, so large organisations give their files numbers, and they are stored in number order. Clearly, a numerical system needs to have an index system so that a person's name can be attached to the appropriate number.

A hospital is likely to give a patient a hospital number, which will appear on all relevant documentation, so that it is always possible to trace his or her medical notes. However, there still needs to be an overall record to attach that patient's name and address to that particular set of case notes, and these days this is normally kept on a central computer.

Computerised systems

If your organisation uses a computerised system, there will be very clear procedures to be followed by everyone who accesses the system. The procedures will vary depending on the system used, but usually involve accessing files through a special programme: this may well have been written especially for your organisation, or may be one specifically for record keeping in health and care settings.

You are unlikely to be able to delete or alter any information in a patient's file on a computer. It is possible that you will only be able to add information in very specific places, or it could be that files are 'read only' and you cannot add any information to them. This process, because it will not allow people to change or alter files, does have the advantage that information is likely to remain in a clear format. It is less likely to become lost or damaged in the way that manual files are.

Evidence in action (KS 17)

Find out about the filing system used in your workplace and ask if you could visit where all the health records are kept. Check how much information is kept in files, and how much on computer. Find out if the system is alphabetical or numerical, and ask someone who understands it to show you how it is used. Make notes for your portfolio.

Other types of records

Most organisations maintain electronic records for accounts, suppliers, personnel and all essential business records. There will be a back up for any electronically held information; this may be a paper system or off-site electronic back up.

Useful information about advice and support services in the area could be maintained in a resource area or filing system. An electronic index of useful websites, with links, can be very valuable for patients and their families if they have computer access and are comfortable accessing information in this way.

Some basic rules about filing

Do	Don't
Leave a note or card (or something similar) when you borrow a file from a manual filing system	Remove an index card from a system
Return files as soon as possible	Keep files lying around after you have finished with them
Enter information clearly and precisely	Alter or move around the contents of a file, or take out or replace documents which are part of someone's file
Make sure that you access electronic files strictly within your permitted level of access	Make any changes to files unless permitted to do so
Keep your password safe and private	Copy any part of an electronic record system Share your password with anyone
Make sure you log in and out correctly	Forget to log out

Further reading and research

In this section you have covered aspects of communication to help you build and develop relationships as well as ways to improve your practice as a health care assistant. Opposite are details of further opportunities to research this subject. The list is not exhaustive and some you may find more interesting and useful than others.

Websites

- www.directgov.co.uk (UK government: Data Protection Act 1998, Rights and Responsibilities)
- www.dh.gov.uk (Department of Health: Data Protection Act 1998, Patient choice, Sensory impairment)
- www.arcos.org.uk (ARCOS: Association for Rehabilitation of Communication and Oral Skills)
- www.scie.org.uk (SCIE: Social Care Institute for Excellence)
- www.rnib.org.uk (RNIB: Royal National Institute of Blind People)
- www.sense.org.uk (Sense – UK deafblind charity)
- www.deafblind.org.uk, www.deafblindscotland.org.uk (Deafblind)
- www.rnid.org.uk (RNID: Royal National Institute for the Deaf)
- www.alzheimers.org.uk (Alzheimer's Society)
- www.askmencap.info (Mencap: fact sheets on communication and people with learning disabilities)

Publications

- Butler, S. (2004) *Hearing and Sight Loss*, Age Concern and RNIB
- Caldwell, P., Stevens, P. (2005) *Creative Conversations: Communicating with People with Learning Disabilities*, Pavilion Publishers
- Malone, C., Forbat, L., Robb, M., Seden, J. (2004) *Relating Experience: Stories from Health & Social Care: An Anthology about Communication and Relationships*, Routledge
- Moss, B. (2007) *Communication Skills for Health & Social Care*, Sage Publications Ltd
- Thomson, H., Meggitt, C. (2007) *Human Growth and Development*, Hodder Headline

Promote, monitor and maintain health, safety and security in the working environment

Introduction

This unit is about the way you can contribute to making your workplace a safe, secure and healthy place for people who use it to meet their care needs, for those who work alongside you, and for yourself.

In the first section, you will need to learn about what needs to be done to ensure a safe workplace environment. In the second element, you will be looking at how you may need to adapt the way you work to become more safety conscious, and think about the way in which your work can affect others. The third element in this unit is about how to respond appropriately in an emergency.

What you need to learn

- What is safety?
- How to maintain security
- The legal framework for health, safety and security
- Dealing with hazardous waste
- How to promote a safe work environment
- Safe manual handling
- How to contribute to infection control
- Challenging inappropriate practice
- How to maintain personal safety
- Fire safety
- Health emergencies

What evidence you need to generate for your portfolio

For your award you will mainly be required to produce observations of you carrying out tasks in your workplace. Your assessor will observe you undertaking real life activities to cover the performance criteria. This can be supported by witness testimonies from colleagues who have seen you working.

In addition to this, you will need to demonstrate your knowledge and understanding. You can do this by providing written accounts that identify how you integrate theory with practice, answering verbal or written questions. Having an understanding of health and safety issues is imperative and a legislative requirement when undertaking any task. Therefore evidence can be derived from many work situations.

The knowledge specifications identified under the headers of each section are intended as a guide.

HSC 32 Monitor and maintain the safety and security of the working environment

What is safety?

(KS 1, 3, 4, 6, 11, 12, 13, 14)

It sounds very simple and straightforward to make sure that the workplace is safe and secure. But this is a complex subject and includes all areas of the day-to-day work of a health care assistant. All health care assistants are required to attend mandatory safety and security training, including regular updating sessions, and they are also required to put what they learn into practice.

It may help if you think about safety and security in respect of the areas of responsibility shown in the table below.

Responsibilities for safety and security in the workplace

Employer's responsibilities	Employee's responsibilities	Shared responsibilities
Planning safety and security	Using the systems and procedures correctly	Safety of individuals using the facilities
Providing information about safety and security	Reporting flaws or gaps in the systems, equipment or procedures in use	Safety of the environment
Updating systems and procedures	Ensuring all practice is current, up to date and relevant	Employer to ensure appropriate training is available; employee to ensure mandatory training is undertaken

Safety in the working environment

You and other employees share responsibility with your employer for the safety of all the patients and internal customers who use your service. There are many hazards that can cause injury to patients, and health care assistants need to be aware of the following types of hazards.

Environmental hazards
These include:
- wet or slippery floors
- cluttered passageways or corridors
- re-arranged furniture
- worn carpets
- electrical flexes.

Hazards connected with equipment and materials
Examples of such hazards include:
- faulty brakes on beds
- worn or faulty electrical equipment
- worn or damaged moving and handling equipment
- worn or damaged mobility aids
- incorrectly labelled substances, such as cleaning fluids
- leaking or damaged containers
- faulty waste-disposal equipment.
- overloaded equipment e.g. laundry skips, sharps containers.

Hazards connected with people
This category of hazards includes:
- handling procedures
- visitors to the building
- intruders
- violent and aggressive behaviour.

The health care assistant's role

All health care assistants have a responsibility to contribute to a safe working environment. This means more than simply being aware of the potential **hazards**. A health care assistant must also take steps to check and deal with any sources of **risk**.

If your role involves supervising staff, you must also ensure that these staff are aware of the possible risks and hazards and know how to deal with them, or how to ask for help or advice from a senior member of staff. Although it is ultimately the employer's responsibility, all health care assistants have a duty to ensure the safety of any staff under their supervision.

As part of a health care assistant's contract, there is a responsibility to ensure that you regularly update your knowledge and practice, as well as attending mandatory training.

Health care assistants can fulfil their role in two ways: by dealing directly with the hazard, or by reporting it to a manager.

Dealing directly with the hazard

This means that the health care assistant has taken individual responsibility. It could apply to obvious hazards such as:

- trailing flexes – roll them up and store them safely
- wet floors – dry them as far as possible and put out warning signs.

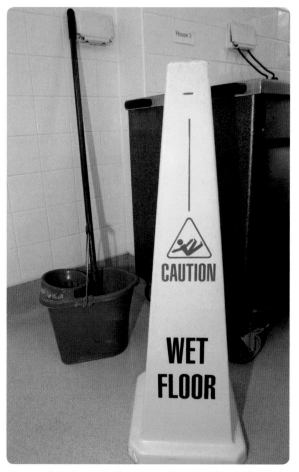

After washing floors dry them as much as possible, and set out warning signs.

- cluttered doorways and corridors – remove objects and store them safely or dispose of them appropriately; if items are heavy, use assistance or mechanical aids
- visitors to the building – challenge anyone you do not recognise; asking 'Can I help you?' is usually enough to establish whether a person has a good reason to be there
- fire – follow the correct procedures to raise the alarm and assist with evacuation.

Informing your manager

You should report hazards that are beyond your role and competence, such as:

- faulty equipment
- worn floor coverings
- loose or damaged fittings
- obstructions too heavy to move safely
- damaged or faulty aids – hoists, bed brakes, bathing aids, etc.
- people acting suspiciously on the premises
- fire.

Once reported, the hazard becomes an organisational responsibility.

How to maintain security

(KS 1, 3, 4, 6, 14, 15, 16)

Most workplaces where care is provided are not secure, as people come and go freely. This is an inevitable part of ensuring that people have choice and that their rights are respected. However, people also have a right to be secure.

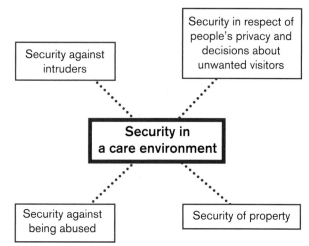

Security against intruders

When working for a large organisation, such as an NHS Trust, all employees should be easily identifiable by identity badges with photographs. Some of these even contain a microchip, which allows the card to be 'swiped' to gain access to secure parts of the building. This makes it easier to identify people who do not have a right to be on the premises. Those visiting the premises to undertake work will need to establish their right to entry and access security or visitor passes.

In a smaller workplace, there may be a system of issuing visitors' badges to visitors who have reasons to be there, or it may simply rely on the vigilance of the staff.

Some workplaces operate electronic security systems, but less sophisticated systems may also be used, such as a keypad with a code number known only to staff and those who are legitimately on the premises. It is often difficult to maintain security with such systems, as codes are forgotten or become widely known. In order to maintain security, it is necessary to change the codes regularly, and to make sure everyone is aware.

Some workplaces still operate with keys, although the days of staff walking about with large bunches of keys attached to a belt are fast disappearing. If mechanical keys are used, there will be a list of named key holders and there is likely to be a system of handover of keys at shift change. However, each workplace has its own system and all health care assistants need to be sure they understand which security system operates in their own workplace.

The more dependent individuals are, the greater the risk to their safety and security. When working with babies, high-dependency or unconscious patients, people with a severe learning difficulty or the confused, health care assistants need to be extremely vigilant in protecting these patients from any breaches in safety and security arrangements.

Workplaces where most or all patients are in individual rooms can also be difficult to make secure, as it is not always possible to check every room if patients choose to close the door. A routine check can be very time-consuming, and can affect patients' rights to privacy and dignity.

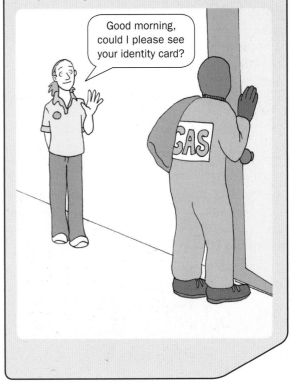

Best practice: Protecting against intruders

✔ Be aware of everyone you come across. Get into the habit of noticing people and thinking, 'Do I know that person?'

✔ Challenge anyone you do not recognise or who does not have an identity badge or visitors pass.

✔ The challenge should be polite. 'Can I help you?' is usually enough to find out if a visitor has a reason to be on the premises.

✔ If a person says that he or she is there to see someone:
   • ask them who they have come to see.
   • don't give directions – escort him or her.

If the person is a genuine visitor, he or she will be grateful.

Good morning, could I please see your identity card?

Ward areas are easier to check, but can present their own problems; it can be difficult to be sure who is a legitimate visitor and who should not be there. Some establishments provide all visitors with badges, but while this may be acceptable in a large institution or an office block, it is not compatible with creating a comfortable and relaxed atmosphere in a ward environment. Extra care must be taken to check that you know all the people in a communal area. If you are not sure, ask. It is better to risk offending someone by asking 'Can I help you?' or 'Are you waiting for someone?' than to leave an intruder unchallenged.

Restricting access

People have a right to choose who they see. This can often be a difficult area to deal with. If there are relatives or friends who wish to visit and an individual does not want to see them, you may have to make this clear. This can be difficult, but you can only be effective if you are clear and assertive. You should not make excuses or invent reasons why visitors cannot see the person concerned. You could say something like: 'I'm sorry, Mr Price has told us that he does not want to see you. I understand that this may be upsetting, but it is his choice. If he does change his mind, we will contact you. Would you like to leave your phone number?' However, it may be more appropriate to hand this over to the practitioner in charge.

Do not allow yourself to be drawn into passing on messages or attempting to persuade – that is not your role. Your job is to respect the wishes of the person you are caring for. If you are asked to intervene or to pass on a message, you must refuse politely but firmly.

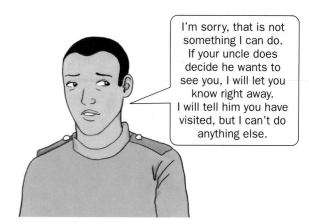

If you are asked to make any intervention that is outside your role, you must refuse politely but firmly.

There may also be occasions when access is restricted for other reasons, possibly because someone is seriously ill and there are medical reasons for limiting access, or because of a legal restriction such as a court order. In such a case, it should be clearly recorded on the patient's notes and your supervisor will advise you about the restrictions. If you are working in a supervisory capacity, it will be part of your role to ensure that junior staff are aware of these restrictions.

Evidence with a case study (KS 8, 9, 10)

A patient has explained that she does not want any visitors as she is feeling too unwell. Make notes for your portfolio about the correct procedure for ensuring visitors' rights to enter your workplace, and explain how you would resolve the conflict of the patient not wanting to see anyone.

Abuse is dealt with in depth in Unit HSC 35 (see page 120), but always remember that patients have a right to be protected from abuse, and you must report immediately any abuse you see or suspect.

Evidence through reflection (KS 4, 8, 11, 12, 14, 15, 16)

Thinking about your work environment, and the individuals you care for, reflect on an incident which may have occurred which had a negative impact on the safety and security provision of your patients. Make notes for your portfolio.

Key term

Abuse Physical, psychological or sexual maltreatment of a person.

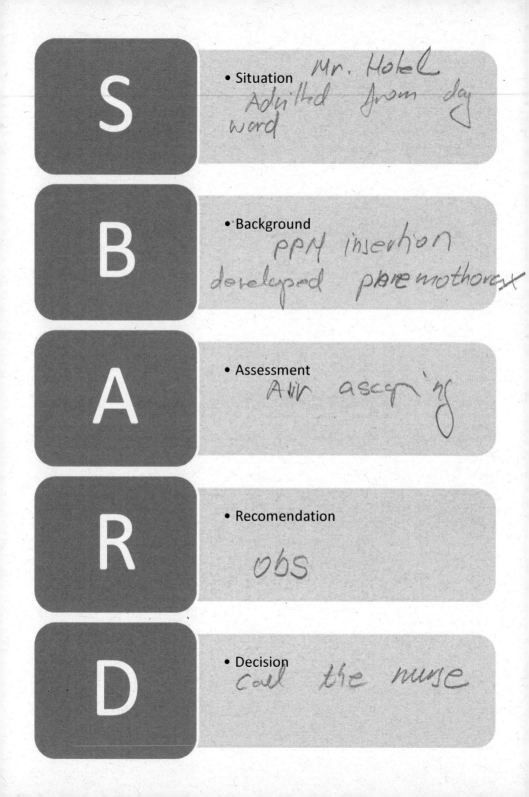

S • Situation — Mr. Hotel Admitted from day ward

B • Background — PPM insertion developed pneumothorax

A • Assessment — Air escaping

R • Recomendation — obs

D • Decision — call the nurse

Security of property

Property and valuables belonging to patients in care settings should be safeguarded. Your organisation will have a property book in which records of all valuables and personal possessions are entered.

There may be particular policies within your organisation, but as a general rule you are likely to need to:

- make a record of all possessions on admission
- record valuable items separately
- describe items of jewellery by their colour, for example 'yellow metal' not 'gold'
- ensure that individuals sign for any valuables they are keeping, and that they understand that they are liable for their loss
- inform your manager if an individual is keeping valuables or a significant amount of money.

It is always difficult when items go missing in a care setting, particularly if they are valuable. It is important that you check all possibilities before calling the police.

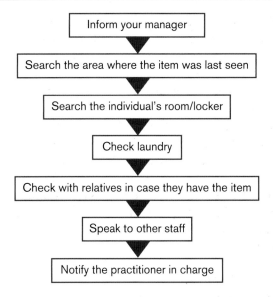

Action stages when property goes missing.

The legal framework for health, safety and security

(KS 1, 3, 4)

The settings in which you provide care are generally covered by the Health and Safety at Work Act (HASAWA) (1974). This Act has been updated and supplemented by many sets of regulations and guidelines, which extend it, support it or explain it. The regulations most likely to affect your workplace are shown in the diagram.

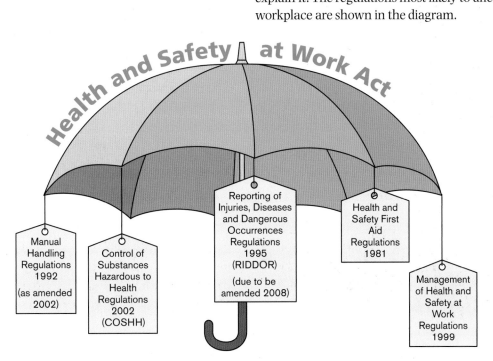

The Health and Safety at Work Act is like an umbrella.

The healthcare assistant and the law

There are many regulations, laws and guidelines dealing with health and safety. Although you do not need to know these in detail, health care assistants do need to know where their responsibilities begin and end.

The law places certain responsibilities on both employers and employees. For example, it is up to the employer to provide a safe place in which to work, but the employee also has to show reasonable care for his or her own safety.

Employers have to:

- provide a safe workplace
- ensure that there is safe access to and from the workplace
- provide information on health and safety
- provide health and safety training in accordance with minimum standards
- undertake **risk assessment** for all hazards.

Employees must:

- take reasonable care for their own safety and that of others
- co-operate with the employer in respect of health and safety matters
- not intentionally damage any health and safety equipment or materials provided by the employer.

Both the employee and employer are jointly responsible for safeguarding the health and safety of anyone using the premises.

Key term

Risk assessment A formal evaluation of a particular risk.

Evidence through reflection (KS 6, 18)

Check that all your mandatory training is up to date. Write a reflective account to identify how you have put information gained from the training sessions into practice.

Each workplace where there are five or more employees must have a written health and safety policy. The policy must include:

- a statement of intention to provide a safe workplace
- the name of the person responsible for implementing the policy
- the names of any other individuals responsible for particular health and safety hazards
- a list of identified health and safety hazards and the procedures to be followed in relation to them
- procedures for recording accidents at work
- details for evacuation of the premises.

The Health and Safety Executive

Britain's Health and Safety Commission (HSC) and the Health and Safety Executive (HSE) are responsible for the regulation of almost all the risks to health and safety arising from work activity in Britain. The Health and Safety Commission is sponsored by the Department of Work and Pensions and is accountable to the Minister of State for Work. The HSE's job is to help the HSC ensure that risks to people's health and safety from work activities are properly controlled.

The Health and Safety Executive (http://www.hse.gov.uk) states:

'Our mission is to protect people's health and safety by ensuring risks in the changing workplace are properly controlled'.

The HSC believes in the prevention of accidents, and its key roles include providing information and support to ensure that workplaces are safe and the enforcement of the law in order to ensure that legislation is adhered to. The HSE has the power to prosecute employers who fail in any way to safeguard the health and safety of people who use their premises.

The Management of Health and Safety at Work Regulations Act (1999) states that employers have to assess any risks that are associated with the workplace and any work activities – this means *all* activities, from walking on wet floors to dealing with violence. Having carried out a risk assessment, the employer must then apply risk control measures – actions must be taken to reduce the risks. For example, alarm buzzers may need to be installed or extra staff employed to deal with intruders, as well as steps such as providing extra training for staff or written guidelines on how to deal with a particular hazard.

Risk assessments are vitally important in order to protect the health and safety of both staff and patients. A health care assistant should always check that a risk assessment has been carried out before undertaking any task, and then follow the steps identified in the assessment in order to reduce the risk. However, risk assessment should be an ongoing procedure and should be taken into consideration before any aspect of care is undertaken.

Remember

Do not forget that you must balance the wishes and preferences of each individual who uses your service with your own safety and the safety of others. Some examples of this principle are discussed in the section on manual handling later in this chapter (page 58).

Control of Substances Hazardous to Health (COSHH) (2002)

There are many substances hazardous to health – nicotine, many drugs, alcohol – and the COSHH Regulations (2002) relate to substances that have been identified as toxic, corrosive or irritant. This includes cleaning materials, pesticides, acids, disinfectants and bleaches, and naturally occurring substances such as blood and bacteria. Workplaces may have other hazardous substances that are particular to the nature of the work carried out.

The Health and Safety Executive states that employers must take the following steps to protect employees from hazardous substances.

Step 1: Find out what hazardous substances are used in the workplace and the risks these substances pose to people's health.

Step 2: Decide what precautions are needed before any work starts with hazardous substances.

Step 3: Prevent people being exposed to hazardous substances or, where this is not reasonably practicable, control the exposure.

Step 4: Make sure control measures are used and maintained properly, and that safety procedures are followed.

Step 5: If required, monitor exposure of employees to hazardous substances.

Step 6: Carry out health surveillance where assessment has shown that this is necessary, or where COSHH makes specific requirements.

Step 7: If required, prepare plans and procedures to deal with accidents, incidents and emergencies.

Step 8: Make sure employees are properly informed, trained and supervised.

Every workplace must have a COSHH file, which should be easily accessible to all staff. This file lists all the hazardous substances used in the workplace. It should detail:

- where hazardous substances are stored
- how hazardous substances are labelled
- the effects of hazardous substances
- the maximum amount of time it is safe to be exposed to the hazardous substance
- how to deal with an emergency involving one of the hazardous substances.

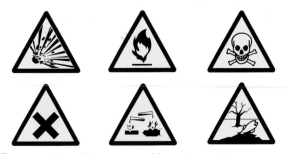

These symbols, which warn you of hazardous substances, are always yellow.

If you have to work with hazardous substances, make sure that you take the precautions detailed in the COSHH file. This may be wearing protective personal equipment (PPE), such as gloves, aprons or protective goggles, or it may involve limiting the time you are exposed to the hazardous substance or only using the substance in certain prescribed circumstances. Health care assistants are required by law to wear the protective personal equipment provided for them by their employer.

The COSHH file should also give you information about how to store hazardous substances. This will involve using the correct containers as supplied by the manufacturers. All containers must have safety lids and caps, and must be correctly labelled.

Never use the container of one substance for storing another, and *never* change the labels.

The symbols in the following illustration indicate hazardous substances. They are there for your safety and for the safety of those you care for and work with. Before you use *any* substance, whether it is liquid, powder, spray, cream or aerosol, take the following simple steps:

- check the container for the hazard symbol
- if there is a hazard symbol, go to the COSHH file
- look up the precautions you need to take with the substance
- make sure you follow the procedures, which are intended to protect you.

If you are concerned about a substance being used in your workplace that is not in the COSHH file, or if you notice incorrect containers or labels being used, report this to your manager. Once you have informed your manager, it becomes his or her responsibility to act to correct the problem.

Reporting of Injuries, Diseases and Dangerous Occurrences (RIDDOR) (1995)

Reporting accidents and ill health at work is a legal requirement. All accidents, diseases and dangerous occurrences should be reported to the RIDDOR Incident Contact Centre. The Centre was established on 1 April 2001 as a single point of contact for all RIDDOR incidents in the UK. The information is important because it means that risks and causes of accidents, incidents and diseases can be identified across the country. All notifications are passed on to either the local authority Environmental Health department, or the Health and Safety Executive, as appropriate.

Your employer needs to report:

- deaths
- major injuries (see the next page)
- accidents resulting in more than three days off work
- diseases
- dangerous occurrences (near misses).

Reportable major injuries and diseases

The following injuries need to be reported:

Reportable major injuries and diseases

Reportable injuries	Reportable diseases
fracture other than to fingers, thumbs or toes	certain poisonings
amputation	
dislocation of the shoulder, hip, knee or spine	some skin diseases such as occupational dermatitis, skin cancer, chrome ulcer, oil folliculitis acne
loss of sight (temporary or permanent)	
chemical or hot metal burn to the eye or any penetrating injury to the eye	lung diseases including occupational asthma, farmer's lung, pneumoconiosis, asbestosis and mesothelioma
injury resulting from an electric shock or electrical burn leading to unconsciousness or requiring resuscitation or admittance to hospital for more than 24 hours	
any other injury which leads to hypothermia (getting too cold), heat-induced illness, or unconsciousness; requires resuscitation; or requires admittance to hospital for more than 24 hours	infections such as leptospirosis, hepatitis, tuberculosis, anthrax, legionellosis (Legionnaires' disease) and tetanus
unconsciousness caused by asphyxia (suffocation) or exposure to a harmful substance or biological agent	
acute illness requiring medical treatment, or leading to loss of consciousness, arising from absorption of any substance by inhalation, ingestion or through the skin	other conditions such as occupational cancer, certain musculoskeletal disorders, decompression illness and hand-arm vibration syndrome.
acute illness requiring medical treatment where there is reason to believe that this resulted from exposure to a biological agent or its toxins or infected material.	

Did you know?

If something happens which does not result in a reportable injury, but which clearly *could* have done, then it may be a dangerous occurrence which must be reported immediately.

Evidence through reflection (KS 3)

Make sure you know your hospital's injury reporting system where the accident report forms or the accident book are kept, and who is responsible for recording accidents, this is likely to be your manager.

Think of an incident you may have been involved in and make notes in your portfolio on the actions that were taken and by whom.

Accidents at work

If accidents or injuries occur at work, either to you, to other staff or to an individual you are caring for, then the details must be recorded. For example, someone may have a fall, or slip on a wet floor. You must record the incident regardless of whether there was an injury.

Your employer will have procedures in place for making a record of accidents – either an accident book or an accident report form – and this is required by the RIDDOR (1992) regulations.

Any medical treatment or assessment that is necessary should be arranged without delay. If a patient has been involved in an accident, you should check if there is anyone they would like to be contacted – perhaps a relative or friend. If the accident is serious, and you cannot consult the patient – because they are unconscious, for example – the next of kin should be informed as soon as possible.

Complete a report, and ensure that all witnesses to the accident also complete reports.

Date: 24.6.08   Time: 14.30 hrs   Location: Main ward

Description of accident:

PH got out of her chair and began to walk across the main ward with the aid of her stick. She turned her head to continue the conversation she had been having with GK, and as she turned back again she appeared not to have noticed that MP's handbag had been left on the floor. PH tripped over the handbag and fell, banging her head on a footstool.

She appeared shaken and, although she said that she was not hurt, there was a large bump on her head. PH appeared pale and shaky. I asked J to fetch a blanket and to call Mrs J, the practitioner in charge. Covered PH with a blanket. Mrs J arrived immediately. Dr was sent for after PH was examined by Mrs J.

Dr arrived after about 20 mins and said that she was bruised and shaken, but did not seem to have any injuries.

She wanted to go and lie down. She was helped to bed.

Incident was witnessed by six patients who were in the ward at the time: GK, MP, IL, MC, CR and BQ.

Signed: Name:

An example of an accident report form.

Checklist: completing an accident report

You should include the following in any accident report (see the example above):

- date, time and place of accident
- person/people involved – bearing in mind the Data Protection Act (1998)
- circumstances and details of exactly what you saw
- anything which was said by the individuals involved
- the condition of the individual after the accident
- steps taken to summon help, time of summoning help and time when help arrived
- names of any other people who witnessed the accident
- any equipment involved in the accident.

Dealing with hazardous waste

(KS 3, 4, 6, 11, 12, 14)

As part of providing a safe working environment, employers have to put procedures in place to deal with waste materials and spillages. There are various types of waste, which must be dealt with in particular ways. The types of hazardous waste you are most likely to come across are shown in the table on the next page, alongside a list of the ways in which each is usually dealt with. Waste can be a source of infection, so it is very important that you follow the procedures your employer has put in place to deal with it safely.

Type of waste	Method of disposal
Clinical waste – used dressings	Yellow bags, clearly labelled with contents and location. This waste is incinerated.
Needles, syringes, cannulas ('sharps')	Yellow sharps box. Never put sharps into anything other than a hard plastic box. This is sealed and incinerated when two thirds full.
Spillages – e.g. urine, vomit, blood, sputum, faeces	Area to be cleaned and disinfected as per hospital policy. All clinical waste to be disposed of in yellow bag.
Soiled linen	Red bags, direct into laundry; bags disintegrate in wash.
Recyclable instruments and equipment	Blue bags, to be returned to the Central Sterilisation Services Department (CSSD) for recycling and sterilising.

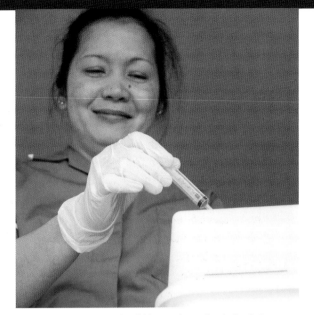

Needles and syringes should be put into a hard plastic box, which is sealed and incinerated.

Evidence in action (KS 3, 4, 11, 12)

1 Find the needle stick injury policy for your workplace. Write notes for your portfolio on how this policy could reduce the risk of contamination and infection to a health care assistant.

2 Look at the picture below. How many possible hazards and risks can you find in the picture?
   • List at least six.
   • Which of these are the responsibility of the employer?
   • Which should you do something about?

3 Name three types of waste and their methods of disposal.

4 How should hazardous substances be stored?

5 What are the employer's responsibilities in respect of hazardous substances?

6 What are the employee's responsibilities for hazardous substances?

Discuss the answers with your assessor and make notes for your portfolio.

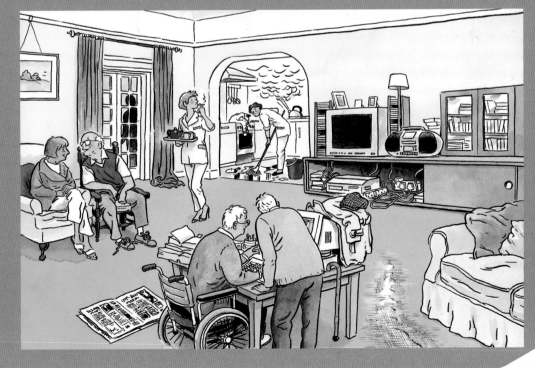

In the previous section, we examined the polices and procedures which have to be put in place to protect staff and people who use health services, and the laws which govern health and safety. In this section, we examine what the health care assistant actually does to promote health and safety in the work environment and the steps to follow to ensure that the laws and policies work in practice.

How to promote a safe work environment

(KS 1, 2, 3, 6, 9, 11, 12, 13, 14, 15, 16, 18)

Health care environments are places where accidents can quite often happen, not because staff are careless or fail to check hazards, but because of the vulnerability of the patients who use the health care facilities.

Patients are often ill, frail or have physical conditions that affect mobility, such as arthritis or Parkinson's disease, where the patient may be susceptible to falls and trips because they are unsteady, and the slightest change in surface or level can upset their balance. Increasing age can also result in less flexibility of muscles and joints, meaning that people are less able to compensate for a loss of balance or a slip and are more likely to fall than younger people, who may be better able to save themselves by reacting more quickly.

Age is not the only factor to increase risk. Other factors, such as impaired vision, can increase the risk of accidents from trips, falls, and knocking into objects. Hearing loss can increase the risk of accidents where people have not heard someone, or perhaps something such as a trolley, approaching around a corner. Dementia can increase risks because people fail to remember to take care when they move about. They can also forget where they have put things down and fail to understand the consequences of actions such as pulling on cupboard doors.

Supporting individuals to assess and manage risks

It is important that you support patients in your care to ensure their own health and well-being. Wherever possible, encourage them to:

- express their needs and preferences about their own health and well-being
- understand and take responsibility for promoting their own health and care
- assess and manage risks to their health and well-being
- identify and report any factors that may put themselves or others at risk.

It is important that you develop an awareness of health and safety risks and that you are always aware of any risks in any situation you are in. If you get into the habit of making a mental checklist, you will find that it helps. The checklist will vary from one workplace to another, but could look like this.

Checklist for a safe work environment

Hazards	Check
Environment	
Floors	❏ Are they dry?
Carpets	❏ Are they worn or curled at the edges?
Doorways and corridors	❏ Are they clear of obstacles?
Electrical flexes	❏ Are they trailing?
Equipment	
Beds	❏ Are the brakes on? ❏ Is the bed at a safe height?
Electrical appliances	❏ Are cables worn? ❏ Have they been safety checked?
Lifting equipment	❏ Is it worn or damaged?
Mobility aids	❏ Are they worn or damaged? ❏ Are they of the correct size/height?
Substances such as cleaning fluids	❏ Are they correctly labelled and stored?
Containers	❏ Are they leaking or damaged?
Waste disposal equipment	❏ Is it faulty? If so, why?

People	
Visitors to the building	❏ Should they be there?
	❏ Do they have identification?
Handling procedures	❏ Have they been assessed for risk?
Intruders	❏ Have security been called/notified?
Violent and aggressive behaviour	❏ Has it been dealt with?
Staff	❏ Have they been cleared by occupational health as fit to work?

Evidence in action (KS 14)

Using a checklist, access an area of your workplace for health safety and security risks. Keep the checklist in your portfolio as evidence.

One of the other factors to consider in your checklist may be what your colleagues do about health and safety issues. It is very difficult if you are the only person following good practice. You may be able to encourage others by trying some of the following options:

- always showing a good example yourself by being a role model
- explaining why you are following procedures
- accessing some health and safety leaflets from your trades union, environmental health office or online and leaving them in the staffroom for people to see
- work shadowing the risk manager.

What you wear

There are several reasons why what staff wear has an impact on health and safety, and why employers issue a uniform policy (code of dress) to their employees. The uniform should be comfortable and well fitting with plenty of room for movement. Inappropriate clothing can be restrictive and prevent free movement when working with patients.

High-heeled or poorly supporting shoes are a risk to health care assistants in terms of foot injuries, and they also present a risk to the patients you care for because, if you overbalance or stumble, so will they.

Staff should tie up long hair. Hair can contain substantial amounts of bacteria, which could cause infection. In addition, loose long hair could be a safety hazard. Agitated or confused patients may grab at an assistant's hair, or it might get caught in equipment.

There are restrictions on wearing jewellery or carrying things in your pocket that could cause injury – to yourself or the patient. Wristwatches should not be worn because, apart from the possibility of scratching a patient when providing personal care, wearing a watch can harbour bacteria and prevent good hand-washing technique. Fob watches that pin onto the uniform are convenient and easy to obtain.

Many workplaces do not allow the wearing of rings with stones. Not only are they a possible source of infection, but they can also scratch patients or tear protective gloves.

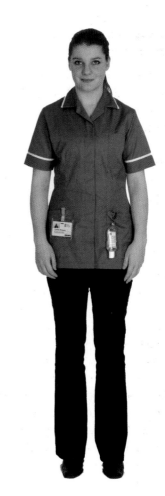

It is essential for health and safety that all staff dress appropriately for work and follow their workplace uniform policy.

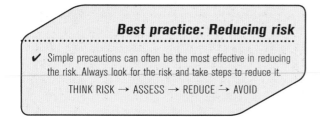

Best practice: Reducing risk

....

✔ Simple precautions can often be the most effective in reducing the risk. Always look for the risk and take steps to reduce it.

THINK RISK → ASSESS → REDUCE → AVOID

Safe manual handling

(KS 1, 2, 3, 4, 6, 8, 9, 11, 12, 13, 14)

Moving and handling patients is the single largest cause of injuries at work in health care settings. One in four health care workers takes time off because of a back injury sustained at work.

The Manual Handling Operations Regulations (1992) require employers to avoid all manual handling where there is a risk of injury 'so far as it is reasonably practical'. All health care assistants must understand and follow the procedures and polices laid down by the organisation they work for.

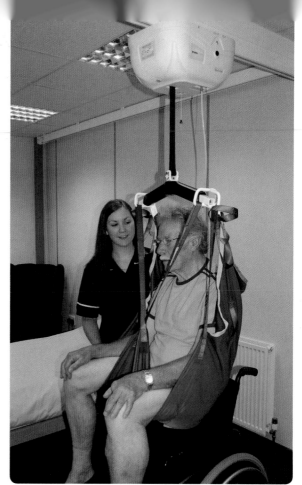

Make sure the patient feels safe and comfortable throughout the move.

Lifting Operations and Lifting Equipment Regulations (1992) (LOLER)

These regulations apply to all workplaces and refer to employers. Employers have a duty under LOLER to ensure that all the equipment provided in their workplace is:

- sufficiently strong and stable for the particular use and marked to indicate safe working loads
- positioned and installed to minimise any risks
- used safely – that is, the work is planned, organised and performed by competent people
- subject to ongoing thorough examination and, where appropriate, inspection by competent people.

In addition employers must ensure that:

- lifting operations are planned, supervised and carried out in a safe way by competent people
- equipment for lifting people is safe
- lifting equipment and accessories are thoroughly examined
- a report is submitted by a competent person following a thorough examination or inspection.

Lifting equipment designed for lifting and moving loads must be inspected at least annually, but any equipment that is designed for moving and handling people must be inspected at least every six months. A nominated competent person may draw up an examination scheme for this purpose.

Under the Management of Health and Safety at Work Regulations (1999), employees have a duty to ensure that they take reasonable care of themselves and others who may be affected by the actions that they undertake – this includes using equipment such as hoists and turning boards provided by the employer to reduce the risk of manual handling.

When manual lifting is necessary

There is almost no situation in which manual moving and handling could be considered acceptable, but the views and rights of the individual being moved must be taken into account and a compromise achieved. On the rare

You have a patient on the ward who is bed bound. In the course of a day this patient will require bathing, sitting on the commode, sitting in the chair for meals and sitting up in bed. Identify for your portfolio the different techniques, procedures and equipment you might need or use in order to move this person safely and write notes.

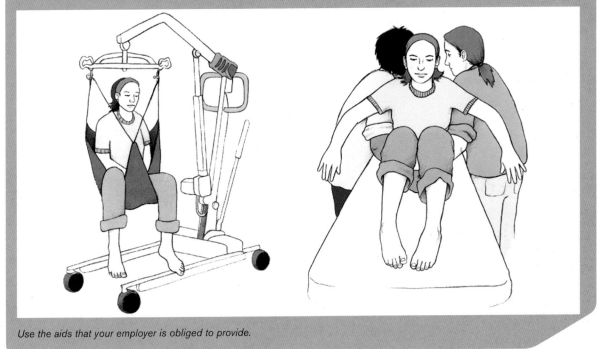

Use the aids that your employer is obliged to provide.

occasions when it is still absolutely necessary for manual lifting to be done, the employer has to make a 'risk assessment' and put procedures in place to reduce the risk of injury to the employee. This could involve ensuring that sufficient staff are available to move or handle someone safely, which can often mean that four people are needed.

Your employer will arrange for all staff to attend a mandatory moving and handling course with regular updates.

From the patient's point of view

It is paramount that patients are encouraged to help themselves as much as possible. Patients can become dependent on the people providing their care for them – this is called 'learned helplessness'. This can occur when health care assistants find it is quicker and easier to do things themselves, rather than allowing the patient to do it. If patients accept that someone else will take over all their care, they may stop making the effort to maintain their independence – in short, they learn how to become helpless.

Write notes for your portfolio on how you would encourage a post-operative patient to take responsibility for their own mobility.

It is also essential that the views of the person being moved are taken into account. While you and your employer need to make sure that you and other staff are not put at risk by moving or handling, it is also important that the person needing assistance is not caused pain, distress or humiliation. Groups representing disabled people have pointed out that policies excluding any lifting may infringe the human rights of individuals needing mobility assistance. For example, individuals may in effect be confined to bed unnecessarily and against their will by a lack of lifting assistance. A High Court judgement (A & B vs East Sussex County Council, 2003) found in favour of two disabled women who had been denied access to lifting because the local authority had a 'blanket ban' on lifting, regardless of circumstances. Such a ban was deemed unlawful. It is likely that similar cases will be brought under the Human Rights Act (1998), which gives people protection against humiliating or degrading treatment.

The Disability Discrimination Act (1995) was introduced to ensure that providers of services make reasonable adjustments to the way they deliver their services so that disabled people can use them. The new duties apply to all service providers where physical features make access to their services impossible or unreasonably difficult for disabled people. This could include the entrance to a hospital being up some steps making it impossible for a person in a wheelchair to get up them; now a ramp would have to be provided as a result of the Disability Discrimination Act (1995).

Remember

You will need to relate the information covered in this unit to Unit CHS 12.

How to contribute to infection control

(KS 3, 4, 8, 11, 12, 14, 15, 18)

The very nature of work in a care setting means that great care must be taken to control the spread of infection. A health care assistant will come into contact with a number of people during the working day and this is an ideal opportunity for infection to spread. Infection that spreads from one person to another is called 'cross-infection'. If you work in a hospital setting, infection control is essential.

There are various steps you can take in terms of the way you carry out your work (wherever you work) which can help to prevent the spread of infection.

No one knows what viruses or bacteria an individual may be harbouring, so it is important that you take precautions when dealing with everyone. These precautions are called 'standard precautions' because health care assistants need to follow them with everyone they deal with. All staff must be familiar with standard precautions and adhere to them.

Infection control is covered in greater depth in Topic 1 on page 137.

Wear gloves

When	Any occasion when you will have contact with body fluids (including body waste, blood, mucus, sputum, sweat or vomit), or when you have any contact with anyone with a rash, pressure sore, wound, bleeding or any broken skin. You must also wear gloves when you clear up spills of blood or body fluids or have to deal with soiled linen or dressings.
Why	Because gloves act as a protective barrier against infection.
How	Check gloves before putting them on to make sure they are not cracked or faded. When you pull them on, make sure that they fit properly. If you are wearing a gown, pull them over the cuffs. Take them off by pulling from the cuff and remember to dispose of them in the correct waste disposal container then wash and dry your hands thoroughly.

How to use gloves properly

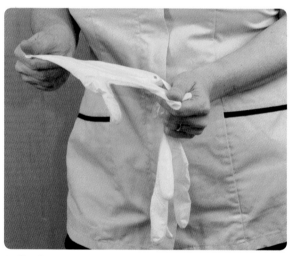

1 *Check gloves before putting them on. Never use gloves with holes or tears. Check that they are not cracked or faded.*

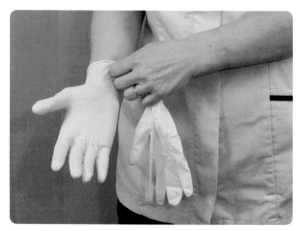

2 *Pull gloves on, making sure that they fit properly. If you are wearing a gown, pull them over the cuffs.*

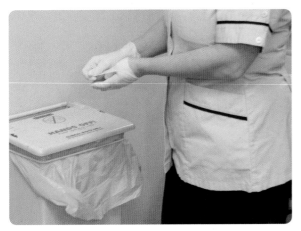

3 *Take them off by pulling from the cuff – this turns the glove inside out. Pull off the second glove while still holding the first, so that the two gloves are folded together inside out.*

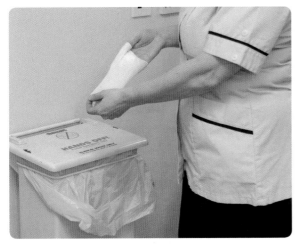

4 *Dispose of them in the correct waste disposal container and wash your hands.*

Wash and dry your hands thoroughly

When	Before and after carrying out any procedure which has involved contact with an individual, or with any body fluids, soiled linen or clinical waste. You must wash your hands even though you have worn gloves. You must also wash your hands before you start and after you finish your shift, before and after eating, after using the toilet and after coughing, sneezing or blowing your nose.
Why	Because hands are a major route to spreading infection. When tests have been carried out on people's hands, an enormous number of bacteria have been found.
How	Wash hands in running water, in a basin deep enough to hold the splashes and with either foot pedals or elbow bars rather than taps, because you can re-infect your hands from still water in a basin, or from touching taps with your hands once they have been washed. Use the soaps and disinfectants supplied. Make sure that you wash thoroughly following the correct procedure, including between your fingers. This should take between 10 and 20 seconds.

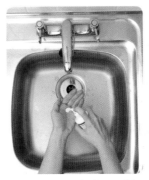

1 *Wet your hands thoroughly under warm running water and squirt liquid soap onto the palm of one hand.*

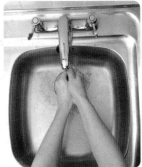

2 *Rub your hands together to make a lather.*

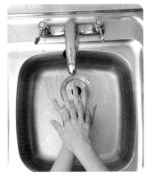

3 *Rub the palm of one hand along the back of the other and along the fingers. Then repeat with the other hand.*

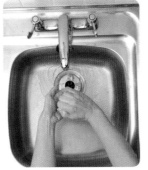

4 *Rub in between each of your fingers on both hands and round your thumbs.*

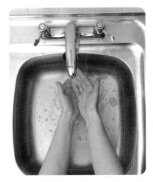

5 *Rinse off the soap with clean water.*

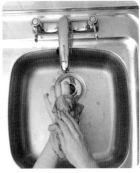

6 *Dry hands thoroughly on a disposable towel.*

Alcohol hand rub

Alcohol hand rubs can be useful when hands are socially clean and if you are not near a source of water. A small amount should be used and rubbed into the hands, using the same technique as for washing with water. The hand rub should be rubbed in until the hands are completely dry.

Wear protective clothing

When	You should always wear a plastic apron for any procedure that involves bodily contact or is likely to deal with body waste or fluids.
Why	Because it will reduce the spread of infection by preventing infection getting on your clothes and spreading to the next person you come into contact with.
How	The plastic apron should be disposable and thrown away at the end of each procedure. You should use a new apron for each patient you come into contact with.

Tie up hair

Why	Because if it hangs over your face, it is more likely to come into contact with the patient you are working with and could spread infection. It could also become entangled in equipment and cause a serious injury or a patient may pull/grab on your hair which may cause injury.

Clean equipment

Why	Because infection can spread from one person to another on instruments, linen and equipment just as easily as on hands or hair.
How	By washing large items like trolleys with antiseptic solution. Small instruments must be sterilised. Do not shake soiled linen or leave it on the floor. Keep it held away from you. Place linen in the proper bags or hampers for laundering.

Deal with waste

Why	Because it can then be processed correctly, and the risk to others working further along the line in the disposal process is reduced as far as possible.
How	By placing it in the proper bags. Make sure that you know the system in your workplace. It is usually: • clinical waste – yellow • soiled linen – red • recyclable instruments and equipment – blue

Take special precautions

When	There may be occasions when you have to deal with a patient who has a particular type of infection that requires **universal precautions**. This can involve things like hepatitis, some types of food poisoning or highly infectious diseases.
How	Your workplace will have infection control procedures to follow. They may include such measures as gowning, double gloving or wearing masks. Follow the procedures strictly. They are there for your benefit and for the benefit of the other individuals you care for.

Key term

Universal precautions Standard infection control practices used universally in health care settings to minimise the risk of exposure to pathogens. Also known as standard precautions.

Evidence through reflection (KS 11, 12)

Make notes of three ways in which infection can be spread. Then note down three effective ways to reduce the possibility of cross-infection and keep the notes for your portfolio.

Prevention of infection is everyone's responsibility, so you must ensure that colleagues follow the appropriate guidelines.

Challenging inappropriate practice

(KS 10, 16, 18)

You may have to deal with the situation where one of your colleagues is misusing equipment or behaving in an inappropriate way towards patients or other health care assistants, in a way that fails to minimise risks to health, safety or security.

If you are faced with the situation where a colleague is behaving inappropriately or bad practice is being allowed to occur, you can respond in several ways. Depending on the severity of the problem, you should:

- challenge the behaviour, or the source of the bad practice
- have a one-to-one discussion with the colleague in question
- act as a mentor with whom your colleague can share problems and difficulties
- act as a role model of good practice
- always report problems to your manager.

Best practice: Steps to personal safety

✔ Attend mandatory training provided by your employer in techniques to combat aggression and violence. It is foolish and potentially dangerous to go into risky situations without any training.

✔ Try to defuse potentially aggressive situations by being as calm as possible and by talking quietly and reasonably. But if this is not effective, leave and summon help as per your organisation's procedure.

✔ Raise the alarm if you find you are in a threatening situation.

✔ Do not tackle aggressors, whoever they are – raise the alarm.

✔ Use an alarm or panic button if you have it – otherwise shout, very loudly.

Evidence with a case study (KS 3, 4, 6)

Inappropriate behaviour

Consider incidences of inappropriate practice that you may have been involved in with a member of staff within your workplace. Reflect on how the situation was dealt with and make notes for your portfolio.

How to maintain personal safety

(KS 2, 3, 4, 10, 15, 16, 17, 18)

There is always an element of risk in working with people. There is little doubt that in recent years there has been an increase in the level of personal abuse suffered by those working in the health care services.

However, there are some steps you can take to assist with your own safety.

HSC 32c Minimise risks arising from incidents and emergencies

Fire safety

(KS 3, 4, 12, 15, 16, 17, 18)

Your workplace will have procedures that must be followed in the case of an emergency. All workplaces must display information about what action to take in case of fire. The fire procedure is likely to be similar to the one shown on the next page.

Make sure that you know where the appropriate fire extinguishers or fire blankets are in your workplace, and also where the fire exits are.

Your employer will have installed fire doors to comply with regulations – never prop them open.

Your employer must provide fire lectures for all health care assistants each year. All staff must attend and make sure that they are up to date with the procedures to be followed.

The Fire Precautions (Workplace) (Amendment) Regulations (1999) require that all workplaces should be inspected by the fire authority to check means of escape and firefighting equipment and warnings. A fire certificate must also be issued. A breach of fire regulations could lead to a prosecution of the employer, the responsible manager, or other staff members.

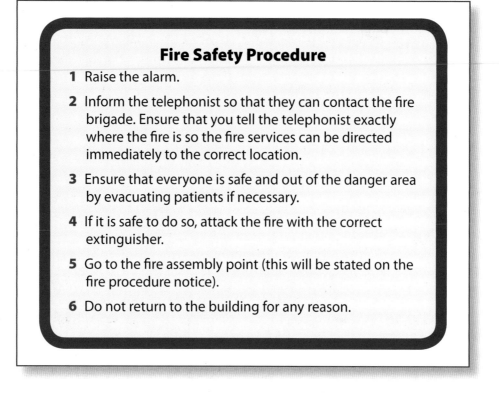

Fire Safety Procedure

1 Raise the alarm.

2 Inform the telephonist so that they can contact the fire brigade. Ensure that you tell the telephonist exactly where the fire is so the fire services can be directed immediately to the correct location.

3 Ensure that everyone is safe and out of the danger area by evacuating patients if necessary.

4 If it is safe to do so, attack the fire with the correct extinguisher.

5 Go to the fire assembly point (this will be stated on the fire procedure notice).

6 Do not return to the building for any reason.

Which extinguisher?

There are specific fire extinguishers for fighting different types of fire. It is important that you know this. You do not have to memorise them as each one has clear instructions on it, but you do need to be aware that there are different types and make sure that you read the instructions before use.

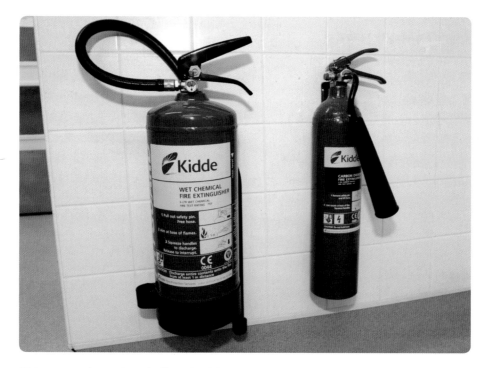

Make sure you know where the fire extinguishers are in your workplace.

Extinguisher type and patch colour	Use for	Danger points	How to use	How it works
Red Water	Wood, cloth, paper, plastics, coal, etc. Fires involving solids.	Do not use on burning fat or oil, or on electrical appliances.	Point the jet at the base of the flames and keep it moving across the area of the fire. Ensure that all areas of the fire are out.	Mainly by cooling burning material.
Blue Multi-purpose dry powder	Wood, cloth, paper, plastics, coal, etc. Fires involving solids. Liquids such as grease, fats, oil, paint, petrol, etc. but **not** on chip or fat pan fires.	Safe on live electrical equipment, although the fire may re-ignite because this type of extinguisher does not cool the fire very well. Do **not** use on chip or fat pan fires.	Point the jet or discharge horn at the base of the flames and, with a rapid sweeping motion, drive the fire towards the far edge until all the flames are out.	Knocks down flames and, on burning solids, melts to form a skin smothering the fire. Provides some cooling effect.
Blue Standard dry powder	Liquids such as grease, fats, oil, paint, petrol, etc. but **not** on chip or fat pan fires.	Safe on live electrical equipment, although does not penetrate the spaces in equipment easily and the fire may re-ignite. This type of extinguisher does not cool the fire very well. Do **not** use on chip or fat pan fires.	Point the jet or discharge horn at the base of the flames and, with a rapid sweeping motion, drive the fire towards the far edge until all the flames are out.	Knocks down flames.
Cream AFFF (Aqueous film-forming foam) (multi-purpose)	Wood, cloth, paper, plastics, coal, etc. Fires involving solids. Liquids such as grease, fats, oil, paint, petrol, etc. but **not** on chip or fat pan fires.	Do **not** use on chip or fat pan fires.	For fires involving solids, point the jet at the base of the flames and keep it moving across the area of the fire. Ensure that all areas of the fire are out. For fires involving liquids, do not aim the jet straight into the liquid. Where the liquid on fire is in a container, point the jet at the inside edge of the container or on a nearby surface above the burning liquid. Allow the foam to build up and flow across the liquid.	Forms a fire-extinguishing film on the surface of a burning liquid. Has a cooling action with a wider extinguishing application than water on solid combustible materials.
Cream Foam	Limited number of liquid fires.	Do **not** use on chip or fat pan fires. Check manufacturer's instructions for suitability of use on other fires involving liquids.	Do not aim jet straight into the liquid. Where the liquid on fire is in a container, point the jet at the inside edge of the container or on a nearby surface above the burning liquid. Allow the foam to build up and flow across the liquid.	

continued

Black Carbon dioxide CO2	Liquids such as grease, fats, oil, paint, petrol, etc. but **not** on chip or fat pan fires.	Do **not** use on chip or fat pan fires. This type of extinguisher does not cool the fire very well. Fumes from CO_2 extinguishers can be harmful if used in confined spaces: ventilate the area as soon as the fire has been controlled.	Direct the discharge horn at the base of the flames and keep the jet moving across the area of the fire.	Vaporising liquid gas smothers the flames by displacing oxygen in the air.
Fire blanket	Fires involving both solids and liquids. Particularly good for small fires in clothing and for chip and fat pan fires, provided the blanket **completely** covers the fire.	If the blanket does not completely cover the fire, it will not be extinguished.	Place carefully over the fire. Keep your hands shielded from the fire. Take care not to waft the fire towards you.	Smothers the fire.

Security issues

As noted in the previous section, you need to be vigilant about security risks, such as fires, and know who to report any problems to.

Evacuating buildings

In an extreme case it may be necessary to help evacuate buildings if there is a fire, or for other security reasons, such as:

- a bomb scare
- the building has become structurally unsafe
- an explosion
- a leak of dangerous chemicals or fumes.

The evacuation procedure you need to follow will be laid down by your workplace. The information will be the same whatever the emergency is: the same exits will be used and the same assembly point. It is likely to be along the following lines.

- Stay calm, do not shout or run.
- Do not allow others to run.
- Organise people quickly and firmly without panic.
- Direct those who can move themselves and assist those who cannot.
- Use wheelchairs to move people quickly.
- Move a bed with a person in, if necessary.

Health emergencies

(KS 2, 3, 4, 5, 6, 7, 8, 14, 15, 16, 17)

Helping in a health emergency is about first aid, and you need to understand the actions you should take if a health emergency arises. The advice that follows is not a substitute for a first aid course, and will only give you an outline of the steps you need to take. Reading this part of the chapter will not qualify you to deal with these emergencies. You should be careful about what you do, because the wrong action can cause more harm to the casualty. Always summon help immediately.

What you can safely do

Most people have a useful role to play in a health emergency, even if it is not dealing directly with the ill or injured person. It is also vital that someone:

- summons help as quickly as possible
- offers assistance to the competent person who is dealing with the emergency, i.e. fetches the resuscitation trolley, defibrilator and drip stand to the site of the emergency
- clears the immediate environment and makes it safe – for example, if someone has fallen through a glass door, the glass must be cleared

away as soon as possible before there are any more injuries

- offers help and support to other people who have witnessed the illness or injury and may have been upset by it such as closing the curtains around other patients or alternatively evacuate laterally. Clearly this can only be dealt with once the ill or injured person is being helped.

> **Evidence through reflection (KS 6, 8, 16, 17, 18)**
>
> Think about an emergency situation you have been involved in and the role you played within that. Identify aspects of this emergency that you were able to deal with and those that you were not, and the reasons why. Make notes for your portfolio.

How you can help the casualty in a health emergency

It is important that you are aware of the initial steps to take when dealing with the commonest health emergencies. You may be involved with any of these emergencies when you are at work. If you are working in a hospital, skilled assistance is likely to be available, so the likelihood of your having to act in an emergency, other than to summon help, is remote. However, you will be expected to instigate help until assistance arrives.

This section gives a guide to recognising and taking initial action in a number of health emergencies:

- severe bleeding
- cardiac arrest
- shock
- loss of consciousness
- epileptic seizure
- choking and difficulty with breathing
- fractures and suspected fractures
- burns and scalds
- poisoning
- electrical injuries.

Severe bleeding

Severe bleeding can be the result of a fall or injury. The most common causes of severe cuts are glass, as the result of a fall into a window or glass door, or knives from accidents in the kitchen.

Symptoms

There will be apparently large quantities of blood from the wound. In some very serious cases where an artery has been injured, blood may appear/pump out. Even small amounts of blood can be alarming, both for you and the casualty. Severe bleeding requires urgent medical attention in hospital. Although people rarely bleed to death, extensive bleeding can cause shock and loss of consciousness.

Aims

- To bring the bleeding under control
- To limit the possibility of infection
- To arrange urgent medical attention.

Action

1 You will need to apply pressure to a wound that is bleeding. If possible, use a sterile dressing. If one is not readily available, use any readily available absorbent material, or even your hand. Observe universal precautions if possible (see *Protect Yourself*). You will need to apply direct pressure over the wound for 10 minutes (this can seem like a very long time) to allow the blood to clot.

2 If there is any object in the wound, such as a piece of glass, do not try to remove it. Simply apply pressure to the sides of the wound.

3 Lay the casualty down and raise the affected area if possible.

4 Make the person comfortable, secure and covered to control temperature – ensure privacy and dignity is maintained at all times.

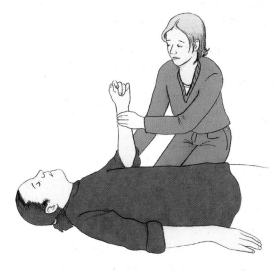

Lay the casualty down and raise the affected part.

Protect yourself

You should take steps to protect yourself when you are dealing with casualties who are bleeding. Your skin provides an excellent barrier to infections, but you must take care if you have any broken skin such as a cut, graze or sore. Seek medical advice from your workplace Occupation Health Advisor if blood comes into contact with your mouth, nose or gets into your eyes. **Blood-borne** viruses (such as HIV or hepatitis B or C) can be passed only if the blood of someone who is already infected comes into contact with broken skin or is absorbed through nucleus membranes.

Key term

Blood-borne Carried in the blood.

Did you know?

The number of HIV positive people in Eastern Europe increased 25 per cent in 2007 to 1.7 million (Source: www.thewellproject.org).

- If possible, wear disposable gloves and goggles.
- If this is not possible, cover any areas of broken skin with a waterproof dressing.
- If possible, wash your hands thoroughly in soap and water before and after treatment.
- Take care with any needles or broken glass in the area and ensure a sharps bin is to hand.
- Use a mask for mouth-to-mouth resuscitation if the casualty's nose or mouth is bleeding.

Memory jogger

What is the correct procedure for washing your hands? Refresh your memory by looking at page 61.

Cardiac arrest

Cardiac arrest occurs when a person's heart stops. Cardiac arrest can happen for various reasons, the most common of which is a heart attack, but a person's heart can also stop as a result of shock, electric shock, a convulsion or other illness or injury.

Symptoms

- No pulse
- No breathing.

Aims

- To obtain medical help as a matter of urgency
- It is important to give oxygen, using mouth-to-mouth resuscitation, and to stimulate the heart, using chest compressions. This procedure is called cardio-pulmonary resuscitation or CPR. You will attend a mandatory training session to learn how to resuscitate with mandatory annual updates within your workplace.

Action

1 Ensure the area is safe and free of danger before approaching the patient, i.e if the patient has been electrocuted, check that the current has been turned off.

2 Check whether the patient has a pulse and whether they are breathing.

3 If not, call for urgent help from a registered nurse who will assess the need for summoning help.

4 Start methods of resuscitation if you have been taught how to do it.

5 Keep up resuscitation until help arrives.

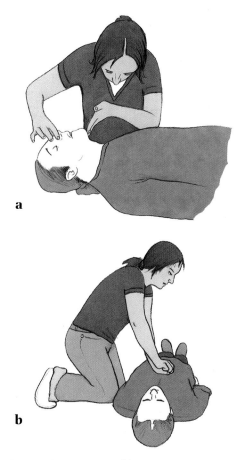

Mouth-to-mouth resuscitation (a) and chest compressions (b).

Shock

Shock occurs because blood is not being pumped around the body efficiently. This can be the result of loss of body fluids through bleeding, burns, severe vomiting or diarrhoea, or a sudden drop in blood pressure or a heart attack.

Symptoms

The signs of shock are easily recognised. The patient:

- will look very pale, almost grey
- will be very sweaty, and the skin will be cold and clammy
- will have a very fast pulse
- may feel sick and may vomit
- may be breathing very quickly.

Aims

- To obtain medical help as a matter of urgency
- To improve blood supply to heart, lungs and brain.

Action

1 Summon expert medical or nursing assistance.

2 Lay the person down on the floor or place the bed to arrest position. Try to raise their feet off the ground (or the foot of the bed) to help the blood supply to the important organs.

3 Loosen any tight clothing.

4 Watch the person carefully. Check the pulse and breathing regularly.

5 Keep the person warm and comfortable.

Do not:

- allow the casualty to eat or drink
- leave the casualty alone, unless it is essential to do so briefly in order to summon help.

Loss of consciousness

Loss of consciousness can happen for many reasons, from a straightforward faint to unconsciousness following a serious injury or illness.

Symptom

A reduced level of response and awareness. This can range from being vague and 'woozy' to total unconsciousness.

Aims

- To summon expert medical help as a matter of urgency
- To keep the airway open
- To note any information which may help to find the cause of the unconsciousness.

Action

1 Make sure that the person is breathing and has a clear airway.

2 Maintain the airway by lifting the chin and tilting the head backwards.

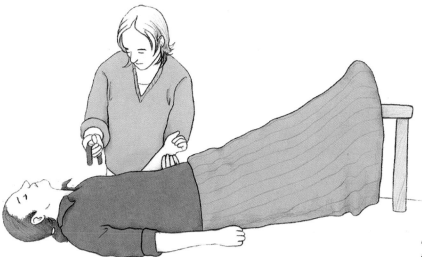

Raise the feet off the ground and keep the casualty warm.

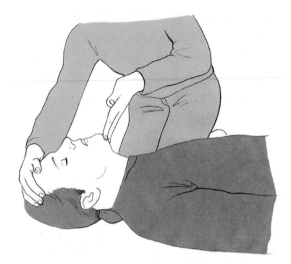

Open the airway.

1. Kneel at one side of the casualty, at about waist level.

2. Tilt back the person's head – this opens the airway. With the casualty on his or her back, make sure that limbs are straight.

3. Bend the casualty's near arm as in a wave (so it is at right angles to the body). Pull the arm on the far side over the chest and place the back of the hand against the opposite cheek (**a** in the diagram).

4. Use your other hand to roll the casualty towards you by pulling on the far leg, just above the knee (**b** in the diagram). The casualty should now be on his or her side.

5. Once the casualty is rolled over, bend the leg at right angles to the body. Make sure the head is tilted well back to keep the airway open (**c** in the diagram).

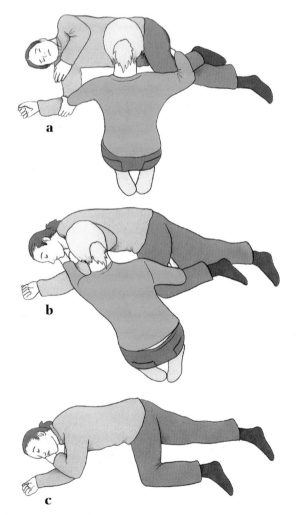

The recovery position.

3. Look for any obvious reasons why the person may be unconscious, such as a wound or an ID band telling you of any condition he or she may have. For example, many people who have medical conditions that may cause unconsciousness, such as epilepsy or diabetes, wear special bracelets or necklaces giving information about their condition. If in a hospital setting, ask a colleague to check the patient's care plan for any conditions that could cause the patient to become unconscious.

4. Place the casualty in the recovery position (see below), *but not if you suspect a back or neck injury*, until expert medical or nursing help or the emergency services arrive.

Do not:
- attempt to give anything by mouth
- attempt to make the casualty sit or stand
- leave the casualty alone, unless it is essential to leave briefly in order to summon help.

The recovery position

Many of the actions you need to take to deal with health emergencies will involve you in placing someone in the recovery position. In this position, a casualty has the best chance of keeping a clear airway, not inhaling vomit and remaining as safe as possible until help arrives. This position should not be attempted if you think someone has back or neck injuries and it may not be possible if there are fractures of limbs.

Epileptic seizure

Epilepsy is a medical condition which causes disturbances in the brain that result in sufferers becoming unconscious and having involuntary contractions of their muscles. This contraction of the muscles produces the fit or seizure. People who suffer with epilepsy do not have any control over their seizures, and may do themselves harm by falling when they have a seizure. However, some people may be aware of an 'aura' before they have an epileptic seizure: if this is the case, the casualty can be put into a safe position before the seizure begins.

Key term

Aura A sensation that precedes the onset of certain disorders.

Aims
- To ensure that the person is safe and does not injure themselves during the fit
- To offer any help needed following the fit.

Action
1 Try to make sure that the area in which the person has fallen is safe.

2 Loosen all clothing.

3 Once the seizure has ended, make sure that the person has a clear airway and place in the recovery position.

4 Make sure that the person is comfortable and safe and that dignity is maintained. Particularly try to prevent head injury.

5 If the fit lasts longer than five minutes, or you are not aware that the casualty is a known epileptic, call the emergency team.

Do not:
- attempt to hold the casualty down, or put anything in the mouth
- move the casualty until he or she is fully conscious, unless there is a risk of injury in the place where he or she has fallen.

Choking and difficulty with breathing (in adults and children over 8 years)

This is caused by something (usually a piece of food) stuck at the back of the throat. It is a situation that needs to be dealt with, as people can quickly stop breathing if the obstruction is not removed.

Symptoms
- Red, congested face at first, later turning grey
- Unable to speak or breathe, may gasp and indicate throat or neck.

Aims
- To remove obstruction as quickly as possible
- To summon medical assistance as a matter of urgency if the obstruction cannot be removed.

Action
1 Try to get the person to cough. If that is not immediately effective, move on to step 2.

2 Bend the person forwards. Slap sharply on the back between the shoulder blades up to five times (**a** in the diagram).

3 If this fails, stand behind the person with your arms around him or her. Join your hands just below the breastbone. One hand should be in a fist and the other holding it (**b** in the diagram).

4 Sharply pull your joined hands upwards and into the person's body at the same time. The force should expel the obstruction.

5 You should alternate backslaps and abdominal thrusts until you clear the obstruction.

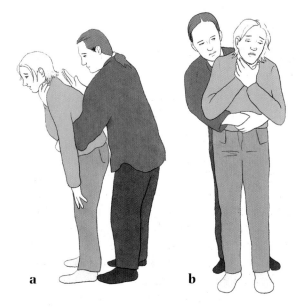

a   b

Dealing with an adult who is choking.

Fractures and suspected fractures

Fractures are breaks or cracks in bones. They are commonly caused by a fall. The casualty will need to go for an x-ray as soon as possible to have a fracture diagnosed correctly.

Symptoms

- Acute pain around the site of the injury
- Swelling and discoloration around the affected area
- Limbs or joints may be in odd positions
- Broken bones may protrude through the skin.

Action

1 The important thing is to support the affected part. Help the casualty to find the most comfortable position.

2 Support the injured limb in that position with as much padding as necessary – towels, cushions or clothing will do.

3 Summon medical help.

Do not:

- try to bandage or splint the injury
- allow the casualty to have anything to eat or drink.

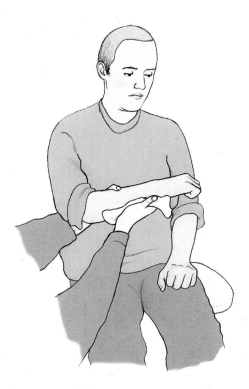

Support the injured limb.

Burns and scalds

There are several different types of burn; the most usual are burns caused by heat or flame. Scalds are caused by hot liquids. People can also be burned by chemicals or by electrical currents such as diathermy used in operating theatres.

Symptoms

- Depending on the type and severity of the burn, skin may be red, swollen and tender, blistered and raw or charred
- Usually severe pain and possibly shock.

Aims

- To obtain immediate medical assistance if the burn is over a large area (as big as the casualty's hand or more) or is deep.
- Call for medical assistance if the burn is severe or extensive. If the burn or scald is over a smaller area, the casualty could be transported to hospital by car.
- To stop the burning and reduce pain.
- To minimise the possibility of infection.

Action

1 For major burns, summon immediate medical assistance.

2 Cool down the burn. Keep it flooded with cold water for 10 minutes. If it is a chemical burn, this needs to be done for 20 minutes. Ensure that the contaminated water used to cool a chemical burn is disposed of safely.

3 Remove any jewellery, watches or clothing that are not sticking to the burn.

4 Cover the burn if possible, unless it is a facial burn, with a sterile or at least clean non-adhesive dressing. If this is not possible, leave the burn uncovered. For a burn on a hand or foot, a clean plastic bag will protect it from infection until it can be treated by an expert.

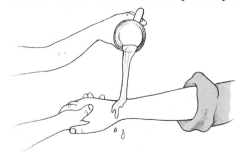

Cool the burn with water.

If clothing is on fire, remember the basics: *stop*, *drop*, *wrap* and *roll* the person on the ground.

Do not:

- remove anything which is stuck to a burn
- touch a burn, or use any ointment or cream
- cover facial burns – keep pouring water on until help arrives.

> ### Did you know?
> Approximately 250 people die from burns and 130,000 require treatment for burns in the UK each year (Source: www.nhsdirect.nhs.uk).

Poisoning

People can be poisoned by many substances: drugs, plants, chemicals, fumes or alcohol.

Symptoms

Symptoms will vary depending on the poison.

- The person could be unconscious
- There may be acute abdominal pain
- There may be blistering of the mouth and lips.

Aims

- To remove the casualty to a safe area if he or she is at risk, and it is safe for you to move the casualty
- To summon medical assistance as a matter of urgency
- To gather any information which will identify the poison
- To maintain a clear airway and breathing until help arrives.

Action

1 If the casualty is unconscious, place him or her in the recovery position to ensure that the airway is clear, and that he or she cannot choke on any vomit.

2 Call for medical assistance.

3 Try to find out what the poison is and how much has been taken. This information could be vital in saving a life.

4 If a conscious casualty has burned mouth or lips, he or she can be given small frequent sips of water or cold milk.

Do not try to make the casualty vomit.

> ### Did you know?
> Around 50,000 people require treatment for poisoning in the UK each year this includes accidental poisoning, particularly in children, and overdoses (Source: www.nhsdirect.nhs.uk).

Electrical injuries

Electrocution occurs when an electrical current passes though the body.

Symptoms

Electrocution can cause cardiac arrest and burns where the electrical current entered and left the body.

Aims

- To remove the casualty from the current when you can safely do so
- To obtain medical assistance as a matter of urgency
- To maintain a clear airway and breathing until help arrives
- To treat any burns.

Action

There are different procedures to follow depending on whether the injury has been caused by a high or low voltage current.

Injury caused by high voltage current

This type of injury may be caused by overhead power cables or rail lines, for example.

1 Contact the emergency services immediately.

2 *Do not* touch the person until all electricity has been cut off.

3 If the person is unconscious, clear the airway.

4 Treat any other injuries present, such as burns.

5 Place in the recovery position until help arrives.

Injury caused by low voltage current

This type of injury may be caused by electric kettles, computers, drills, lawnmowers, etc.

1 Break the contact with the current by switching off the electricity, at the mains if possible.

2 It is vital to break the contact as soon as possible but, if you touch a person who is 'live' (still in contact with the current), you too will be injured. If you are unable to switch off the electricity, then you *must* stand on something dry which can insulate you – such

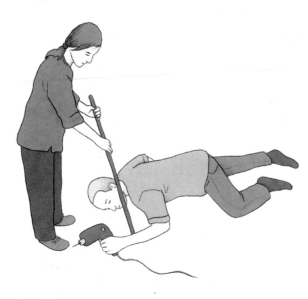

Move the casualty away from the current.

as a telephone directory, rubber mat or a pile of newspapers – and then move the casualty away from the current as described below.

3 Do not use anything made of metal, or anything wet, to move the casualty from the current. Try to move him or her with a wooden pole or broom handle, even a chair.

4 Alternatively, pull the casualty with a rope or cord or, as a last resort, pull by holding any of the person's dry clothing that is *not* in contact with the casualty's body.

5 Once the person is no longer in contact with the current, you should follow the same steps as with a high voltage injury.

Did you know?

Approximately 50 people are killed by and 4,000 require treatment for electricity-related injuries every year in the UK (Source: www. nhsdirect.nhs.uk).

Other ways to help

Summon assistance

Out of a hospital setting, in the majority of cases, this will mean telephoning 999 and requesting an ambulance. It will depend on the setting in which

you work and clearly is not required if you work in a hospital! But it will mean calling for a colleague with medical qualifications, who will then be able to make an assessment of the need for further assistance.

If you need to call an ambulance, try to keep calm and give clearly all the details you are asked for. Do not attempt to give information until it is asked for – this wastes time. Emergency service operators are trained to find out the necessary information, so let them ask the questions, and then answer calmly and clearly. Follow the action steps outlined in the previous section while you are waiting for help to arrive.

Assist the person dealing with the emergency

A second pair of hands is invaluable when dealing with an emergency. If you are assisting someone who has first aid or medical expertise, follow all of his or her instructions, even if you don't understand why. An emergency situation is not the time for a discussion or debate – that can happen later. You may be needed to help to move a casualty, or to fetch water, blankets or dressings, or to reassure and comfort the casualty during treatment.

Make the area safe

An accident or injury may have occurred in an unsafe area, or that accident may have made the area unsafe for others. For example, if someone has tripped over an electric flex, there may be exposed wires or a damaged electric socket. Alternatively, a fall against a window or glass door may have left shards of broken glass in the area, or there may be blood or other body fluids on the floor. You may need to make the area safe by turning off the power, clearing broken glass or dealing with a spillage.

It may be necessary to redirect people away from the area of the accident in order to avoid further casualties.

Maintain the privacy of the casualty

You may need to act to provide some privacy for the casualty by asking onlookers to move away or stand back. If you can erect a temporary screen this may help to offer some privacy. It may not matter to the casualty at the time, but he or she has a right to privacy if possible.

Make accurate reports

You may be responsible for making a report on an emergency situation you have witnessed or for filling in records later. Concentrate on the most important aspects of the incident and record the actions of yourself and others in an accurate, legible and complete manner.

> **Evidence through reflection**
> **(KS 15, 16, 17)**
>
> Write a list of some of the security, health incidents and emergencies that could happen in your workplace. Remember to include issues such as safe waste disposal, accident reporting, visitor's policy as well as emergencies like cardiac arrests. Having completed the list, write down the appropriate action to take for each issue on the list, including when it is appropriate to ask for help. Keep your notes in your portfolio.

How to deal with distress

People who have witnessed accidents can often be very distressed by what they have seen. The distress may be as a result of the nature of the injury, or the blood loss. It could be because the casualty is a friend or relative, or simply because seeing accidents or injuries is traumatic. Some people can become upset because they feel helpless and do not know how to assist, or they may have been afraid and then feel guilty later.

You may need to reassure people about the casualty and the fact that they are being cared for appropriately. However, do not give false reassurance about things you may not be sure of.

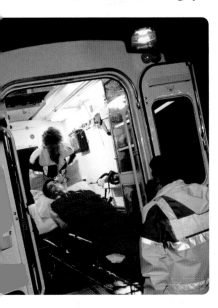

You may need to allow individuals to talk about what they saw. One of the commonest effects of witnessing a trauma is that people need to repeat over and over again what they saw.

Witnessing accidents is often distressing.

What about you?

You may feel very distressed by the experience you have gone through. You may find that you need to talk about what has happened, and that you need to look again at the role you played. You may feel that you could have done more, or you may feel angry with yourself for not having a greater knowledge about what to do. It is often useful to 'debrief' with other members of your working team in situations such as this. The chaplaincy can offer support in these circumstances. Remember to maintain confidentiality.

There is a whole range of emotions that you may experience; Unit HSC 35 covers in detail the different ways to cope with such feelings (page 130). You should be able to discuss them with your supervisor and use any support provided by your employer.

Further reading and research

Workplace health, safety and security is an important and complex issue. This section has dealt with the key factors and below are details of opportunities to find out more.

Websites

- www.dh.gov.uk (Department of Health: Health and safety, Emergency planning)
- www.hse.gov.uk (HSE: Health and Safety Executive)
- www.healthandsafetytips.co.uk (Health and Safety for Beginners)
- www.nric.org.uk (NRIC: National Resource for Infection Control)
- www.neli.org.uk (NeLI: National electronic Library of Infection)
- www.nice.org.uk (NICE: National Institute for Health and Clinical Excellence)

Publications

- Bowmen R. C., Emmett R. C. (1998) *A Dictionary of Food Hygiene*, CIEH
- Hartropp H. (2006) *Hygiene in Health and Social Care*, CIEH
- Horner J. M. (1993) *Workplace Environment, Health and Safety Management: A Practical Guide*, CIEH

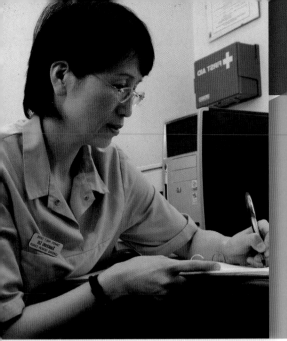

Reflect on and develop your practice

Introduction

The knowledge and skills addressed in this unit are the key to working effectively in all aspects of your practice as a health care assistant. In order to work effectively, it is essential to know how to evaluate your work, how you can improve on what you do, and understand the factors that have influenced your attitudes and beliefs.

The care sector is constantly benefiting from new research, developments, policies and guidelines. In order to offer the best possible level of service to those you care for, you need to make sure that you are up to date in work practices and knowledge, and aware of current thinking. As an assistant in a care setting, you have a responsibility to constantly review and improve your practice in compliance

with your job description and Knowledge and Skills Framework (KSF) post outline. It is the right of patients to expect the best possible quality of care from those who provide it, and high quality care requires all health care assistants to regularly reflect on their own practice and look at ways of improving.

Each organisation and each individual owes a duty of care to patients; this means that it is your responsibility to make sure that the service provided is the best it can possibly be. This is not an option, but a duty that you accept when you choose to become a health care assistant. The information in this unit will help you to identify the best ways to develop and update your own knowledge and skills.

What you need to learn

- How to explore your own values, interests and beliefs
- How your values, interests and beliefs influence your practice
- Reflective practice
- Support networks
- Learning from work practice
- Making good use of training/development opportunities
- Developing your own personal effectiveness
- Understanding new information
- How to ensure your practice is up to date
- Preparing a development plan

What evidence you need to generate for your portfolio

For your award you will mainly be required to produce observations of you carrying out tasks in your workplace. Your assessor will observe you undertaking real life activities to cover the performance criteria and scope. This can be supported by witness testimonies from colleagues who have seen you working.

In addition to this, you will need to demonstrate your knowledge and understanding. You can do this by providing written accounts that identify how you integrate theory with practice, answering verbal or written questions. Having an understanding of the principles of reflection will develop your practice in an appropriate way. You will find many opportunities to reflect within your day-to-day support.

The knowledge specifications identified under the headers of each section are intended as a guide.

HSC 33 Reflect on your practice

How to explore your own values, interests and beliefs

(KS 2, 5, 6, 7, 8, 9, 10, 11)

Everyone has their own **values**, **beliefs** and preferences. They are an essential part of who you are. What you believe in, what you see as important and what you see as acceptable or desirable are as much a part of your personality as whether you are shy, outgoing, funny, serious, friendly or reserved.

> ### Key terms
>
> **Values** Principles or standards which underpin the way individuals behave.
>
> **Beliefs** Mental acceptance of something as being true or real.

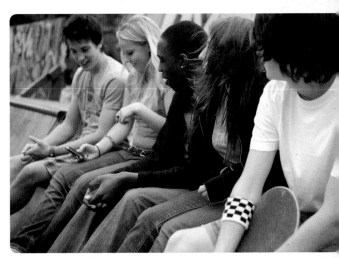
Everyone is different!

People whose work involves caring for others need to be aware of their own values. You may work with vulnerable people, so it is important to be able to make them feel safe and to be able to meet their self-esteem needs. The way in which you respond to people is linked to what you believe in, what you consider important and the things that interest you. You may find you react positively to people who share your values and less warmly to people who have different priorities. When you develop friendships, it is natural to spend time with people who share your interests and values, those who are 'on your wavelength'.

Choosing your friends and meeting with others who share your interests is one of life's joys and pleasures; however, the professional relationships you develop with people you care for are another matter. As a professional carer, you are required to provide the same quality of care for all, not just for those who share your views and beliefs. This may seem obvious, but knowing what you need to do and achieving it successfully are not the same thing.

Working in the health care sector, you are bound to come across patients and colleagues whose views you don't agree with, and who never seem to understand your point of view. Awareness of differences, your reaction to them and how they affect the care you give is a crucial part of personal and workplace development.

Read and make notes for your portfolio on your feelings and responses to the table below. How do you manage to make the right responses when there is a clash between your views and those of the people you are working with?

Your beliefs/values/interests	Situation	Possible effect
People have a responsibility to look after their health	You are caring for someone with heart disease who continues to smoke and eats a diet high in fried foods and cream cakes	You find it difficult to be sympathetic when someone complains about their condition and you make limited responses
War and violence are wrong and people who fight should not be glorified as heroes	An elderly patient constantly recalls tales of his days as a soldier and wants you to admire his bravery and that of his comrades	You try to avoid spending time chatting with him and limit your contact to providing physical care
Television	A patient on the ward constantly has the TV on and turned up very loudly	You find it hard not to ask them to turn it down or off. You hurry through your work and your irritation shows in your body language

If you allow your own preferences to dominate your work with patients, you are unlikely to be able to meet your patient's needs satisfactorily. It is not always easy to make the right decisions when there is a clash between your own views and those of the patients you work with. Sometimes the best way to address these problems is to begin by seeking a better understanding of your own views and values.

One way of beginning this process is to make yourself aware of the factors that have influenced the development of your personality. This is not as easy as it sounds: you may feel you know yourself very well, but knowing who you are is not the same as understanding how your beliefs are influencing your reactions.

1 Take a range of items from a newspaper – about six or seven – about issues in health care. Make a note of your views on each of them: say what your feelings are on each one – does it shock or disgust you, make you sad, or angry, or grateful that it hasn't happened to you?

2 Try to think about why you reacted in the way you did to each of the items in the newspaper. Think about what may have influenced you to feel that way. The answers are likely to lie in a complex range of factors, including your upbringing and background, experiences you had as a child and as an adult, and relationships you have shared with others. Make notes for your portfolio.

Unravelling these influences is never easy, and you are not being asked to carry out an in-depth analysis of yourself – simply to begin to realise how your development has been influenced by a series of factors.

Factors which influence our development

Everyone's values and beliefs are affected to different degrees by the same range of factors.

Each of us will be influenced to a greater or lesser degree by these layers of influence. As each individual is different, the extent of the influences will be different for each person. It is therefore important that you have considered and reflected on the influences on your development so that you understand how you became the person you are.

Key influences on development

The following are some of the key factors associated with differences between people – the factors that can result in different people having different values.

You should be able to begin to trace some of the influences from your past environment on the development of your own attitudes and values.

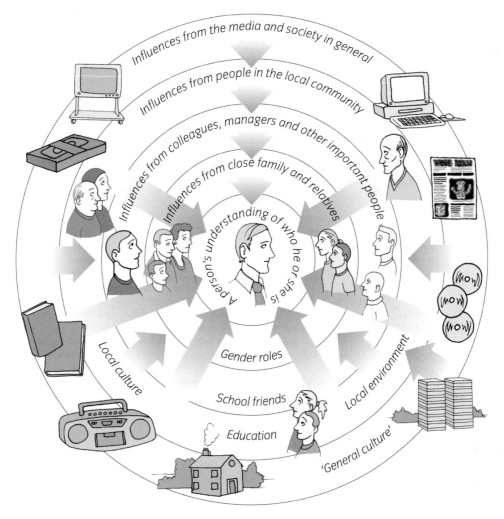

Circles of influence.

We are strongly influenced by our contact with other people. But different people live very different lives and mix with communities that have very different beliefs. People have different cultures, family values, religions, social class backgrounds, and so on. Men often grow up with very different expectations and experience of life from women. Older people are likely to have had different life experiences from those of younger people.

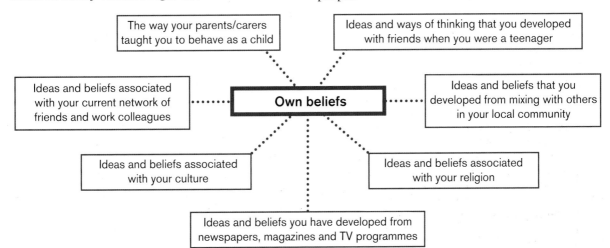

Some ways in which people are different from each other

Age	People may be classified as being children, teenagers, young adults, middle aged or old. Discrimination can creep into our thinking if we see some age groups as being 'the best', or if we make assumptions about the abilities of different age groups.
Gender	In the past, men often had more rights and were seen as more important than women. Assumptions about gender, such as what is women's work and what is men's work, can still result in wrong assumptions and discrimination.
Race	People understand themselves in terms of ethnic categories such as being black or white, as European, African or Asian. Many people have specific national identities such as Polish, Nigerian, English or Welsh. Assumptions about racial characteristics and beliefs, or thinking that some groups are superior to others, result in discrimination.
Class	People differ in their upbringing, the kind of work they do and the money they earn. People also differ in the lifestyles they lead and the views and values that go with different levels of income and spending habits. People may discriminate against others because their class or lifestyle is different.
Religion	People grow up in different traditions of religion. For some people, spiritual beliefs are at the centre of their understanding of life. For others, religion influences the cultural traditions that they celebrate; for example, many Europeans celebrate Christmas even though they might not see themselves as practising Christians. Discrimination can take place when people assume that their customs or beliefs should apply to everyone else.
Sexuality	Many people see their sexual orientation as very important to understanding who they are. Gay and lesbian relationships are often discriminated against. Heterosexual people sometimes judge other relationships as 'wrong' or abnormal.
Ability	People may make assumptions about what is 'normal'. People with physical disabilities or learning difficulties may become labelled, stereotyped and discriminated against as damaged versions of 'normal' people.
Relationships	People choose many different lifestyles and emotional commitments, such as marriage, having children, living in a large family, living a single lifestyle but having sexual partners, or being single and not being sexually active. People live within different family and friendship groups. Discrimination can happen if people start to judge that one lifestyle is 'right' or best.
Politics	People can develop different views as to how a government should act, how welfare provision should be organised and so on. Disagreement and debate are necessary; but it is important not to judge people as bad or stupid because their views are different from ours.

Problems arise because our own culture and life experience may lead us to make assumptions as to what is right or normal. When we meet people who are different it can be easy to see them as 'not right' or 'not normal'. Different people see the world in different ways.

How your values, interests and beliefs influence your practice

(KS 2, 5, 7, 9, 11)

Once you have begun to identify the major factors that have influenced your development, the next stage is to look at how they have affected the way in which you work and relate both to patients and colleagues. This is the basis of developing into a health care assistant who evaluates what they do.

Working in health care requires that, in order to be effective and to provide the best possible service for those you care for, you need to be able to think about and evaluate what you do and the way you work, and to identify your strengths and weaknesses. It is important that you learn to think about your own practice in a constructive way. **Reflection** and **evaluation** should not undermine your confidence in your own work; rather you should use them in a constructive way, to identify areas that require improvement.

Key terms

Reflection Deep and careful thought.
Evaluation Considering something to judge its quality, condition or importance.

The ability to do this is an indication of excellent practice. Any health care assistants who believe that they have no need to improve their practice, or to develop and add to their skills and understanding, are not demonstrating good and competent practice.

Becoming a thoughtful practitioner is not about torturing yourself with self-doubts and examining your weaknesses until you reach the point where you lose your **self-confidence**. But it is important that you examine the work you have done and identify areas where you know you may need to carry out additional personal development. A useful tool in learning to become a **reflective practitioner** is to develop a series (or cycle) of thought processes that you can use, either after you have dealt with a difficult situation or at the end of each shift or day's work, to look at your own performance.

Key terms

Self-confidence Belief in your own abilities.

Reflective practitioner Someone who evaluates the work they do.

Reflective practice

(KS 2, 3, 4, 7, 8, 9, 11)

The purpose of reflective practice is to improve and develop your work by thinking carefully about what you are doing and this involves thinking things over.

Reflection involves discovering new ideas or new relationships between ideas, and this helps us to make new sense of practice issues. Reflection is something we all do all the time without realising it – reflective practice organises this process. There will be many occasions when you have thought through what happened during a shift on your ward. You may have sat on the bus going home thinking (reflecting) about the things that have gone well during a shift and the things that have not gone so well. By organising these thoughts, we can improve the way we work, and we can study closely things that have not gone according to plan. When we organise this process, we call it a reflective cycle.

What is a reflective cycle?

Theorists have described different sorts of reflective cycles, each of which has a number of clear stages.

Here are the stages of Gibbs' reflective cycle.

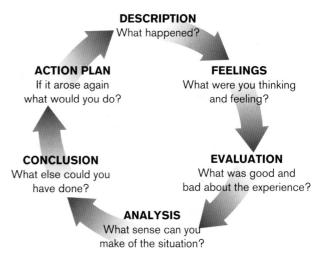

Gibbs' model of reflection (© University of Northampton).

Stage 1: Description of the event

Describe in detail the event you are reflecting on. Just write the facts – not your opinion.

Include: where you were; who else was there; why you were there; what you were doing; what other people were doing; what was the context of the event; what happened; what your part was in this; what parts the other people played; and what was the result.

Stage 2: Feelings

Try to recall and explore the things that were going on inside your head, e.g. why does this event stick in your mind? Include: how you were feeling when the event started; what you were thinking about at the time; how it made you feel; how other people made you feel; how you felt about the outcome of the event; what you think about it now.

Stage 3: Evaluation

Try to evaluate or make a judgement about what has happened. Consider what was good about the experience and what was bad about the experience or did not go so well.

Stage 4: Analysis

Break the event down into its component parts so they can be explored separately. You may need to ask more detailed questions about the answers to the last stage. Include: what went well; what you did well; what others did well; what went wrong or did not turn out how it should have done; in what way you or others contributed to this.

Stage 5: Conclusion

This differs from the evaluation stage in that now you have explored the issue from different angles and have a lot of information to base your judgement on. It is here that you are likely to develop insight into your own and other people's behaviour in terms of how they contributed to the outcome of the event. Remember: the purpose of reflection is to learn from an experience. Without the detailed analysis and honest exploration that occurs during all the previous stages, it is unlikely that all aspects of the event will be taken into account – and valuable opportunities for learning can be missed. During this stage, you should ask yourself what you could have done differently.

Stage 6: Action plan

Think yourself forward into encountering the event again and plan what you would do – would you act differently or would you be likely to do the same?

Here the cycle is tentatively completed and suggests that should the event occur again it will be the focus of another reflective cycle.

Another cycle of reflection is detailed below.

Johns' reflective cycle

Here are the stages of Johns' (1995) reflective cycle. This cycle encourages the user to firstly describe and then think carefully about the incident that happened. Next the user is asked to think about what influenced their decision and how they have dealt with the situation better. Lastly the person thinks about what they have learned from the experience and how this may change what they may do in the future. Johns is reputed to have encouraged the link between theory and practice with the use of his cycle.

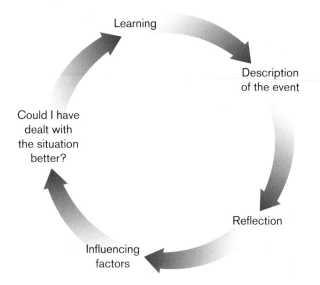

Johns' (1995) cycle of reflection.

Stage 1: Description of the event

Describe in detail the event you are reflecting on. Just write the facts – not your opinion.

Include: where you were; who else was there; why you were there; what you were doing; what other people were doing; what was the context of the event; what happened; what your part was in this; what parts the other people played; and what was the result.

Stage 2: Reflection

Include here what you were trying to achieve, the factors that led you to behave as you did, and what were the consequences of your actions. How did this make you and your patient feel?

Stage 3: Influencing factors

Think about the things that influenced what you did. For example, do you feel you had sufficient training to deal with this situation? Did you receive enough support from your practitioner in charge?

Stage 4: Could I have dealt with the situation better?

Think about what else you could have done. If you had done things differently, what would have been the outcome?

Stage 5: Learning

Describe how this whole experience made you feel. Has it changed the way you think and how you would behave in the future?

Source: Johns, C. (1995) 'Framing Learning Through Reflection with Carpers Fundamental Ways of Knowing' in *Nursing Journal of Advanced Nursing* 22:226–234

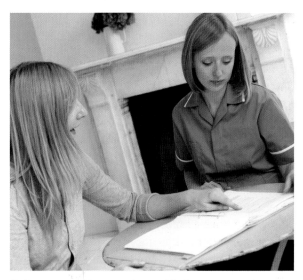

Reflecting can help you understand feelings and the wider issues involved.

Learning

The final stage of Johns' cycle refers to learning, so when you have identified the skills you may need to improve your practice, you will need to find out your own learning style. One of the best-known theories about the way in which people learn is the Lewin/Kolb cycle of experiential learning.

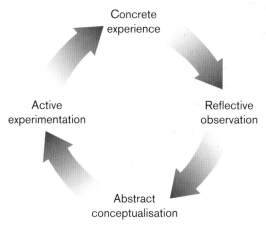

Kolb's cycle (1984).

Basically, this cycle means the following.

- Something happens to you or you do something; it can be an unusual event or something you do every day (**concrete experience**).
- You think about it (**reflective observation**).
- You work out some general rules about it, or you realise that it fits into a theory or pattern you already know about (**abstract conceptualisation**).

- Next time the same situation occurs, you apply your rules or theories (**active experimentation**).
- This will make your experience different from the first time, so you will have different factors to think about and different things to learn – so the cycle continues. You never stop learning.

Imagine that you are working with a man who has a learning difficulty. It is the first time you have met him and you are offering him a drink at lunchtime. You offer a glass of orange squash by placing it in front of him. He immediately pushes the glass away with a facial expression that you take to express disgust.

Within Kolb's learning cycle you have had a concrete experience.

Stage 1

Stage 1 of the learning cycle is the experience that this service user has rejected your offer of orange squash. But why has he reacted in this way?

Stage 2

Stage 2 involves thinking through some possible reasons for the reaction. Perhaps he doesn't like orange squash? Perhaps he doesn't like the way you put it in front of him? Perhaps he doesn't like to take a drink with his meal? Could it be an issue to do with social group membership? For example, could a cold drink symbolize childhood status for this individual? Does he see adult status as defined by having a hot drink? Reflection on the non-verbal behaviour of the service user may provide a range of starting points for interpreting his actions.

Stage 3

Kolb's third stage involves trying to make sense of our reflections. What do we know about different cultural interpretations of non-verbal behaviour? What are the chances that the way we placed the drink in front of the person has been construed as an attempt to control or dominate him? We didn't intend to send this message but the service user may have interpreted our behaviour on an emotional level as being unpleasant. The more we know about human psychology and social group membership the more we can analyse the service user's reaction. We need to choose the most likely explanation for the service user's behaviour using everything we know about people.

Stage 4

Kolb's fourth stage involves 'experimenting', or checking out ideas and assumptions that we may have made. The worker might attempt to modify his or her non-verbal behaviour to look supportive. The worker might show the service user a cup and saucer to indicate the question: 'Is this what you would like?' If the service user responds with a positive non-verbal response, the worker would have been around the four stages of the cycle and would have solved the problem in a way that valued the individuality and diversity of the individual.

Workers might expect to have to go round this 'learning cycle' a number of times before they were able to correctly understand and interpret a service user's needs.

How quickly can you work through these four stages? Would you be able to think through these issues while working with the service user, or would you need to go away and reflect on practice? The answer to this question might depend on the amount of experience you have had in similar situations.

What is your learning style?

Honey and Mumford (1982) developed a theory of a four-stage process of learning from experience. They believed that some people develop a preference for a particular type of learning style. Some people enjoy the activity of meeting new people and having new experiences, but these 'activists' may

not get so much pleasure from reflecting, theorising and finding answers to individual needs. Some people mainly enjoy sitting down and thinking things through. These are 'reflectors'. Some people enjoy analysing issues in terms of established theoretical principles; these people are 'theorists'. Finally, some people prefer trying out new ideas in practice – these people are 'pragmatists'.

Honey and Mumford have argued that the ideal way to approach practical learning is to balance all the different components of these learning styles. Some people can achieve this more **holistic** approach, whereas others find it more difficult.

> ### Key term
>
> **Holistic** Considering a person as a whole.

The diagram shows how Honey and Mumford's theory of learning styles fits the four-stage learning cycle.

You can test your own learning style preference or obtain further details of tests based on this theory at www.peterhoney.com.

This cycle of learning from experience is just one model of learning. This model may be useful in practice, especially as a way of approaching complicated non-routine problem solving. There are many other ways in which health care assistants might undertake personal development.

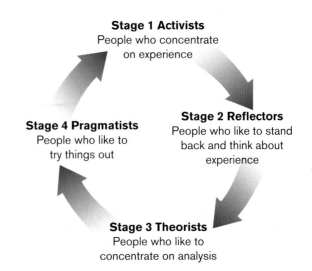

Stage 1 Activists
People who concentrate on experience

Stage 2 Reflectors
People who like to stand back and think about experience

Stage 3 Theorists
People who like to concentrate on analysis

Stage 4 Pragmatists
People who like to try things out

Honey and Mumford's theory of learning styles.

Different ways of learning

Formal training and development are not the only ways you can learn and expand your knowledge and understanding. There are plenty of other ways to keep up progress towards the goals you have set yourself.

Not everyone learns best from formal training. Other ways people learn are from:

- being shown by more experienced colleagues – this is known as 'sitting next to Nellie'
- working and discussing things as a team or group
- reading textbooks, journals and articles
- following up information on the Internet
- asking questions and holding professional discussions with colleagues and managers
- alternative work shadow, i.e. tissue viability, dementia care, Macmillan stoma nurses.

Support networks

(KS 5, 6, 7, 8, 9, 11)

Undertaking reflection alone is very difficult, so it is important to make use of your manager or mentor in order to get feedback on what you have done. Support networks, whether they are formal or informal, are one of the most effective means of identifying areas of your own practice that need further development. They will also help you to deal with any dilemmas or conflicts that you have identified.

Formal networks

These networks of support may be put in place by your employer. They are likely to consist of your immediate manager and possibly other more senior members of staff on occasion. You are likely to have a regular system of feedback and support meetings, or **appraisal** sessions with your manager. These could be at differing intervals depending on the system in your particular workplace, but are unlikely to be less frequent than once a month.

These systems are extremely useful in giving you the opportunity to benefit from feedback from your manager, who will be fully aware of the work you have been doing, and able to identify areas of practice that you may need to improve and areas in which you have demonstrated strength.

The appraisal or supervision system in your workplace may also be the point at which you identify a programme of development you need to undertake. Some employers identify this at 6-monthly or 12-monthly intervals, and some more frequently. Your manager is likely to identify which of the available training programmes are appropriate for the areas of your practice identified as needing development.

This process should link to your identified personal Knowledge and Skills Framework outcomes.

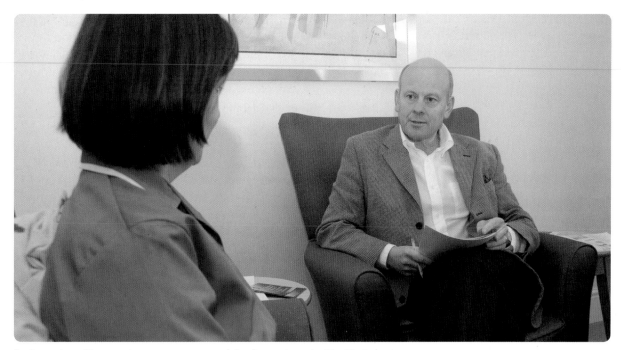

In discussion with your manager, programmes of development can be identified.

Getting the most out of management

Make sure that you are well prepared for sessions with your manager so that you can get maximum benefit from them. This will mean bringing together your reflections on your own practice, using examples and case notes where appropriate. You will need to demonstrate to your manager that you have reflected on your own practice and that you have begun identifying areas for development. If you can provide evidence through case notes and records to support this, it will assist your manager greatly.

You will also need to be prepared to receive feedback from your manager. While feedback is likely to be given in a positive way, this does not mean that it will be uncritical. Many people have considerable difficulty in accepting criticism in any form, even where it is intended to be supportive and constructive. If you are aware that you are likely to have difficulty accepting criticism, try to prepare yourself to view feedback from your manager as valuable and useful information that can add to your ability to reflect effectively on the work you are doing.

Evidence in action (KS 8)

Ask a colleague or, if you don't feel able to do that, ask a friend or family member to offer some constructive criticism on a task you have undertaken – a practical activity such as cooking a meal, or work you have undertaken in the garden or in the house, would be suitable.

If you are able to practise receiving **constructive feedback** on something which is relatively unthreatening, you are likely to be able to use the same techniques when considering feedback on your working practices. Make notes for your portfolio.

Key term

Constructive feedback Helpful response.

Your response to feedback should not be to defend your actions or to reject the feedback. You must try to accept and value it. A useful reply would be: 'Thank you, that's very helpful. I can use that next time to improve.' If you are able to achieve this you are likely to be able to make the maximum use of opportunities to improve your practice.

On the other hand, if criticism of any kind undermines your confidence and makes it difficult for you to value your own strengths, you should ask your manager to identify areas in which you did well, and use the positive areas to help you respond more constructively to any feedback.

Your manager's role

Your manager's role is to support and advise you in your work and to make sure that you know and understand:

- your rights and responsibilities as an employee
- what your job involves and the procedures your employer has in place to help you carry out your job properly
- the philosophy of care where you work – that is, the beliefs, values and attitudes of your employer regarding the way that patients are cared for – and how you can demonstrate values of care in the way you do your work
- your career development needs – the education and training requirements for the job roles you may progress into, as well as for your current job.

> ### Evidence in action
> ### (HSC 33: KS 5, 6, 9; HSC 35: KS 5, 9)
>
> Ask your manager for a copy of the relevant policy or plan at work on the supervision of staff.
>
> Read the plan and note down what it covers: for example, why and how you will be supervised, how often you can expect to be formally supervised and what kinds of things your manager will be able to help you with in your work role and career.
>
> If the plan is not clear, make a list of the things on which you would like your manager's support and agree a time and place to discuss these items with him or her. Keep your notes as evidence for your portfolio.

Training and development sessions

One of the other formal and organised ways of reflecting on your own practice and identifying strengths, weaknesses and areas for development is during training opportunities. On a course, or at a training day, aspects of your practice and areas of knowledge that are new to you will be discussed, and this will often open up avenues that you had not previously considered. This is one of the major benefits of making the most of all the training and education opportunities that are available to you. Training may also give you the opportunity in other work areas. You see the patients journey through the service rather than simply the area you work.

See page 90 for more about making the most of training opportunities.

> ### Evidence through reflection (KS 9)
>
> Identify any training sessions you have recently attended and document how you have integrated what you have learned into your practice. Write notes for your portfolio.

Informal networks

Informal support networks are likely to consist of your work colleagues and are helpful arenas to debrief and informally reflect. These can be major sources of support and assistance. Part of the effectiveness of many teams in many workplaces is their ability to provide useful ideas for improving practice, and support when things go badly.

Some staff teams provide a completely informal and ad-hoc support system, where people give you advice, guidance and support as and when necessary. Other teams will organise this on a more regular basis, and they may get together to discuss specific situations or problems that have arisen for members of the team. You need to be sure that you are making maximum use of all opportunities to gain support, advice and feedback on your practice. It is of course possible that you do not receive support when you require it. If you feel unsupported, as a responsible worker you should seek out support from an appropriate member of staff.

> ### Evidence through reflection (KS 6, 8)
>
> Identify the formal and informal support networks in your workplace. Note down the ways in which you use the different types of network and how they support your development. If you identify any gaps or areas where you feel unsupported, discuss this with your manager. Make notes for your portfolio.

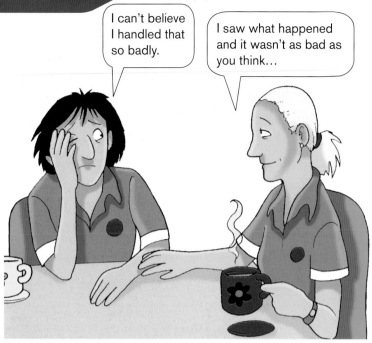

Informal networks can be important sources of support and assistance.

HSC 33 Take action to enhance your practice

Learning from work practice

Everything you do at work is part of a process of learning. Even regular tasks are likely to be important for learning because there is always something new each time you do them. A simple task like taking a patient a hot drink may result in a lesson – if, for example, you find that the patient tells you he or she doesn't want tea, but would prefer coffee this morning. You will have learned a valuable lesson about never making assumptions that everything will be the same.

Learning from working is also about using the huge amount of skills and experience your colleagues and manager will have. Not only does this mean they will be able to pass on knowledge and advice to you, but you have the perfect opportunity to discuss ideas and talk about day-to-day practice in the service you are delivering.

Finding time to discuss work with colleagues is never easy; everyone is busy and you may feel that you should not make demands on their time. You may be in a position where you have to prioritise your time to provide supervision for others, and your manager has to prioritise time for your supervision.

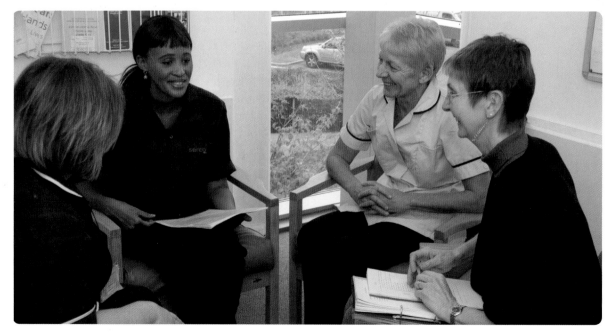

Finding time to discuss work with colleagues is never easy.

Most supervision will take place at scheduled times, but you may also be able to discuss issues in the course of hand-over meetings or team meetings, and other day-to-day activities. Use supervision time or quiet periods to discuss situations which have arisen, problems you have come across or new approaches you have noticed other colleagues using.

Evidence through reflection (KS 11)

Over the next week, make notes about periods of time that seem to provide a good opportunity to talk to a senior colleague or manager. When you have worked out the opportunities, take the initiative and raise a question about work you have been doing. You may have straightforward questions, or more complicated issues to do with appropriate decisions about rights, risks and choices: for example, 'How did you make the decision that it was safe enough for Mr Jackson to get out of bed and go to the toilet on his own when there are obvious risks involved?'

Try this with different experienced colleagues – you may be surprised at what you learn. Keep your notes as evidence for your portfolio.

Using your mistakes

Everyone makes mistakes – they are one way of learning. It is important not to waste your mistakes, so if something has gone wrong, make sure you learn from it. Discuss problems and mistakes with your manager, and work out how to do things differently next time. It is important to reflect on both success and failure, and you can use reflective skills to learn from situations that have not worked out the way you planned.

However, it is important that you consider carefully why things turned out the way they did and think about how you will ensure that they go according to plan next time. Unfortunately, there are real people on the receiving end of our mistakes in care, and learning how not to do it again is vitally important.

Using your successes

Talking to colleagues and managers is equally useful when things work out really well. It is just as important to reflect on why something worked, so that you can repeat it.

A key factor is to be organised in your approach to your development. Thompson (1996) emphasises 'being **systematic**' as an important skill in care work. Practice is systematic when you know:

- what you are trying to achieve
- how you are you going to achieve it
- how you will tell when you have achieved it.

Source: Thompson, N. (1996) *People Skills* Macmillan

Key term

Systematic Orderly.

If, for example, you were planning to develop your communication skills, you might have the aim of establishing a degree of trust with a patient. You would not be able to plan a set strategy to produce trust – it is a feeling that might grow and develop within a caring relationship. But you could list some of the skills you would be using in your communication that would contribute to the development of a caring relationship.

You would have to have an understanding of relationships and trust in order to be able to explain the degree to which you have established a trusting relationship. You should use theory during the planning stage of your work to identify how you will know if you have achieved your aim.

Thompson argues that vague, unfocused care work can result in poor quality care and also in stress for the health care assistant. Some benefits of planned, systematic work, based on Thompson's analysis, are shown on the next page.

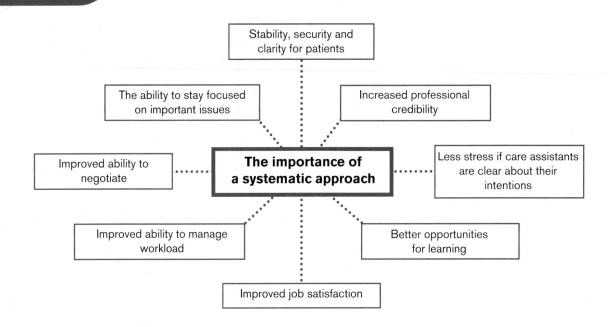

Making good use of training/ development opportunities

(KS 3, 4, 5, 6, 8, 9)

Personal development is to do with developing the personal qualities and skills that everyone needs in order to live and work with others, such as understanding, empathy, patience, communication and relationship building. It is also to do with the development of **self-confidence**, self-esteem and **self-respect**.

If you look back on the ways in which you have changed over the past five years, you are likely to find that you are different in quite a few ways. It is worth reviewing your learning style on a regular basis as this may change as you become more experienced. Most people change as they mature and gain more life experience. Important experiences such as changing jobs, moving home, illness or bereavement can change people. It is inevitable that your personal development and your development at work are linked – your personality and the way you relate to others are the major tools you use to do your job. Taking advantage of every opportunity to train and develop your working skills will also have an impact on you as a person.

Development at work is to do with developing the qualities and skills that are necessary for the workplace. Examples are teamwork, the ability to communicate with different types of people, time management, organisation, problem solving, decision making and, of course, the skills specific to the job.

Key terms

Personal development Developing the personal qualities and skills needed to live and work with others.

Self-confidence A personal judgement of capability.

Self-respect Overall appraisal of one's own worth.

Development at work Developing the qualities and skills necessary for the workforce.

Continuous development involves regularly updating the skills you need for work. You can achieve this through attending training sessions both on and off the job, and by making the most of the opportunities you have for training by careful planning and preparation.

Legal requirements for training

The Health and Social Care (Community Health and Standards) Act (2003) established the Healthcare Commission as the independent inspection body for both the NHS and independent healthcare. The Healthcare Commission applies core standards with the intention of improving the way healthcare is provided. This includes standards relating to staff training and personal and professional development.

All staff are required to undertake **induction** and **mandatory** training when they first start working in health care and subsequent annual updates.

Key terms

Induction Being taught about general principles at the beginning of a new job.

Mandatory Required by law.

How to get the best out of training

Your manager should work with you to decide on the types of training and development that will benefit you most. This will depend on the stage you have reached with your skills and experience. This can be identified at your annual appraisal meeting to discuss your personal development plan.

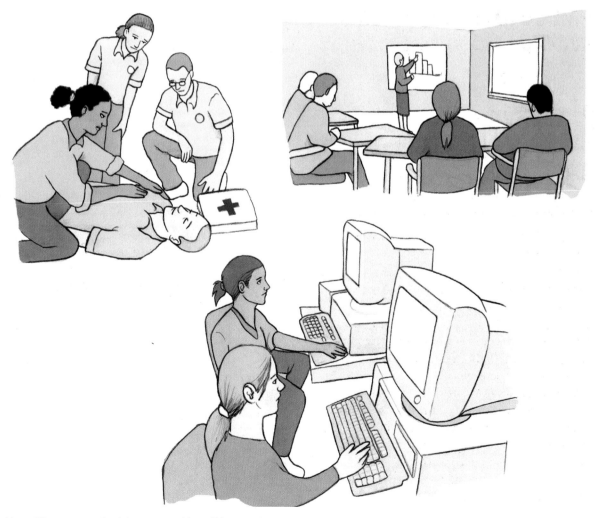

Many different types of training opportunities will be open to you.

It may be that not all the training you want to do is appropriate for the work you are currently assigned to – you may think that a course in advanced therapeutic activities sounds fascinating, but your manager may suggest that a course in basic moving and handling is what you need right now. You will only get the best out of training and development opportunities if they are the right ones for you at the time. There will be opportunities for training throughout your career, and it is important that you work out which training is going to help you to achieve your goals. However, not all development is necessarily from training undertaken at work. Night classes specialising in creative writing may develop your communication skills in writing; leading a group of Brownies may develop your organisational skills.

Evidence with a case study (KS 2)

Choosing appropriate training

Michelle is a health care assistant in a large hospital, on a busy ward. She was very aware of the fact that she lacked assertiveness in the way she dealt with both her colleagues and many of her patients. Michelle was always the one who agreed to run errands and to cover additional tasks that others should have been doing. She knew that she ought to be able to say no, but somehow she couldn't and then became angry and resentful because she felt she was doing far more work than many others on her team.

Her manager raised the issue during an appraisal and supervision session and suggested that Michelle should consider attending assertiveness training. Although initially reluctant, Michelle decided to take the opportunity. After six weeks of attending classes and working with the supportive group she met there, Michelle found that she was able to deal far more effectively with unfair and unreasonable requests from her colleagues and to deal in a firm but pleasant way with her patients.

1 What difference is Michelle's training likely to make a) to the patient she works with, and b) to herself?

2 Have you ever said 'yes' to extra work or additional responsibility when you wanted to say 'no'? How did this make you feel?

3 What could you have done about it?

Make notes for your portfolio.

How to use training and development

You should work with your manager to prepare for any training you receive, and to review it afterwards. You may want to prepare for a training session by:

- reading any materials which have been provided in advance

- talking to your manager or a colleague who has attended similar training, about what to expect
- thinking about what you want to achieve as a result of attending the training.

Best practice: Training

Make the most of training by:

✔ preparing well

✔ taking a full part in the training and asking questions about anything you don't understand

✔ collecting any handouts and keeping your own notes and reflections on the training.

Think about how to apply what you have learned to your work by discussing the training with your manager later. Review the ways in which you have benefited from the training and how you can apply this to practice.

Evidence through reflection (KS 9, 11)

Think about the last training or development session you took part in and write a short reflective report for your portfolio.

- Describe the preparations you made beforehand so that you could benefit fully from it.

- Describe what you did at the session: for example, what and how did you contribute, and what did you learn? Do you have a certificate to show that you participated in the session? Do you have a set of notes?

- How did you follow up the session? Did you review the goals you had set yourself, or discuss the session with your manager?

- Describe how you have used what you learned at the session: for example, how has the way you work changed, and how have your patients and colleagues benefited from your learning?

Developing your own personal effectiveness

(KS 2, 6, 10, 11)

The health and social care sector is one which constantly changes and moves on. New standards reflect the changes in the profession, such as the emphasis on quality services, the focus on tackling exclusion, and the influence of the culture of rights and responsibilities. There has been a huge increase in understanding in all parts of the sector, and a recognition of the satisfaction that comes from working alongside patients as partners and directors of their own care, rather than as passive receivers of services.

Developments in technology have brought huge strides towards independence for many patients, thus promoting a changing relationship with health care assistants; at the same time, technological developments have brought different approaches to the way in which work in care is carried out and the administration and recording of service provision.

Legislation and the resulting guidelines are a feature of the work of the sector. Sadly, many of the new guidelines, policies and procedures result from inquiries and investigations following tragedies, errors and neglect, such as the case of Victoria Climbie.

Evidence in action (KS 10)

Find out what you can about the following inquiries. Write notes on what happened and how they have changed health care practice.

- Harold Shipman inquiry
- Victoria Climbie inquiry
- Alder Hey inquiry
- Clothier Report

The BBC News website is a good source of information for this activity.

Despite all this, much of what we do in the care sector will remain the same: the basic principles of caring, treating people with dignity and respect, ensuring they have choice and promoting independence will continue, and the skills of good communication remain as vital as ever.

Being aware of new developments

There are many ways in which you can ensure that you keep up to date with new developments in the field of care, and particularly those that affect your own area of work. You should not assume that your workplace will automatically inform you about new developments, changes and updates

which affect your work – you must be prepared to actively maintain your own knowledge base and to ensure that your practice is in line with current thinking and new theories. The best way to do this is to incorporate an awareness of the need to constantly update your knowledge into all of your work activities. If you restrict your awareness of new developments to specific times, such as a monthly visit to the library, or a training course every six months, you are likely to miss out on a lot of information. It is useful to read regularly nursing journals and periodicals that will be accessible from your hospital library.

Sources of information

The media

The area of health and care is always in the news, so it is relatively easy to find out information about new studies and research. You will need to pay attention when watching television and listening to radio news bulletins to find out about new developments, legislation, guidelines and reports related to the health and care service.

Evidence in action (KS 6)

For one week, keep a record of every item which relates to health and care services that you hear on a radio bulletin, see in a television programme, or read in a newspaper article. You are likely to be surprised at the very large number of references you find. Discuss these with your manager and make notes for your portfolio.

Articles in newspapers and professional journals are excellent sources of information. When reporting on a recently completed study, they usually give information about where to obtain a copy of it.

Reports and reviews

You can read the findings of inquiries into the failures experienced within social work, health and social care, and this might provide you with a focus for reflection. In the past, there have been many cases where children and adults have been neglected or abused and social services have failed to protect vulnerable people adequately. Currently there is great national concern about the cleanliness and safety of hospital wards. While you may not be involved in policy-making decisions with respect to these services, there may be many principles such as 'whistle blowing' that are relevant in your own work setting. Many past serious failings might have been preventable if people had been able to identify the issues and take action earlier.

Remember: as well as reflecting on failures of the service, it is just as important to reflect on positive practice.

Conferences

Professional journals such as the British Journal of Healthcare Assistants also carry advertisements for conferences and training opportunities. You may also find such information in your workplace accessed through your training department. There is often a cost involved in attending these events, so the restrictions of the training budget in your workplace may mean that you cannot attend. However, it may be possible for one person to attend and pass on the information gained to others in the workplace, or to obtain conference papers and handouts without attending.

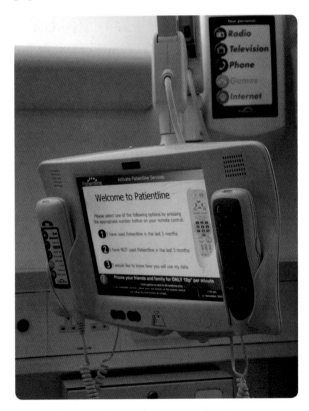

Information accessed on the Internet can be a great benefit to patients, but can raise concerns too.

The Internet

The development of information technology, and in particular the Internet, has provided a vast resource of information, views and research, all of which is available to patients, sometimes by their bedside.

There are clearly some limitations to using the Internet: for example, many people are reluctant to look for information through that route because they are not confident about using computers. However, the use of computers in the hospital environment is widespread and important. If you have access to a computer, using the Internet is a simple process that you could easily learn.

Another disadvantage is that you need to be wary of the information you obtain on the Internet, unless it is from accredited sources such as a government department, a reputable university or college, or an established research centre. Make every effort to check the validity of what you are reading. The World Wide Web provides free access to vast amounts of information, but it is an unregulated environment – anyone can publish information, and there is no requirement for it to be checked or approved. People can publish their own views and opinions, which may not be based on fact. These views and opinions from a wide range of people are valuable and interesting in themselves, but be careful that you do not assume anything to be factually correct unless it is from a reliable source, for example from a reputable UK website.

Treated with care, the Internet can prove to be one of the speediest and most useful tools in obtaining up-to-date information.

Your manager and colleagues

Never overlook the obvious: one of the sources of information which may be most useful to you is close at hand – your own workplace manager and colleagues. They may have many years of experience and accumulated knowledge that they will be happy to share with you. They may also be updating their own practice and ideas, and may have information that they would be willing to share.

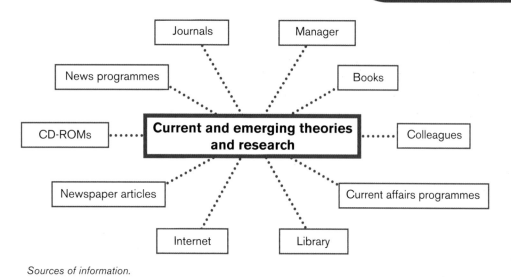

Sources of information.

Understanding new information

(KS 6, 9, 11)

Reading and hearing about new studies and pieces of research is all very well, but you must understand what it is that you are reading. It is important that you know how new theories are developed and how research is carried out.

Reliability and validity

There are specific methods of carrying out research to ensure the results are both reliable and valid. Research is judged on both of these factors, and you need to be able to satisfy yourself that the reports you read are based on reliable and valid research.

Reliability means the results would be repeated if someone else were to carry out the same piece of research in exactly the same way. **Validity** means that the conclusions that have been drawn from the research are consistent with the results, consistent with the way in which the research was carried out, and consistent in the way in which the information has been interpreted.

The research process

You will need to understand some of the basic terms used when discussing research in any field.

Primary research refers to information or data obtained directly from the research carried out, not from books or previously published work.

Secondary research refers to information obtained from books, previously published research and reports, CD-ROMs, the Internet, etc. – any information obtained from work carried out by others. For example, if you were asked to write an assignment, you are most likely to find the information from secondary sources such as textbooks or the Internet, rather than carry out a research project yourself in order to establish the information you need.

The information obtained from research is often referred to as **data**. It is called data regardless of whether it is in numbers or in words.

There are two broad areas of approach to research and they determine both the way in which the research is carried out and the type of results that are obtained. The first is referred to as **quantitative**; the second is **qualitative**.

Quantitative research

This approach has developed from the way in which scientists carry out laboratory experiments. The method produces statistical and numerical information. It provides hard facts and figures – quantities – and uses statistics and numbers to draw conclusions and make an analysis.

Many researchers in the field of health care use quantitative approaches and produce quantitative data. They may carry out 'experiments' using many of the rules of scientific investigation. In general, if you are reading research that provides statistics and numerical information and is based purely on facts, it is likely to have used one of the quantitative approaches.

Many government publications are good examples of quantitative research – they give statistics in relation to the National Health Service, such as the numbers of patients on waiting lists or the numbers having a particular operation.

Qualitative research

A qualitative approach looks at the 'quality' rather than the 'quantity' of something. It would be used to investigate the feelings of people who have remained on the waiting list for treatment, or people's attitudes towards residential care, or the quality of hospital food. Generally, qualitative data is produced in words rather than figures and will consist of descriptions and information about people's lives, experiences and attitudes.

Evidence through reflection (KS 6, 9, 11)

By using any of the methods for finding up-to-date information, such as newspapers, journals, reports, television, the Internet or textbooks, find two pieces of research carried out within the past two years. One should be quantitative and one qualitative. Read the results of both pieces of research. Make notes for your portfolio of the differences in the type of information provided.

How to ensure your practice is up to date

(KS 6, 8, 9, 10, 11)

There is little point in reading articles, watching TV programmes and attending training days if your work practice is not updated and improved as a result.

With the enormous pressures on everybody in the health and care services, it is often difficult to find time to keep up to date and to change the practices you are used to. Any form of change takes time and is always a little uncomfortable or unusual to begin with. So when we are under

pressure because of the amount of work we have to do, it is only normal that we tend to rely on practices, methods and ways of working which are comfortable, familiar and can be done swiftly and efficiently.

You will need to make a very conscious effort to incorporate new learning into your practice. You need to allocate time to updating your knowledge, and incorporating it into your practice. You could try the ways shown under *Best practice* to ensure that you are using the new knowledge you have gained. Discuss this with your manager; a good time to do this is at your personal KSF development review.

Best practice: Applying new skills and knowledge in practice

✔ Plan out how you will adapt your practice on a day-to-day basis, adding one new aspect each day. Do this until you have covered all the aspects of the new information you have learned.

✔ Discuss with your manager and colleagues/assessor what you have learned and how you intend to change your practice, and ask for feedback on how it is going.

✔ Write a checklist for yourself and check it at the end of each day.

✔ Give yourself a set period of time – for example, one month – to alter or improve your practice, and review it at the end of that time.

New knowledge is not only about the most exciting emerging theories. It is also often about mundane and day-to-day aspects of your practice, which are just as important and can make just as much difference to the quality of care you provide for your service users.

Evidence through reflection (KS 2, 7, 8, 9, 11)

Think about an occasion when you have been able to reflect on an area of your own practice or knowledge that needed improvement. Identify how you found the time to undertake this and the steps you took to achieve the improvement. Record what you did and also how you incorporated the new knowledge into your practice. Once you have identified this and recorded it in detail, include it in your portfolio.

Preparing a development plan

(KS 1, 5, 9, 11)

It is a requirement of many organisations that their staff have personal development plans. A **personal development plan (PDP)** is a very important document as it identifies your training and development needs and, because the plan is updated when you have taken part in training and development, it also provides a record of participation.

> ### Key term
>
> **Personal development plan (PDP)** Document used to summarise work activities and identify aims and goals over a defined period.

A personal development plan should be worked out and negotiated with your manager, but it is essentially your plan for your career. You need to think about what you want to achieve, and discuss with your manager the best ways of achieving your goals. Goals and targets are important as they can help motivate employees to focus on specific aims over a period of time, which will hopefully improve the way they work. Any goals or targets should be SMART.

Specific – be clear about what you want to achieve.
Measurable – make sure you can show you have achieved your goal.
Achievable – make sure you are capable of achieving your goal.
Realistic – make sure your goals are possible.
Time-based – be clear about the time you give yourself to achieve your goal.

Timescales must be realistic: for example, if you were to decide that you needed to achieve competence in managing a team in six months, this would be unrealistic and unachievable. You would inevitably fail to meet your target and would therefore be likely to become demoralised and demotivated. But if your target was to attend a training and development programme on team building during the next six months and to lead perhaps two team meetings by the end of the six months, those goals and targets would be realistic and you would be likely to achieve them.

There is no single right way to prepare a personal development plan, and each organisation is likely to have its own way. However, it should include different development areas, such as practical skills and communication skills, linked to the **Knowledge and Skills Framework**.

When you have set your targets, you need to review how you are progressing towards achieving them. This should happen every six months or so. You need to look at what you have achieved and how your plan needs to be updated with your manager.

> ### Memory jogger
>
> Look back to page 85 where the Knowledge and Skills Framework is explained.

What type of PDP?

Development plans can take many forms, but the best ones are likely to be developed in conjunction with your manager. You need to carefully consider the

Development plan		
Area of competence	**Goals**	**Action plan**
Time management and workload organisation	Learn to use computer recording and information systems	Attend 2-day training and use study pack. Attend follow-up training days. Use computer instead of writing reports by hand.
Review date: 3 months		
Professional development priorities	IT and computerised record systems	
My priorities for training and development in the next 6 months are:		
My priorities for training and development in the next 6-12 months are:	As above and keping up to date with mandatory training.	
Repeat this exercise in: 6 months and review the areas of competence and priorities.		

'areas of competence' and understand which ones you need to develop for your work role. Identify each as an area in which you feel fully confident, one where there is room for improvement and development, or one where you have very limited current ability. The headings in the table are suggestions only.

Once you have completed your plan, you can identify the areas on which you need to concentrate. You should set some goals and targets, and your manager should be able to help you ensure they are realistic. Only you and your manager can examine the areas of competence and skills you need to achieve. This is a personal development programme for you and you must be sure that it reflects not only the objectives of your organisation and the job roles they may want you to fulfil, but also your personal ambitions and aspirations.

When you have identified the areas in which you feel competent and chosen your target areas for development, you will need to design a personal development log which will enable you to keep a record of your progress. This can be put together in any way that you find effective.

Evidence in action (KS 1, 9)

Your task is to prepare a personal development plan. You should use a computer to do this, even if you print out a hard copy in order to keep a personal portfolio.

1 Use the model on the following pages to prepare your plan.

2 Complete the plan as far as you can at the present time. Note where you want your career to be in the short, medium and long term. You should also note down the training you want to complete and the skills you want to gain. You should do this on a computer if possible, otherwise complete a hard copy and keep it in a file.

3 Update the plan regularly. Keep on reviewing it with your manager.

Completed PDP

Name: A. Assistant

Workplace: Another Hospital Trust

Manager: A. Boss

Long-term goals (1-5 years)
To complete my NVQ level 3

Medium-term goals (6-12 months)
To complete my first aid training
To learn how to use the hospital computer system

Short-term goals
To admit my first patient without supervision

Areas of strength
I am good at talking to and caring for patients

Areas of weakness
I do not like to bother the senior members of staff when I do not understand something

In your plan, you may wish to include things as varied as learning sign language or learning a particular technique for working with patients with dementia. You could also include areas such as time management and stress management. All of these are legitimate areas for inclusion in your personal development plan.

Training and development

This section of your plan helps you to look at what you need to do in order to reach the goals you recorded in the first section. You should make a note of the training and development you need to undertake in order to achieve what you have identified.

Short-term goals	Development needed
To admit my first patient without supervision	To ask my manager if I can watch her admit a patient and then have her watch me until she is happy I can do it alone.

Medium-term goals	Development needed
To complete my first aid training	To gain permission from my manager to enrol on the in-house first aid training course
To learn how to use the hospital computer system	When the ward is quiet to ask my colleagues to show and let me use the system.
	Enrol on a free 'computers for the terrified' evening class

Long-term goals	Development needed
To complete my NVQ 3	To apply for Trust sponsorship to do the NVQ
	To research what is required to complete the NVQ
	To organise my personal life to allow me to achieve this NVQ

Milestones and timescales

In this section, you should look at the development you have identified in the previous section and plan some timescales.

Evidence through reflection (KS 7, 8, 9, 11)

Decide what the **milestones** will be on the way to achieving your goal. Make sure that your timescales are realistic. Make notes for your portfolio.

Key term

Milestones Indicators for short-term objectives.

Development	Milestone	By when
To admit my first patient without supervision	To ask my manager if I can watch her admit a patient	Within the next 3 months
	To have my manager watch me until she is happy I can do it alone.	Within the next 6 months
To complete my first aid training	To ask my manager to enrol me on the in house first aid training course	On the next available course – within 6 months
To learn how to use the hospital computer system	Ask my colleagues to show and let me use the system.	Within the next 6 months
	Enrol on a free 'computers for the terrified' evening class.	Within the next 6 months
To complete my NVQ 3	To apply for Trust sponsorship to do the NVQ.	Within the next year
	To research what is required to complete the NVQ.	Within the next 6 months
	To organise my personal life to allow me to achieve this NVQ.	Before the start of the NVQ

Reviews and updates

This section helps you to stay on track and to make the changes that will be inevitable as you progress. Not all your milestones will be achieved on target – some will be later, some earlier. All these changes will affect your overall plan, and you need to keep up to date and make any alterations as you go along.

Milestone	Target date	Actual achievement
To ask my manager if I can watch her admit a patient. To have my manager watch me until she is happy I can do it alone.	Within the next 3 months Within the next 6 months	Achieved within a week Achieved within a month
To ask my manager to enrol me on the in-house first aid training course.	On the next available course – within 6 months	Next course full – name on waiting list for next available one.
Ask my colleagues to show and let me use the system. Enrol on a free 'computers for the terrified' evening class.	Within the next 6 months Within the next 6monthns	Achieved within a month Enrolled on course to start next September
To apply for Trust sponsorship to do the NVQ. To research what is required to complete the NVQ. To organise my personal life to allow me to achieve this NVQ.	Within the next year Within the next 6 months Before the start of the NVQ	Applied but no funding from Trust. Looking into funding myself to start next January. Achieved within a month. After school club arranged within a month.

Further reading and research

The introduction to this section highlights your duty to make sure that the service provided is the best it can possibly be. In order to do this it is essential that you are constantly reflecting on your practice and striving to develop the way you work. Here are some suggestions of further reading and research to help you to do this.

Websites

- www.gscc.org.uk (GSCC: General Social Care Council – training and learning)
- www.dh.gov.uk (Department of Health: human resources and training)
- www.skillsforcare.org.uk (Skills for Care: workforce development for UK social care sector)
- www.skillsforhealth.org.uk (Skills for Health: workforce development for UK health sector)
- www.cwdcouncil.org.uk (Children's Workforce Development Council)
- www.scie.org.uk (SCIE: Social Care Institute for Excellence)

Publications

- Hawkins R., Ashurst A. (2006) *How to be a Great Care Assistant*, Hawker Publications
- Knapman J., Morrison T. (1998) *Making the Most of Supervision in Health & Social Care*, Pavilion Publishers
- Shakespeare P. (journal) *Learning in Health and Social Care*, Blackwell Publishing

Promote choice, well-being and the protection of all individuals

Introduction

Caring for patients is about making sure that you value everyone you work with as an individual, and that you treat them with respect and make sure they can enjoy life with the dignity that every individual deserves. It is also about making sure you promote patients' rights and preferences, and promote choice and well-being.

Well-being is about much more than just health; it is about every part of people's lives including feeling safe, valued and respected. Choice, as much independence as possible and the opportunity to reach your own potential are the key factors in achieving individual well-being.

Everyone has the right to be protected from abuse and harm. You have an important role in noticing and reporting any signs of abuse, neglect or other harm.

The World Health Organisation (WHO) identifies health as 'a state of complete physical, mental and social well-being and not merely absence of disease or infirmity' (WHO 1948).

What you need to learn

- Relationships
- Choice and empowerment
- Individuals' rights
- Providing support to meet the needs and preferences of individuals
- Active support
- Dealing with conflicts
- Treating people as individuals
- How to recognise your own prejudices and deal with them
- Anti-discriminatory practice
- Forms of abuse
- Signs and symptoms which may indicate abuse
- Where abuse can happen
- How to respond to abuse and neglect
- The effects of abuse
- How the law affects what you do

What evidence you need to generate for your portfolio

For your award you will mainly be required to produce observations of you carrying out tasks in your workplace. Your assessor will observe you undertaking real life activities to cover the performance criteria and scope. This can be supported by witness testimonies from colleagues who have seen you working.

In addition to this you will need to demonstrate your knowledge and understanding. You can do this by providing written accounts that identify how you integrate theory and practice, answering verbal or written questions. Promoting choice, well-being and protection for all your patients is a core role for health care workers and should be seen as an integral aspect of practice. Therefore evidence for this unit will be derived from all work situations.

The knowledge specifications identified under the headers of each section are intended as a guide.

HSC 35 Develop supportive relationships that promote choice and independence

Relationships

(KS 22, 23)

Being able to develop effective working relationships with patients is an essential skill for a health care assistant. Developing a working relationship with a patient is about using all your communication skills, but it also means establishing a two-way process and making a connection with the other person and all experience many types of relationships.

Different types of relationships

Everyone has a wide range of relationships with different people, ranging from family to work colleagues. Each of the different types of relationship is important and plays a valuable role in contributing to the overall well-being of each of us. The needs and demands of different types of relationships are varied. Evidence through reflection identifies the different roles you have in both your working and personal lives. How has each had an impact on how you care for patients?

Professional caring relationships

As a health care assistant, the relationships you form with patients and work colleagues are essential to providing an effective service.

You will need to make use of all the communication skills you have learned in order to develop relationships that make patients feel valued as individuals, respected and treated with dignity. The caring relationship must provide support and, most importantly, should empower the individual to become as independent as possible.

Working relationships with colleagues should be based on a respect for the skills and work of others, and consideration for the demands that work roles place on others. Workloads and responsibilities should be shared as appropriate.

Evidence through reflection (KS 4, 8, 15)

Think about the responsibilities and workload of yourself and the people you work with. Identify how you could best support your colleagues in the workplace. Make notes for your portfolio.

The government is concerned that patients should be treated as individuals. The Department of Health has established a National Service Framework for Older People (2001). This is a 10-year programme aimed at improving the delivery of health and care services for older people. Standard 2 of this framework is entitled 'Person-centred care', which stresses the importance of choice, respect and dignity in meeting the needs of patients.

Choice and empowerment

One of the vitally important aspects of building relationships in your job is making sure that patients are able to make informed choices and take control over as much of their lives as possible – this is referred to as **empowerment**.

Key term

Empowerment Helping people make choices, promoting self-esteem and confidence, and encouraging individuals to take action for themselves when possible.

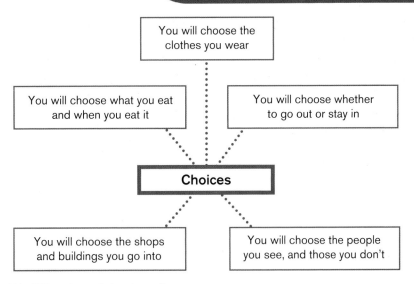

You will choose the clothes you wear

You will choose what you eat and when you eat it

You will choose whether to go out or stay in

Choices

You will choose the shops and buildings you go into

You will choose the people you see, and those you don't

We all like to have choices in our lives.

You will find more information on how you can actively support individuals to maintain their independence later in this unit, on page 111.

Many people who receive care services are often unable to make choices about their lives. This can be because of a range of different circumstances, but it can be because of the way health care services are provided.

In our own daily lives we take many things for granted. You can usually make basic choices in your life without even having to think about them.

Most of the time you give little thought to these choices. However, if you consider the patients in your own setting, you will realise that not all of them have the same options and choices as you do.

Evidence through reflection (KS 2, 3)

For a couple of days, keep a list of the choices you make about everyday aspects of your life.

Now, think about the patients in your work setting. Write down next to each item on your list the initials of patients who are also able to make the same choices as you every day. Do these patients have all the same choices as you and if not, why not?

Now explain how this exercise has helped you to understand how to better support patient choice.

Keep your notes for your portfolio.

In order to understand the importance of the effects of empowerment, you must understand what can happen to people who feel that they are

powerless in relation to the care they are receiving. How much we value ourselves – our **self-esteem** – is a result of many factors, but a very important one is the extent of control, or power, we have over our lives.

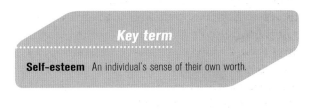

Key term

Self-esteem An individual's sense of their own worth.

Of course, many other factors influence our self-esteem, such as:

- the amount of encouragement and praise we have had from certain people in our lives, such as parents and teachers
- whether we have positive and happy relationships with other people
- the amount of stimulation and satisfaction we get from our work – paid or unpaid.

Patients who are unable to exercise choice and control may very soon suffer lower self-esteem and lose confidence in their own abilities. Unfortunately, this means they may become convinced that they are unable to do many tasks for themselves, and that they need help in most areas of their day-to-day lives. It is easy to see how such a chain of events can result in patients becoming dependent on others and less able to do things for themselves. Once this downward spiral has begun it can be difficult to stop, so it is far better to avoid the things that make it begin.

Self-esteem has a major effect on people's health and well-being. People with a confident, positive view of themselves, who believe that they have value and worth, are far more likely to be happy and healthy than someone whose self-esteem is poor and whose confidence is low.

People who have a positive and confident outlook are far more likely to be interested and active in the world around them, while those lacking confidence and belief in their own abilities are more likely to be withdrawn and reluctant to try anything new. It is easy to see how this can affect someone's quality of life and reduce his or her overall health and well-being.

Empowerment for patients

It is often the case that patients are told the level of support they will receive and the days on which they will receive it when they leave hospital. They may even be told the times at which they will receive such help. The reasons for this are obvious: all services have limited budgets and staff resources, and these have to be managed in order to provide the best possible service for the largest number of people. Organisations that plan and deliver services have to respond on a general scale; they will try to take into account individual needs, but the nature of organisations makes it difficult to do so effectively.

Always recognise and encourage achievements.

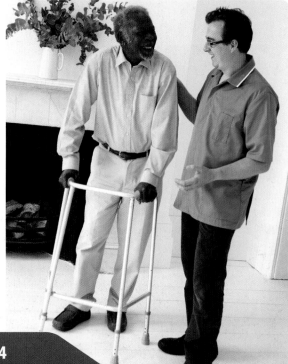

The point at which practices can be adapted to meet needs and empower patients, their families and carers, is when the health care assistant delivering the service meets and interacts with the patient. There are many ways in which you can ensure that your own practice empowers patients as far as possible. These are discussed in detail on page 113.

Evidence with a case study (KS 4, 12, 16)

Empowerment

Elspeth is 78 years old and is recovering in hospital from a total hip replacement. She is mentally alert, but is profoundly deaf. Elspeth has difficulty in undertaking day-to-day personal care as she has severe arthritis, which has made movement difficult and painful. Elspeth will soon be discharged to a nursing home for rehabilitation.

Write notes for your portfolio answering the following questions.

1 How may a 78-year-old's views about life differ from that of a young person?
2 How could the proposed discharge make Elspeth feel?
3 How will you ensure that Elspeth is made aware of the proposed discharge?
4 What steps will you take to allow her to express her views about the discharge?
5 How will you make sure that Elspeth's views are treated with value and respect?
6 How will you make sure that Elspeth feels valued during the process?
7 How can you empower Elspeth in this situation?

Individuals' rights

(KS 1, 2, 3, 4, 5, 6, 7, 8, 11)

In order to look at rights and responsibilities in terms of how they affect the people you work with and provide care for, it is helpful to discuss them under the following headings:

- rights under National Standards, codes of practice, charters, guidelines and policies
- rights provided by law.

With rights comes responsibilities, and it is impossible to consider one without the other.

Rights under codes of practice, charters, guidelines and policies

These are rights which do not have the force of law, but which are enforceable within health care

Healthcare Assistants: **CODE OF CONDUCT**

You have a right...
- to be valued and respected for the vital contribution that you make to patient care
- to be heard as an equal member of the team
- to personal development and feedback on your role
- to access personal and professional training, to progress and develop your knowledge

- to express concern about patient care
- to an induction programme
- to a mentor to help guide and support you
- to be treated equitably and fairly
- to pay that reflects the role that you are undertaking.

Your responsibilities
- You have a duty of care to your patients, colleagues and self – this means that you should always act in a manner that will promote their best interest.
- You should not undertake any task or duty unless you feel competent to carry it out safely.
- You must always maintain patient confidentiality. If uncertain or concerned about the confidence that you have been asked to keep, seek advice from someone senior.
- Always respect and value every team member's contribution.

- You should always ensure that you communicate effectively with patients in your care. Take time to listen to their concerns and support them during your care.
- Treat every patient as an individual and respect their rights and beliefs, even where they might differ from your own.
- Document care, observations and changes clearly in black ink; ensure that, where appropriate, changes in patients' conditions are reported.

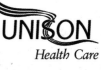

UNISON
Health Care

Designed and produced by UNISON Communications. Published by UNISON, 1 Mabledon Place, London WC1H 9AJ. Printed by Inprint CU/Oct05/15133/2456.

As a health care assistant you have rights as well as responsibilities.

practice and designed to improve the services people receive.

Health care assistants should always refer to their manager and to their job descriptions when seeking guidance on their role in the workplace.

Currently there is no official registration of health care assistants in this country and consequently no official body to issue a Code of Practice. However, the trades union Unison has produced a Code of Conduct which is useful for health care assistants to refer to.

Your employer will also have a range of policy and procedure documents that will define how staff should conduct themselves with patients.

If unsure of your role seek guidance from other members of your team.

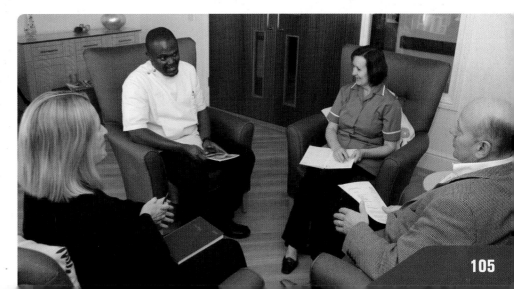

Rights also involve responsibilities. Everyone has the responsibility not to infringe the rights of other people. Some rights and responsibilities are set out below.

Rights provided by law

The United Kingdom's Human Rights Act (1998) means that residents of the UK are now entitled to seek help from the courts if they believe that their human rights have been infringed.

Anyone who works within health care will be working within the provisions of the Human Rights Act (1998), which guarantees the following rights.

- The right to life.
- The right to freedom from torture and inhuman or degrading treatment or punishment.
- The right to freedom from slavery, servitude and forced or compulsory labour.
- The right to liberty and security of person.
- The right to a fair and public trial within a reasonable time.

Rights of patients	Responsibilities
Diversity and the right to be different Including a patient's right to express his or her own identity, culture, lifestyle and interpretation of life.	**Respect for diversity in others** Including an acceptance that other people have a right to interpret life differently. A responsibility not to discriminate against others on the basis that the patient's identity, lifestyle or culture is morally superior to that of others.
Equality and freedom from discrimination Including freedom from discrimination on the basis of race, sex, ability, sexuality or religion.	**Respect for the equality of others** Including respect for, and not discrimination against, members of other social groups.
Control over own life, choice and independence Including the freedom to choose lifestyle, self-presentation, diet and routine.	**Respect for the independence, choice and lifestyle of others** Including arriving at a balance between the impact of the patient's own choices and the needs of other people who may be affected by them – including health care assistants.
Dignity and privacy Including the right to be responded to in terms of the patient's own interpretation of dignity and respect.	**Respect for the dignity and privacy of others** Including issues associated with the identity needs of other users or carers.
Confidentiality Including rights as established in law and codes of practice.	**Respect for the confidentiality of others** Including others' legal rights, and rights established in codes of practice.
Effective communication Including appropriately clear and supportive communication that minimises vulnerability.	**Communication with others which does not seek to cause offence or threaten**
Safety and security Including physical safety, living in an environment that promotes health and emotional safety, security of property, and freedom from physical, social, emotional or economic abuse.	**Contributing to the safety and security of others** Including behaving in a way that does not threaten or abuse the physical or emotional safety and security of others.
The right to take risks Including taking risks as a matter of choice, in order to maintain the patient's own identity or perceived well-being.	**Not to expose oneself or others to unacceptable risks** Including a willingness to negotiate with respect to the impact of risk on others.

- The right to freedom from retrospective criminal law and no punishment without law.
- The right to respect for private and family life, home and correspondence.
- The right to freedom of thought, conscience and religion.
- The right to freedom of expression.
- The right to freedom of assembly and association.
- The right to marry and found a family.
- The prohibition of discrimination in the enjoyment of convention rights.
- The right to peaceful enjoyment of possessions and protection of property.
- The right of access to an education.
- The right of free elections.
- The right not to be subjected to the death penalty.

Evidence in action (KS 1, HSC 33)

Write a piece for your portfolio about how you can incorporate the Human Rights Act (1998) into your practice.

Law, rights and discrimination

Discrimination is a denial of rights. Discrimination can be based on race, gender, disability or sexual orientation. The main Acts of Parliament relating to discrimination are:

- The Equal Pay Act 1970
- The Sex Discrimination Act 1975 (Amended 1986)
- The Race Relations Act 1976 (Amended 2000)
- The Disability Discrimination Act 1995 And Disability Rights Commission Act 1999.

In addition it is important to note the regulations that provide a legal right not to be discriminated against on the basis of sexual orientation or religious belief. These are:

- The Employment Equality (Sexual Orientation) Regulations 2003
- The Employment Equality Regulations (Religion or Belief) Regulations 2003

Evidence in action (KS 5, 6)

Write short notes for your portfolio on the importance of the above Acts of Parliament within your workplace.

Providing support to meet the needs and preferences of individuals

(KS 1, 2, 3, 4, 5, 6, 7, 8, 9, 11, 16)

Patients experience a range of needs. Some older patients may be physically frail; they may need assistance in order to be able to eat, assistance with bathing and personal care, getting dressed, going to bed and mobility. These patients may experience a loss of control over their daily living.

Some patients may perceive themselves as dependent on health care workers when they are in hospital to organise their daily care and ensure their needs are met appropriately. Some older patients may be disorientated, and people with dementia may feel that they are unable to interpret and control their surroundings without appropriate support. Children are often unable to make wise decisions or choices because of limited understanding. It is the responsibility of the health care worker to ensure patients' independence is preserved if not improved while they are in hospital.

Evidence through reflection (KS 12, 14, 15, 16, 22, 23)

Write a reflective account for your portfolio on how you could have improved the independence of one of the patients in your care while meeting their needs and preferences.

As well as vulnerability with respect to needs, patients can also be at risk of exploitation, abuse and physical or emotional damage resulting from unmet needs. It is therefore vitally important that health care assistants are actively concerned with promoting choice and independence in all their interactions with patients.

Maslow's hierarchy of needs

A widely accepted model for interpreting human needs was developed by Abraham Maslow in the 1950s. Although Maslow's hierarchy may be perceived as a simplification, it provides a useful tool for summarising the range of human needs. There was a time when care was thought of as being about only the provision of food, shelter and warmth. Maslow's definition of needs covers social, emotional and intellectual needs, as well as the need to maintain physical health.

Development of full potential — Respect for individuality and support to help people take control of their own lives will often be necessary to help people develop their full potential

Self-esteem needs — Respect for diversity, dignity and privacy will be important in helping people to develop or maintain a sense of self-esteem

Social needs — People need to be able to trust their care assistants and receive effective communication in order to meet their social needs

Feeling safe — People need to be free from discrimination, have a right to confidentiality and be free from risks if they are to feel safe

Physical needs — Freedom from abuse and neglect will be important; as well as food and shelter, in order to meet physical needs

According to Maslow's theory, people might be perceived as being vulnerable on different levels.

Evidence through reflection (KS 12)

Thinking of the patients you care for and Maslow's Hierarchy of Needs, write short notes for your portfolio on the kinds of care needs your patients have.

Best practice: Providing active support for rights

✔ Hold regular staff meetings and have a regular item on your agenda about rights.

✔ Ensure that patients are fully aware of complaints procedures and know how to follow them.

✔ Make sure that you know your organisation's policies and guidelines designed to protect and promote people's rights.

✔ Ensure that you share with your colleagues any information that relates to patients' choices, preferences and rights.

✔ Make sure that you discuss choices and preferences with patients.

✔ Support patients to maintain independence together with other rights if necessary.

✔ Never participate in or encourage discriminatory behaviour.

Supporting individuals to access information

Knowledge is power, and giving people information empowers them. Working as a health care assistant means that you will often work with people who are vulnerable and who feel they have no confidence or power to make decisions. Many people you work with will not have the information they need, because:

- they are unaware that the information exists
- they do not know how to find it
- there are physical barriers to accessing information
- there are emotional barriers to seeking information.

Evidence through reflection (KS 11, 12, 14, 16)

Identify the information that is available to support patients within your workplace. Think about the different ways you could use this information to empower your client group. Identify if the information is adequate and appropriate for your client group. If you feel it is not adequate what can you do to improve it? Make notes for your portfolio.

Best practice: Accessing information

✔ Make sure that your information is up to date. You may have to contact quite a few places to make sure you have the most accurate information possible. Check the dates on any leaflets you have and contact the producer of the leaflet to see whether it has been replaced.

✔ Use advice services such as the Patients Advice Liaison Service (PALS) or alternatively the Patient and Public Involvement Group (PPI), which provide a wide range of information. Make use also of the specialist organisations that represent specific groups, such as Age Concern or Scope.

✔ Check whether the information you are providing has local, regional and national elements. For instance, if you are providing information about Age Concern's services for older people, it is important to provide the local contact as well as national contact points.

✔ The information you provide must be in a format that can be used by the person it is intended for. For example, there is little value in providing an ordinary leaflet to a patient with impaired sight. You will need to obtain large print, audio or Braille versions depending on the way in which the individual prefers to receive information.

✔ Consider the language used and provide information in a language the individual can easily understand. Information is of no value if it is misunderstood.

✔ Provide information at an appropriate time, when the patient can make use of it.

✔ The information you provide must be relevant and useful. For example, if a patient wants to make a complaint about any aspects of their stay in hospital, you will need to find out what the complaints procedure is for your workplace and provide the relevant information and forms to be completed.

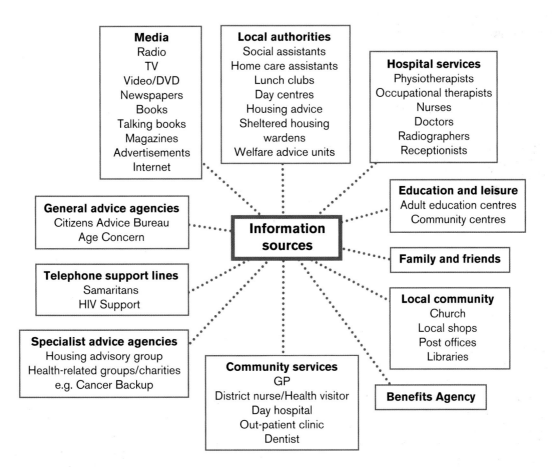

There are many different ways to find out information for patients.

Offering further support where needed

There may be occasions when you have identified a patient's rights and given him or her the information needed. However, the patient may not be able to exercise those rights effectively, because:

- their rights may be infringed by someone else
- there may be physical barriers
- there may be emotional barriers.

When you need to support people to maintain a right to choice and independence, it may be important to involve an outside **advocate**. An advocate is someone who argues a case for another person. An advocate tries to understand a patient's perspective and argue on his or her behalf. Your organisation may have procedures and advice to assist you in gaining the services of people who will act as an advocate for patients.

> **Key term**
>
> **Advocate** A person who is responsible for acting and speaking on behalf of an individual when he or she is unable to do so.

> **Evidence in action (KS 1, 2, 3, 4, 5, 6, 7, 8)**
>
> Find out the roles and responsibilities of an Independent Mental Capacity Advisor. Identify how the use of one of these advocates could promote choice and well-being for your patients. Make notes for your portfolio.

You may also need to defend people's rights in a more informal way during your normal work. For example, people have a right to privacy, and you may need to act to deal with someone who constantly infringes that by discussing other people's circumstances in public. You will have to balance the rights of one person against another, and decide whose rights are being infringed. You may decide that a right to privacy is more important than a right to free speech.

> **Evidence through reflection (KS 3)**
>
> A patient's right to rest may be infringed by someone on the ward who shouts all night. For your portfolio, describe how would you balance the rights of one person not to be disturbed against the rights of another not to be given medication to sedate them and stop them from shouting.

Complaints

An important part of exercising rights is being able to complain if services are poor or do not meet expectations. All public service organisations are required to have a complaints procedure and to make the procedure readily available for people to use. Part of your role may be to assist patients in making complaints, either directly, by supporting them in following the procedure, or indirectly, by making sure that they are aware of the complaints procedure and are able to follow it.

You also need to learn to respond openly and appropriately to any comments or complaints you receive from people about their care. Most complaints procedures will involve an informal stage, where complaints are discussed before they become more formal issues.

Complaints to an organisation are an important part of the monitoring process and they should be considered as part of every review of service provision. If all patients simply put up with poor service and no one complains to an organisation, it will never be aware of where the service needs improvement. Similarly, if complaints are not responded to appropriately, services will never improve.

> **Evidence in action (KS 1, 2, 3, 4, 5, 6, 7, 8)**
>
> Find out the role of the Patient Advice and Liaison Service (PALS). Identify how PALS supports service improvement within the NHS. Make notes for your portfolio.

Active support

The feeling of having achieved something is a feeling everyone can identify with – regardless of the size of the achievement or its significance when viewed from a wider perspective.

Working with patients to help them have a sense of achievement is a key part of caring. It is tempting to undertake tasks *for* people you work with because you are keen to care for them and because you believe that you can make their lives easier. Often, however, you need to hold back from directly providing care or carrying out a task, and look for ways you can enable patients to undertake the task for themselves. This will often involve seeking advice from other members of the multidisciplinary team such as social workers, occupational therapists and physiotherapists.

For example, it may be far easier, less painful and quicker for you to put on people's socks or stockings for them. But this would reinforce the fact that they are no longer able to undertake such a simple task for themselves. Time spent in providing a 'helping hand' sock aid, and showing them how to use it, means that they can put on their own clothing and, instead of feeling dependent, have a sense of achievement and independence.

Sometimes you need to realise that achievement is relative to the circumstances of the patient. Someone recovering from a stroke who succeeds in holding a piece of cutlery for the first time may be achieving something that has taken weeks or even months of physiotherapy, painful exercise and huge determination. The first, supported steps taken by someone who has had a hip replacement represent a massive achievement in overcoming pain, fear and anxiety.

One of the essential aspects of planning health care services is to have a **holistic** approach to supporting people's needs and preferences and this will involve the whole multidisciplinary team. A holistic approach to health care takes into account that all parts of a patient's life will have an impact on their care needs and preferences.

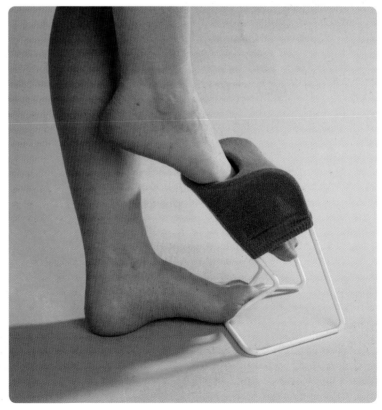

A simple device such as a sock aid can help maintain independence.

What you need to do

Supporting people's independence by encouraging and recognising their achievements is one part of the role of being a health care assistant. Sometimes you may need to spend time guiding patients and encouraging them in order for them to achieve something.

- You may need to steady a patient's hand while they fill in their menu card, but it is far better that you spend time doing this than write it for them.
- You could accompany a patient on many trips to the toilet, and eventually they can go alone.
- You could support a patient with poor motor control to feed themselves by providing the right type of cutlery to aid them.

Make sure you always recognise and celebrate achievements. Your enthusiasm and recognition are important to your patients.

Dealing with conflicts

(KS 1, 2, 3, 4, 5, 6, 7, 8, 11, 15, 17, 18, 19, 20)

As a health care assistant, you can find yourself faced with conflict, arguments, angry people or even potential violence. These situations are always difficult, but you can develop skills in dealing with them.

Most care settings involve living, sharing and working with others. Any situation that involves close and prolonged contact with others has the potential to be difficult. You only have to think about the day-to-day conflicts and difficulties that arise in most families to realise the issues involved when human beings get together in a group.

Conflict resolution is never an easy task, wherever you are and however large or small a scale you

are working on. However, there are some basic guidelines to follow:

- remain calm and speak in a firm, quiet voice – do not raise your voice
- make it clear that neither verbal nor physical abuse will be tolerated
- listen in turn to both sides of the argument – don't let people interrupt each other
- look for reasonable compromises which involve both parties in winning some points and losing others
- make it clear to both sides that they will have to compromise – that total victory for one or the other is not an option.

Sometimes conflicts can arise about behaviour that is not anyone's fault, but is the result of someone's illness or condition. For instance, sometimes patients experiencing some forms of dementia may shout and moan loudly, which may be distressing and annoying to others. These situations require a great deal of tact and explanation. It is simply not possible for the patients concerned to stop their behaviour, so those around them have to be helped to understand the reasons and to cope with the consequences.

HSC 35 Respect the diversity and difference of individuals and key people

If you are going to make sure you always respond to patients in a respectful way which ensures they are treated with dignity, you need to understand the range of ways in which people can fail to be treated with respect or can lose their dignity. It is also important that you recognise the ways in which good practice helps to protect people from discrimination and oppression.

Treating people as individuals

(KS 1, 2, 3, 4, 5, 6, 7, 8, 11, 12, 14, 15, 16, 22, 23)

Memory jogger

Gaining consent is covered in more detail on page 321.

You should always consult the patient and gain their consent before you carry out any procedure explaining everything you do. Everyone should be offered choices wherever possible. Here are examples of the kinds of choices you may be able to offer to people when you provide care.

Care service	Choices
Personal hygiene	Bath, shower or bed bath
	Assistance or no assistance
	Morning, afternoon or evening
	Temperature of water
	Toiletries
Food	Menu
	Timing
	Assistance
	In company or alone

As we have seen, promoting choice and empowerment is about identifying the practical steps you can take in day-to-day working activities to give patients more choice and more opportunities to take decisions about their own lives. Much of this will depend on your work setting and the particular needs of the patients you care for. There are, however, some aspects of empowerment that are common to many settings and most patients. Respecting people's dignity and privacy is always going to be an important factor in promoting their self-esteem.

If self-esteem is about how we *value* ourselves, self-concept (or self-image) is about how we *see* ourselves. These two are different, but both are equally important when you are working. Self-concept is about what makes people who they are. Everyone has a concept of themselves – it can be a positive image overall or a negative one, but a great many factors contribute to an individual sense of identity.

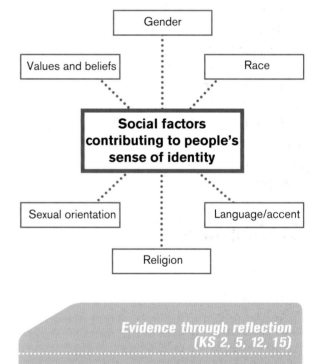

Evidence through reflection (KS 2, 5, 12, 15)

Using the spider diagram above, reflect on how you and the patients you care for will have developed their own sense of identity. Take into consideration the age of your patients, marital status, their family network, their occupation, etc. Make notes for your portfolio.

All of these are aspects of our lives, which contribute towards our idea of who we are. As a health care assistant, it is essential that you consider how each of the patients you work with will have developed a self-concept and individual identity.

As part of empowering patients, you will need to consider how you can promote their own sense of identity. It is about making sure that you recognise that the values, beliefs, tastes and preferences which individuals have – the things that make them who they are – must be supported, nurtured and encouraged, and not ignored and discounted because they are inconvenient or don't fit in with the care system.

In your role as a health care assistant, you will come across situations where a little thought or a small change in practice could give greater opportunities for people to feel that they are valued and respected as individuals. For example, you may need to find out how a patient likes to be addressed. This can be an important way of indicating respect and it is important that you ask a patient their preference on admission to hospital. This information then needs to be documented so all your colleagues are aware.

You will need to give thought to the values and beliefs that patients may have, for example:

- religious or cultural beliefs about eating specific foods
- values about forms of dress which are acceptable
- beliefs or preferences about who should be able to provide personal care.

What you need to do

You need to make sure that people have been asked about religious or cultural preferences and those preferences are recorded so that all health care assistants and others providing care are able to access them.

The National Standards Framework for Older People (2001) requires patient centred planning of care and a single assessment process takes place involving a multidisciplinary, interagency assessment of the needs of patients. This process should result in a documented care plan. It will be important that you know where to find the information for every patient you work with.

How you need to do it

The prospect of having to ask patients questions about their background, values and beliefs can

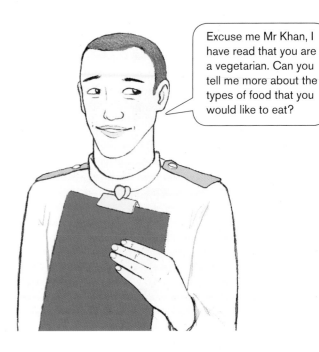

Excuse me Mr Khan, I have read that you are a vegetarian. Can you tell me more about the types of food that you would like to eat?

Patient preferences must be carefully recorded so that all members of the team are aware of the patients' needs.

be quite daunting, but it is rare for patients to be offended by you showing an interest in them. Simple, open questions, asked politely, are usually the best way.

You can obtain some information by observation – looking at someone can tell you a lot about their preferences in dress, for example. Particular forms of clothing worn for religious or cultural reasons are usually obvious (a turban or a sari, for instance, are easy to spot), but other forms of dress may also give you some clues about the person wearing them. Clothes can tell you a lot about someone's age and the type of lifestyle they are likely to be used to. Beware, however – any information you think you gain from this type of observation must be confirmed by checking your facts, do not make assumptions.

Overcoming barriers

Where patients want to make choices about their lives, you should ensure that you do your best to help them to identify any barriers they may meet and then offer support in overcoming them – something which can be a challenge in settings where the needs of other patients must be taken into account.

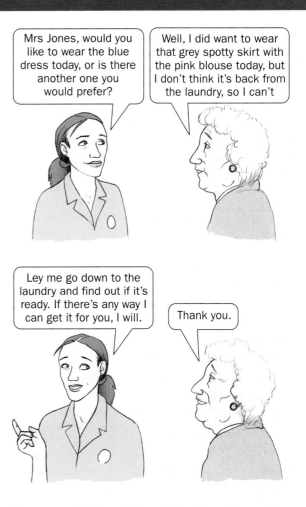

Empowerment includes offering a choice about clothes and supporting patients in their choice.

The health care assistant in the illustration on this page has offered Mrs Jones a choice about clothes. Mrs Jones has indicated that she is not happy with the choice offered, and she has also identified the possible barrier to having the clothes she wants. The health care assistant has looked for a way that the barrier may possibly be overcome. This process can be used in a wide range of situations.

Sometimes patients are not able, because of the nature of a particular condition or illness, to identify choices or to take part in decision making. In these circumstances, it is important that you make every effort to involve them as far as they are able. For example, if a patient communicates differently from you as the result of a particular condition, or there are language differences, it is important that you ensure the communication differences are reduced as far as possible so that the individual can take part in discussions and decisions. This may involve using specific communication techniques, or arranging to have help from an appropriate specialist. Some examples include:

- if you are communicating with a patient with a hearing impairment, you may need to write things down or you may need to arrange for a sign language interpreter. A hearing aid wearer may need access to a loop system.

- if you are communicating with a patient who has speech difficulties following a stroke, you may need to use visual communication, or use cards that show a range of pictures such as food and drink
- if you are communicating with a patient whose first language you do not speak, you will need to use an interpreter.

All of these steps will allow patients to be involved in decisions.

Memory jogger

Do you know what to do when dealing with communication differences? Revisit page 17 to refresh your memory.

In other circumstances, you may be dealing with patients who are not able to fully participate in all decisions about their day-to-day lives because they have a different level of understanding. This could, for example, include patients with learning difficulties, dementia or brain injury.

In this situation, it may be that the individual has an advocate who represents his or her interests and is able to present a point of view to those who are providing services. The advocate may be a professional one such as a solicitor, social assistant or a rights assistant, or it could be a relative or friend. It is essential that you include the advocate in discussions as far as possible to make sure that the patient's point of view is taken into account.

People need to be offered choices because they are all different; don't fall into the trap of stereotyping patients.

The effects of assumptions

'All apples are red.' That statement is clearly silly. Of course they're not – some are green, some are yellow. When it comes to people, everyone is different. However, there is a tendency to make sweeping statements (generalisations) that we believe apply to everyone who belongs to a particular group.

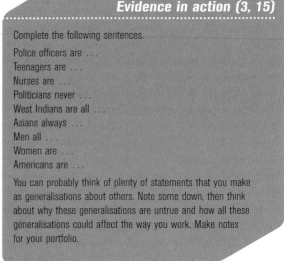

Evidence in action (3, 15)

Complete the following sentences.

Police officers are . . .
Teenagers are . . .
Nurses are . . .
Politicians never . . .
West Indians are all . . .
Asians always . . .
Men all . . .
Women are . . .
Americans are . . .

You can probably think of plenty of statements that you make as generalisations about others. Note some down, then think about why these generalisations are untrue and how all these generalisations could affect the way you work. Make notes for your portfolio.

Avoiding assumptions at work

Take the time and trouble to find out the personal beliefs and values of each of the patients you work with. Think about all the aspects of their lives: diet, clothing, worship, language, relationships with others, bathing. It is your responsibility to find out – not for the patient to have to tell you. It will be helpful for you, and for other assistants, if this type of information is recorded in the patient's personal record.

For example, you may need to know that many Muslims will only accept medical treatment from someone of the same gender, that you will need to enable them to wash in running water rather than a bowl, that they do not eat pork, and that any other meat must have been killed and prepared in a particular way – Halal.

Evidence with a case study (KS 1, 8, 9, 11, 12, 14, 15, 16)

You are providing care for someone who is an Orthodox Jew. As a health care assistant, you need to be aware of their choices relating to food. Research this and make notes for your portfolio.

Although you may hold a different set of values and beliefs from those of the patients you are caring for, you do not have the right to impose your beliefs upon others. There may, in fact, be occasions when you will have to act as an advocate for their beliefs, even if you do not personally agree with them.

Best practice: Valuing diversity

✔ The wide range of different beliefs and values that you are likely to come into contact with, if you work in a health care setting, are examples of the rich and diverse cultures of all parts of the world.

✔ Value each patient as an individual. The best way to appreciate what others have to offer is to find out about them. Ask questions. Patients will usually be happy to tell you about themselves and their beliefs.

✔ The other key is to be open to hearing what others have to say – do not be so sure that your values and beliefs and the way you live are the only ways of doing things.

✔ Think about the great assets which have come to the UK from people moving here from other cultures, including music, food and entertainment, and different approaches to work or relaxation or medicine.

Evidence through reflection (KS 3, 5)

Understanding your values may help you to approach your work in a different way. Make a list, for your portfolio, of the things you believe in as values, and a second list of how they could affect your work. Then go on to explain how you could change to ensure your values do not adversely affect your work.

How to recognise your own prejudices and deal with them

One of the hardest things to do is to acknowledge your own **prejudices** and how they can affect what you do. Prejudices may be the result of your own **beliefs** and **values**, and may come into conflict with work situations. There is nothing wrong with having your own beliefs and values – everyone has them, and they are a vital part of making you the person you are. But you must be aware of your own values and beliefs in order to ensure that they do not stop you working in the way you should.

Key terms

Prejudices Beliefs which are not grounded with any knowledge of what is true or real.

Beliefs A mental acceptance of something as being true or real.

Values Principles or standards which underpin the way individuals behave.

Think about the basic principles that apply in your life. For example, you may have a basic belief that most people are always honest, you may believe that abortion is wrong, you may believe people with disabilities should be looked after and protected; but there will be many others who believe the opposite.

This exercise is very hard, and could take a long time to do – you may find it helps to discuss this task with a work colleague and to do it over a period of time. As you become more aware of your own actions, you will notice how they have the potential to affect your work.

Exploring your own behaviour is never easy, and you need good support from either your supervisor or close friends to do it. You may be upset by what you find out about some of your attitudes, but knowing about them and acknowledging them is the first step to doing something about them.

As a health care assistant, it will be easier to make sure that you are practising effectively if you are confident that you have looked at your own practice and the attitudes that underpin it. Don't forget that you can ask for feedback from patients and colleagues too, not only from your manager.

Beliefs and values of others

Once you are aware of your own beliefs and values, and have recognised how important they are, you must think about how to accept the beliefs and values of others. The patients you work with are all different, and so it is important to recognise and accept that diversity.

Many workplaces now have policies that are about 'managing diversity' rather than 'equal opportunities'. This is because many people have realised that, until diversity is recognised and valued, there is no realistic possibility of any policy about equal opportunities being totally effective.

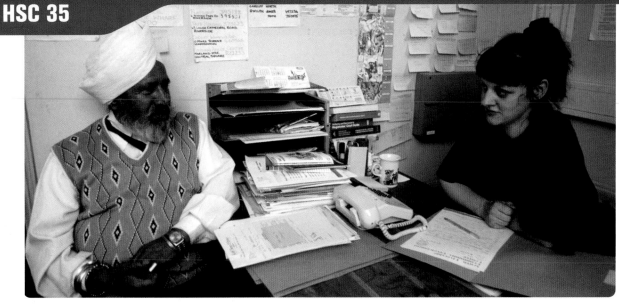

As a health care assistant you must practice in an anti-discriminatory way.

Anti-discriminatory practice

(KS 1, 2, 3, 4, 5, 6, 7, 8, 9, 11, 12, 14, 15, 16, 22, 23)

Receiving an inferior service due to your age, gender, race, sexuality or ability is against the law. Experiencing discrimination can damage a patient's self-esteem and reduce a patient's ability to develop and maintain a sense of identity. As a health care assistant, you must practise in an anti-discriminatory way in your day-to-day work with patients, and challenge any tendency towards the stereotyping or labelling of patients.

Stereotyping	Stereotyping leads to whole groups of people being assumed to be the same. It is often present when you hear phrases such as 'these sorts of people all . . .'. 'Old people love a sing-song' or 'Black people are good athletes' are stereotyping remarks.
Labelling	Slightly more complex than stereotyping, labelling happens when someone thinks the factor that people have in common is more important than the hundreds of factors that make them different.
	For example, the remark 'We should organise a concert for the elderly' makes an assumption that being older is what is important about the people concerned, and that somehow, as you grow older, your tastes become the same as all other people your age. It would be much better to say 'We should organise a concert for older people who like music from the shows' or 'We should organise a concert for older people who like opera', etc.
Discrimination	In care work, discrimination means treating some categories of people less well than others. People are often discriminated against because of their race, beliefs, gender, religion, sexuality or age. Treating everyone the same will result in discrimination because some people will have their needs met and others will not. In order to prevent discrimination, it is important to value diversity and treat people differently in order to meet their different needs.
Anti-discrimination	This means positively working to eliminate discrimination and to challenge it if you see it occurring in your place of work.
	For example, when food is being served, if no account is taken of the religious and cultural needs of patients, you should challenge this and suggest changes.

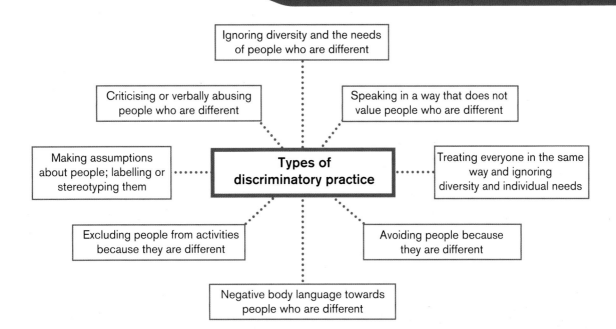

Some obvious types of discriminatory practice are shown above. You should monitor your own and others' behaviour in order to minimise the risk of such practices occurring.

Your day-to-day practice and attitudes are important in how effective your anti-discriminatory practice will be. You should be interested in learning about other people's lifestyle, culture and needs. Finding ways of meeting patients' needs might provide a source of job satisfaction.

Best practice: Anti-discriminatory practice

✔ Be prepared to challenge your own thinking and assumptions.
✔ Don't make judgements about patients – try to gain an understanding about different cultures, beliefs and lifestyles.
✔ Everyone is entitled to their own beliefs and culture. If you don't know about someone's way of life – ask.

Supporting the work of colleagues

You need to support your colleagues, too, to work in ways that recognise and respect patient's beliefs and preferences; your work setting should be a place in which diversity and difference are acknowledged and respected. You need to set a good example and to make it clear that certain behaviour is unacceptable, such as:

- speaking about people in a derogatory way
- speaking to people in a rude or dismissive way
- undermining people's self-esteem and confidence
- patronising and talking down to people
- removing people's right to exercise choice
- failing to recognise and treat people as patients
- not respecting people's culture, values and beliefs.

If you are having difficulty at any time in promoting equality and diversity, you need to seek advice from your manager.

Evidence in action (KS 1, 2, 3, 4, 5, 6, 7, 8, 10, 11, 15, 16, 17, 18, 20)

As a health care assistant, you have a responsibility to ensure that your patient's beliefs and preferences are respected. Identify the steps you would take if you thought a colleague was failing to do this. Make notes for your portfolio.

Steps you can take to reduce discrimination

Think about how you use language. The words and expressions you use are important. Avoid using language that might suggest assumptions, stereotypes or discrimination about groups.

Examples of discriminatory language

Disability	Some words such as 'handicapped' can suggest the discriminatory assumption that disabled people are damaged versions of 'normal' people.
Race	Some words and phrases may be linked to the discriminatory idea that certain ethnic groups (white groups) are superior to others.
Age	Some words and phrases make fun of older people. Do not address an older person as 'pop' or 'granddad' unless you are invited to do so.
Gender	Some words and phrases are perceived as implying that women have a lower social status than men. Addressing women as 'dear', 'petal' or 'flower' may be understood as patronising or insulting.
Sexuality	Gay and lesbian people often object to being catalogued using the biological terminology of 'hetero'- and 'homo'-sexuality. Use the terminology that people would apply to themselves.

Best practice: Helping patients to achieve their full potential

✔ Do not assume that older people are only capable of quiet activities that don't involve too much excitement.

✔ Avoid the temptation to over-protect people and therefore encourage dependence.

✔ Support people in challenging the barriers that stand in their way.

✔ Encourage people to behave assertively but not aggressively and to develop confidence in their own abilities.

✔ Refuse to accept behaviour which you know is discriminatory.

✔ Do not participate in racist or sexist jokes.

✔ If you are uncertain what to do in a particular situation, discuss the problem with the practitioner in charge or your manager.

HSC 35 Contribute to the protection of all individuals

In this element, you will look at some of the most difficult issues that you will face as a health care assistant. Regardless of previous experience, coming face to face with situations where abuse is, or has been, taking place is difficult and emotionally demanding. Knowing what you

are looking for, and how to recognise it, is an important part of ensuring that you are making the best possible contribution to protecting patients from abuse. An understanding of abuse in society, how to recognise it, and what to do about it, is essential for a health care assistant.

It is a tragic fact that almost all disclosures of abuse are true – and you will have to learn to *think the unthinkable*. A health care assistant needs to understand about the different forms of abuse.

If you can learn to consider the possibility of abuse, always to be alert to potentially abusive situations and always to *listen* and *believe* when you are told of abuse, then you will provide the best possible protection for the patients you care for.

Taking the right steps when faced with an abusive situation is the second part of your key contribution to patients who are being, or have been, abused.

Did you know?

2.6 per cent of people aged 66 years or over living in private households, including sheltered housing, reported they had experienced mistreatment involving a family member, friend or care worker during the past year. This represents 1:40 of the population over the age of 66 years (Source: www.natcen.ac.uk).

Forms of abuse

Abuse can take many forms. These are usually classified under five main headings:

- physical
- sexual
- emotional
- financial
- institutional.

Abuse can happen to any patient regardless of their age or service needs. Child abuse is the most well-known and well-recognised type of abuse, but all patient groups can suffer abuse. Abuse of older people and abuse of people with learning difficulties, sensory impairment or physical disabilities is just as common, but often less well recognised.

Physical abuse

Any abuse involving the use of force is classified as physical abuse. This can mean:

- punching, hitting, slapping, pinching, kicking – in fact, any form of physical attack
- burning or scalding
- restraint, such as tying up or tying people to beds or furniture
- refusal to allow access to toilet facilities
- deliberate starvation or force feeding
- leaving patients in wet or soiled clothing or bedding as a deliberate act to demonstrate the power and strength of the abuser
- excessive or inappropriate use of medication
- a carer causing illness or injury to someone they care for.

Sexual abuse

Sexual abuse, whether of adults or children, can also involve abuse of a position of power. Children can never be considered to give informed consent to any sexual activity of any description. For many adults, informed consent is not possible because of a limited understanding of the issues. In the case of other adults, consent may not be given and the sexual activity is either forced on the individual against his or her will or the individual is tricked or bribed into it.

Sexual activity is abusive when informed consent is not freely given. Health care assistants need to be able to recognise situations where abuse is taking place because someone is exploiting their position of relative power.

Sexual abuse can consist of:

- sexual penetration of any part of the body with a penis, finger or any object
- touching inappropriate parts of the body or any other form of sexual contact without the informed agreement of the patient
- sexual exploitation
- exposure to, or involvement in, pornographic or erotic material
- exposure to, or involvement in, sexual rituals
- making sexually related comments or references which provide sexual gratification for the abuser
- making threats about sexual activities.

Emotional abuse

All the other forms of abuse also have an element of emotional abuse. Any situation that means that a patient becomes a victim of abuse at the hands of someone he or she trusted is, inevitably, going to cause emotional distress. However, some abuse is purely emotional – there are no physical, sexual or financial elements involved. This abuse can take the form of:

- humiliation, belittling, putting down
- withdrawing or refusing affection
- bullying
- making threats
- shouting or swearing
- making insulting or abusive remarks
- racial abuse
- constant teasing and poking fun.

Financial abuse

Patients may be vulnerable to financial abuse, particularly those who may have a limited understanding of money matters. Financial abuse, like all other forms of abuse, can be inflicted by family members and even friends as well as health workers or informal carers, and can take a range of forms, such as:

- stealing money or property
- allowing or encouraging others to steal money or property
- tricking or threatening patients into giving away money or property
- persuading patients to take financial decisions which are not in their interests
- withholding money, or refusing access to money
- refusing to allow patients to manage their own financial affairs
- failing to support patients to manage their own financial affairs.

Institutional abuse

Institutional abuse is not only confined to large-scale physical or sexual abuse scandals of the type that are regularly publicised in the media. Of course, this type of systematic and organised abuse goes on in residential and hospital settings, and must be recognised and dealt with appropriately so that patients can be protected. However, patients can be abused in many other ways in settings where they could expect to be cared for and protected. For example:

- patients are not given choice over day-to-day decisions such as mealtimes, bedtimes, etc.
- freedom to go out is limited by the institution – this must be balanced with the needs of each patient's condition
- privacy and dignity are not respected
- personal correspondence is opened by staff
- the setting is run for the convenience of staff, not patients
- excessive or inappropriate doses of sedation/ medication are given
- access to advice and advocacy is restricted or not allowed
- complaints procedures are deliberately made unavailable.

You can probably begin to see that the different types of abuse are sometimes interlinked, and patients can be victims of more than one type of abuse. Abuse is a deliberate act – it is something that someone actively does in order to demonstrate power and authority over another person. It is also done with the motive of providing some sort of gratification or pleasure for the abuser.

Neglect

Neglect happens when care is not given and a patient suffers as a result. The whole area of neglect has many aspects you need to take into

account, but there are broadly two different types of neglect:

- self-neglect
- neglect by others.

Self-neglect

Some people neglect themselves; this can be for a range of reasons. People may be ill, depressed or in pain, or do not feel able to look after themselves. Sometimes people feel that looking after themselves is unimportant. Others choose to live in a way that does not match up to the expectations of other people. Working out when someone is neglecting themselves, given all of these considerations, can be very difficult.

However, what may appear to be self-neglect may, in fact, be an informed choice made by someone who does not regard personal and domestic cleanliness or hygiene as priorities. It is always important to make a professional judgement based on talking with the patient and finding out his or her wishes, before making any assumptions about what may be needed.

Evidence with a case study (KS 1, 2, 3, 4, 5, 6, 7, 8, 11, 12, 16)

Mr Smith is admitted to your ward for surgery in the morning. He lives alone with his cats, has no regard for his personal cleanliness and is refusing to have a bath or shower before surgery.

Make notes for your portfolio on the actions you may take to encourage Mr Smith to have a bath. Make reference to the legislative framework governing patient choice.

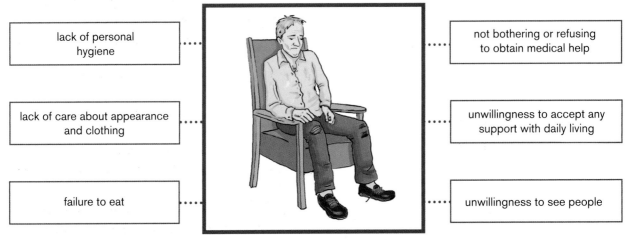

Self-neglect can show itself in a range of ways.

Neglect by others

This occurs when either a health care assistant or an informal carer fails to meet the care needs of a person. Neglect can happen because those responsible for providing the care do not realise its importance, or because they cannot be bothered, or choose not, to provide it. As the result of neglect, patients can become ill, hungry, cold, dirty, injured or deprived of their rights. Neglecting someone you are supposed to be caring for can mean failing to undertake a range of care services: for example:

- not providing adequate food
- not providing assistance with eating food if necessary
- not ensuring that the patient receives personal care
- not ensuring that the patient is adequately clothed
- denying the patient social interaction
- not assisting a patient to meet mobility or communication needs
- failing to obtain necessary medical/health care support
- not supporting social contacts
- not taking steps to provide a safe and secure environment for the patient.

In some care situations, health care assistants may fail to provide some aspects of care because they have not been trained, or because they work in a setting where the emphasis is on cost saving rather than care provision. In these circumstances, it becomes a form of institutional abuse. Health care assistants have a responsibility to report to their practitioner in charge if they ever feel they are being asked to do tasks for which they are not trained.

Unfortunately, there have been NHS Trusts where patients have been found to be suffering from malnutrition as the result of such neglect. Individual health care assistants who are deliberately neglecting patients in spite of receiving training and working in a quality caring environment are likely to be spotted and could be subject to prosecution in a court of law.

However, carers who are supporting people in their own homes are in different circumstances, often facing huge pressures and difficulties. Some may be reluctantly caring for a relative because they feel they have no choice; others may be barely coping with their own lives and may find caring for someone else a burden they are unable to bear. Regardless of the many possible reasons for the difficulties that can result in neglect, it is essential that a suspicion of neglect is investigated and that concerns are followed up so that help can be offered and additional support provided if necessary.

As with self-neglect, it is important that lifestyle decisions made by patients and their carers are respected, and full discussions should take place with patients and carers where there are concerns about possible neglect.

Signs and symptoms that may indicate abuse

(KS 19)

One of the most difficult aspects of dealing with abuse is to admit that it is happening. If you are someone who has never come across deliberate abuse before, it is hard to understand and to believe that it is happening. It is not the first thing you think of when a patient has an injury or displays a change in behaviour. However, you will need to accept that abuse does happen, and is relatively common. Considering abuse should be the first option when a patient has an unexplained injury or a change in behaviour that has no obvious cause.

Abuse happens to children and adults and victims may fail to report abuse for a range of reasons:

- they are too ill, frail or too young
- they don't have enough understanding of what is happening to them
- they are ashamed and believe it is their own fault
- they have been threatened by the abuser or are afraid
- they don't think they will be believed
- they don't believe that anyone has the power to stop the abuse.

Given the fact that relatively few victims report abuse without support, it is essential that those who are working in care settings are alert to the possibility of abuse and are able to recognise possible signs and symptoms.

Signs and symptoms can be different in adults and children and you need to be aware of both because, regardless of the setting you work in, you will come into contact with both adults and children. Your responsibilities do not end with the patient group you work with. If you believe that you have spotted signs of abuse in anyone, you have a duty to take the appropriate action.

Information on signs and symptoms comes with a health warning: none of the signs or symptoms is always the result of abuse, and not all abuse produces these signs and symptoms. They are a general indicator that abuse should be considered as an explanation. You and your colleagues will need to use other skills, such as observation and communication with other professionals, in order to build up a complete picture.

Signs of possible abuse in adults

Abuse can often show as physical effects and symptoms. These are likely to be accompanied by emotional signs and changes in behaviour, but this is not always the case.

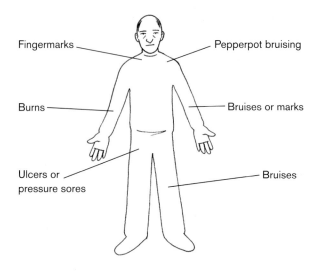

Signs of abuse in adults

Type of sign/symptom	Description of sign/symptom	Possible form of abuse indicated
Physical	frequent or regular falls or injuries	physical
	'pepperpot' bruising – small bruises, usually on the chest, caused by poking with a finger or pulling clothes tightly	physical
	fingermarks – often on arms or shoulders	physical
	bruising in areas not normally bruised such as the inside of thighs and arms	physical
	unusual sexual behaviour	sexual
	blood or marks on underclothes	sexual
	recurrent genital/urinary infections or bleeding	sexual
	marks on wrists, upper arms or legs which could be from tying to a bed or furniture	physical/sexual
	burns or scalds in unusual areas such as soles of feet, inside of thighs	physical
	ulcers, bedsores or rashes caused by wet bedding/clothing	physical
Emotional/behavioural	becoming withdrawn or anxious	all forms of abuse
	loss of interest in appearance	sexual/physical/emotional
	loss of confidence	sexual/physical/emotional
	sudden change in attitude to financial matters	financial
	becoming afraid of making decisions	emotional
	sleeping problems	all forms of abuse
	changes in eating habits	all forms of abuse
	no longer laughing or joking	all forms of abuse
	feeling depressed or hopeless	all forms of abuse
	flinching or appearing afraid of close contact	physical

Any behaviour changes could indicate that the patient is a victim of some form of abuse, but remember that they are only an indicator and will need to be linked to other factors to arrive at a complete picture.

Signs of possible abuse in children

As with abuse in adults, this is not a comprehensive list of every indicator of abuse, and the existence of one of these signs does not by itself mean that abuse has taken place. Each is an indicator that needs to be used alongside your other skills, such as observation and listening. It is a further piece of evidence in building a complete picture.

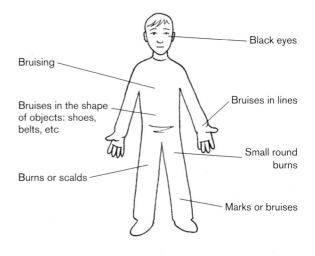

Signs of abuse in children

Type of sign/symptom	Description of sign/symptom	Possible form of abuse indicated
Physical	bruising, or injuries that the child cannot explain	physical
	bruises in the shape of objects – belt buckles, soles of shoes, etc.	physical
	hand marks	physical
	bruises in lines	physical
	injuries to the frenulum (the piece of skin below the tongue), or between the upper and lower lips and the gums	physical
	black eyes	physical
	bruising to ears	physical
	burns, particularly small round burns which could have come from a cigarette	physical
	burns in lines, like the elements of an electric fire	physical
	burns or scalds to buttocks and backs of legs	physical
	complaints of soreness or infections in the genital/anal area	sexual
	frequent complaints of abdominal pain	sexual
	deterioration of personal hygiene	sexual/neglect
Emotional/behavioural	sudden change in behaviour, becoming quiet and withdrawn	sexual/emotional
	change to overtly sexual behaviour, or an obsession with sexual comments	sexual
	problems sleeping or onset of nightmares	sexual/emotional
	a sudden unwillingness to change clothes or participate in sports	sexual/physical
	finding excuses not to go home	physical/sexual/emotional
	appearing tense or frightened with a particular adult	physical/sexual/emotional
	excessive anxiety to please	physical/sexual/emotional

Carer behaviour that should alert you to possible abuse

Sometimes, it is not the behaviour of the patient that is the first noticeable feature of an abusive situation. It can be that the first behaviour you notice is that of the carer. The following are some indications of behaviour that may give cause for concern, although with the usual warning that each is only a *possible* indicator of problems:

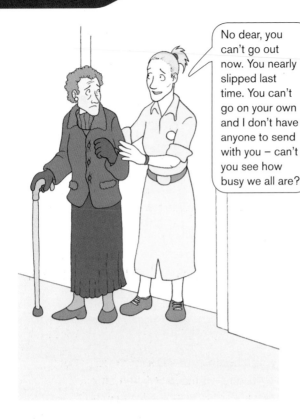

No dear, you can't go out now. You nearly slipped last time. You can't go on your own and I don't have anyone to send with you – can't you see how busy we all are?

closely supported, and you may need to contribute towards activities or therapies that have been planned for the patient. If a patient identifies to you that they are going to harm themselves, it is your responsibility to report this to the practitioner in charge.

Where abuse can happen

(KS 12, 13, 15, 17)

It is not possible accurately to predict situations where abuse will take place – a great deal of misery could be saved if it were. It is possible, however, to identify some factors that seem to make it more likely that abuse could occur. This does not mean that abuse will definitely happen – neither should you assume that all people in these circumstances are potential abusers. But it does mean that you should be aware of the possibility when you are dealing with these situations.

- reluctance to allow visitors to see the patient
- insistence on being present with the patient at all times
- derogatory or angry references to the patient
- excessive interest in financial accounts or assets
- excessive requests for repeat prescriptions.

Up to this point, consideration has been given to abuse by carers, whether parents, informal or professional. But do not forget that in hospital settings, abuse can occur between patients, and it can also happen between visitors and patients. People can also abuse themselves.

Self-harm

The one abuser it is very hard to protect someone from is themselves. Patients who are known to self-harm will be identified in their plan of care, and responses to their behaviour will be recorded. You must ensure that you follow the agreed plan for provision of care to someone who has a history of self-harm. It is usual that an individual who is at risk of harming himself or herself will be

Situations when child abuse can happen

Child abuse can happen in situations where:
- parents are unable to put a child's needs first
- parents or carers feel a need to show dominance over others
- parents or carers have been poorly parented themselves
- parents or carers were abused themselves as children
- families have financial problems (this does not just mean families on low incomes)
- families have a history of poor relationships or of use of violence.

Situations when abuse can happen in a care setting

Abuse can happen in a hospital setting when:
- staff are poorly trained or untrained
- there is little or no management supervision or support
- staff work in isolation
- there are inadequate numbers of staff to cope with the workload
- there are inadequate security arrangements.

Best practice: Helping to stop abuse

If you want to be effective in helping to stop abuse you will need to:

✔ believe that abuse happens

✔ recognise abusive behaviour

✔ be aware of when abuse can happen

✔ understand who abusers can be

✔ know the policies and procedures for handling abuse

✔ follow the patient's plan of care

✔ recognise likely abusive situations

✔ report any concerns or suspicions.

Your most important contribution will be to be *alert*. For example, a patient's plan of care or your organisational policy should specify ways in which the patient's whereabouts are constantly monitored – and if you are alert to where a vulnerable patient is and who they are with, you can do much to help avoid abusive situations.

Abuse in different settings

Abuse can take place at home or in a formal care setting. At home, it could be an informal carer who is the abuser, or it could be a neighbour or regular visitor. It could also be a care worker who is carrying out the abuse. This situation can mean that abuse goes undetected for some time because of the unsupervised nature of a care worker's visits to someone's home.

In a hospital setting, abuse may be more likely to be noticed, although some of the more subtle forms of abuse, such as humiliation, can sometimes be so commonplace that they are not recognised as abusive behaviour.

Key term

Disclosure Giving out information previously hidden.

Abuse in a hospital setting may not just be at the hands of members of staff, but may be institutional abuse. This comes about because of the way in which the organisation is run, where the basis for planning the systems, rules and regulations is not the welfare, rights and dignity of the residents or patients, but the convenience of the staff and management. This is the type of situation where patients can be told when to get up and go to bed, given communal clothing, only allowed medical attention at set times and not allowed to go out.

How to respond to abuse and neglect

(KS 1, 2, 3, 4, 5, 6, 7, 8, 11, 14, 16, 20, 21)

When you find out, or suspect, that a patient is being abused or neglected, you have a responsibility to take action immediately. Concerns, suspicions and firm evidence all require an immediate response.

There are several situations in which you may find yourself in the position of having information to report concerning abuse or neglect.

- A patient may disclose to you that he or she is being abused or neglected.
- You may have clear evidence that abuse or neglect is happening.
- You may have concerns and suspicions, but no definite evidence.

How to respond to disclosure

The correct term for a patient telling you about abuse or neglect is disclosure. If a patient discloses abuse to you, the first and most important response is that you must believe what you are told.

This is often harder than it sounds. If you have never been involved with an abusive situation before, it is hard to believe that such cases arise and that this could really happen.

You must reassure the patient, whether an adult or a child, that you believe what you have been told. Another common fear of people who are being abused is that it is somehow their fault – so you must also reassure them that it is not their fault and that they are in no way to blame for what has happened to them.

When a patient discloses abuse or neglect to you, try not to get into a situation where you are having to deal with a lot of detailed information. After reassuring the patient that you believe him or her, you should report the disclosure immediately to a senior colleague and hand over responsibility. This is not always possible because of the circumstances or location in which the disclosure takes place, or because the patient wants to tell you everything once he or she has started disclosing. If you do find yourself in the position of being given a great deal of information, you must be careful not to ask any leading questions – for example, do not say 'And then did he punch you?' Just ask 'And then what happened?' Use your basic communication and listening skills so that the patient knows he or she can trust you and that you are listening. Make sure you concentrate and try to remember as much as possible so that you can record it accurately. Often it is best to ask the patient if you can recap and make some notes after the disclosure has taken place.

Another common problem that arises with disclosure is that you may be asked to keep the information secret. *You must never make this promise – it is one you cannot keep.* What you can do is promise that you will only tell people who can help.

You may well find yourself in this situation.

The most important first step is to ensure that you know the procedures in your workplace for dealing with abuse and neglect. You should also receive training on abuse as part of your induction and staff development. All workplaces will have policies and procedures and it is vital that you are familiar with them and know exactly who you need to report to. Then you will be in a position to support the patients you work with to understand that you must pass on information about actual or likely danger and abuse. You can also reassure patients about how you can fulfil your responsibilities to protect them from such harm.

Situations where you have evidence

There may be situations where you have evidence of abuse, either because you have witnessed it happening or because you have other evidence. These situations must be reported immediately to your manager, or the person identified in the procedures followed by your workplace for cases of suspected abuse. You should make sure that you provide all the detailed evidence that you have, with full information about how you found the evidence and how and where you have recorded it.

Situations where you have concerns

It is more likely that you will not have evidence but you have noticed some of the signs or symptoms of possible abuse. You must report this as rapidly as you would if you had clear evidence.

It may be tempting to wait until you have more evidence or something happens to confirm your suspicions, but do not do this. You must report

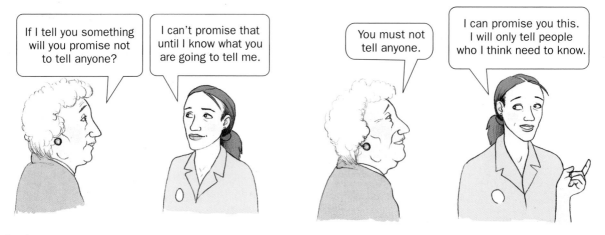

Caption to come.

anything unusual that you notice, even if you think it is too small to be important. It is the small details that make the whole picture. Sometimes, your observations may add to other small things noticed by members of the team, and a picture may start to emerge.

Dealing with abuse in a care setting

One of the most difficult situations to deal with is abuse in a professional care setting, particularly if you believe it to be taking place within your own workplace, or elsewhere in your organisation. If you are concerned about possible abuse or neglect in your workplace, you should follow the same procedures as you would for any other abuse or neglect concerns.

- Report the problem to your manager or practitioner in charge
- If you suspect that your manager is involved, or will not take action, you must refer it to a more senior manager who is likely to be impartial.

Whistle-blowing

Reporting concerns about practice in your workplace is known as 'whistle-blowing'. It is important that you know the details of your organisation's 'whistle-blowing' or 'Speak up' policy.

The law protects your right to express your concerns – it is called the UK Public Interest Disclosure Act (1998). It encourages people to 'blow the whistle' about **malpractice** in the workplace and is designed to ensure that organisations respond by acting on the message rather than punishing the messenger. In addition to employees, it covers trainees, agency staff, contractors, home assistants and every professional in the NHS. The Act means that your employer cannot take any action to victimise you because you have reported genuine concerns.

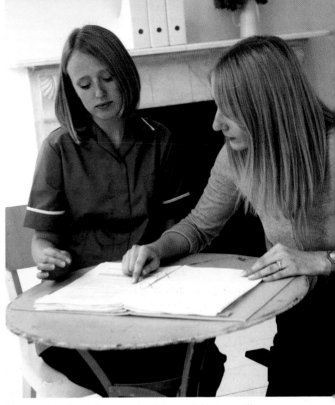
Teamwork and good communication are vital in preventing problems.

Recording information about possible abuse

Any information you have – which could be concerns, hard evidence, or a disclosure – must be carefully recorded. Ideally you should write down your evidence as soon as possible. It is not acceptable to pass on your concerns verbally without backing this up with a recorded report. Verbal information can be altered and can have its meaning changed very easily when it is passed on. Think about the children's game of Chinese Whispers – by the time the whispered phrase reaches the end of it journey, it is usually changed beyond all recognition.

> ### Key term
> **Malpractice** Immoral, unethical or illegal behaviour.

> ### Memory jogger
> Do you remember what best practice is when recording and storing information? Look back at Unit HSC 31 page 40.

Find your workplace policy on whistle blowing or speak up policy. Write notes in your portfolio on how you would do this, if required. Put this policy into action.

Sometimes your information may need to be included in a patient's plan of care or personal records, particularly if you have noticed a change in the way he or she is cared for, or their behaviour could be an 'early warning' that the care team need to be especially observant. Your workplace may have a special report form for recording 'causes for concern'. If not, you should write your report, making sure you include the following:

- everything you have observed
- anything you have been told – but make sure that it is clear that this is not something you have seen for yourself
- any previous concerns you may have had
- what has raised your concerns on this occasion.

Evidence in action (KS 6, 7, 21)

To practise the art of accurate incident reporting, ask a colleague to record an incident that you have both been involved in, while you also do the same thing. Compare your reports and identify how they coincide or differ. Make notes on this exercise and identify how you could improve on your incident writing skills.

In serious cases, your written evidence may be needed by the identified person within your workplace who will investigate the situation. It may be useful for a doctor if he or she has to conduct an examination, or it may be needed for the case conference or for court proceedings. So you must make sure you record all information accurately and factually, avoiding any statements (such as expressions of your personal opinions) that would make it difficult to rely on in future investigations or court proceedings.

The effects of abuse

(KS 10, 12, 13, 15, 17)

Abuse devastates those who suffer it. It causes people to lose their self-esteem and their confidence. Many adults and children become withdrawn and difficult to communicate with. Anger is a common emotion among people who have been abused. This may be directed against the abuser, or at those people around them who failed to recognise the abuse and stop it happening.

One of the greatest tragedies is when people who have been abused turn their anger against themselves, and blame themselves for everything that has happened to them. These are situations that require expert help, and this should be available to anyone who has been abused, regardless of the circumstances.

Some of the behaviour changes that can be signs of abuse can become permanent, or certainly very long lasting. There are very few survivors of abuse whose personality remains unchanged and, for those who do conquer the effects of abuse, it is a long, hard fight.

The abuser, often called the 'perpetrator', also requires expert help, and this should be available through various agencies depending on the type and seriousness of the abuse. People who abuse, whether their victims are children or vulnerable adults, receive very little sympathy or understanding from society. There is little public recognition that some abusers may have been under tremendous strain and pressure, and abusers may find that they have no support from friends or family. Many abusers will face the consequences of their actions alone.

Health care assistants who have to deal with abusive situations will have different emotional reactions. There is no 'right way' to react. Everyone is different and will deal with things in his or her own way. If you have to deal with abuse, these are some of the ways you may feel, and some steps you can take that may help.

Shock

You may feel quite traumatised if you have witnessed an abusive incident. It is normal to find that you cannot get the incident out of your mind, that you have difficulty concentrating on other things, or that you keep having 'flashbacks' and re-enact the situation in your head. You may also feel that you need to keep talking about what happened.

Talking can be very beneficial, but ensure you do this within the safe parameters of your workplace while maintaining confidentiality.

These feelings are likely to last for a fairly short time, and are a natural reaction to shock and trauma. If at any time you feel that you are having difficulty, you must talk to your manager, who should be able to help.

Anger

Alternatively, the situation may have made you feel very angry. While this is understandable, it is not professional and you will have to find other ways of dealing with your anger. Again, your manager should help you to work through your feelings.

Everyone has different ways of dealing with anger, such as taking physical exercise, doing housework, punching a cushion, writing feelings down and then tearing up the paper or crying . It is perfectly legitimate to be angry, but you cannot bring this anger into your relationships at work.

Distress

The situation may have made you distressed, and you may want to go home and have a good cry. This is a perfectly normal reaction. No matter how many years you work, or how many times it happens, you may still feel the same way. Some workplaces will have arrangements in place where assistants are able to share difficult situations and get support from each other. Others may not have any formal meetings or groups arranged, but colleagues will offer each other support and advice in an informal way. You may find that work colleagues who have had similar experiences are the best people with whom to share your feelings.

Memory jogger

Revisit how supervisor networks and supervision may support you. See Unit HSC 33 page 85.

There is, of course, the possibility that the situation may have brought back painful memories for you. There are many avenues of support now available to survivors of abuse. You can find out about the nearest support

confidentially, if you do not want your workplace colleagues or supervisor to know. Remember the occupational health department in your workplace is also there to support you. There is no doubt that dealing with abuse is one of the most stressful aspects of working in care. There is nothing odd or abnormal about feeling that you need to share what you have experienced and looking for support from others. In fact, most experienced managers would be far more concerned about a health care assistant involved in dealing with abuse who appears quite unaffected by it, than about one who comes looking for guidance and reassurance.

Best practice: Dealing with abuse

✔ Feeling upset is normal.

✔ Talk about the incident within your work setting if that helps, but respect the rules of confidentiality.

✔ Being angry is OK, but deal with it sensibly – take physical exercise, do the housework, cry.

✔ Do not let your feelings show to the abuser.

✔ If you are a survivor of abuse and you find it hard to deal with, ask for help.

How the law affects what you do

(KS 1, 2, 3, 4, 5, 6, 7, 8, 21)

Much of the work in caring is governed by legislation, but the only group where legislation specifically provides for protection from abuse is children. Older people and people with a learning difficulty, physical disabilities or mental health problems have service provision, rights and many other requirements laid down in law, but no overall legal framework to provide protection from abuse. The laws which cover your work in the field of care are summarised in the table on page 218.

There are, however, a number of sets of guidelines, policies and procedures in respect of abuse for patients other than children, and you will need to ensure that you are familiar with policies for your area of work, particularly those that apply in your own workplace.

Dealing with abuse is difficult and demanding for everyone, and it is essential that you receive professional supervision from your manager. This may be undertaken in a regular supervision or support meeting if you have one; if not, it will be important that you arrange to meet with your supervisor so that you can ensure you are working in the correct way and in accordance with the procedure in your setting. Your manager will also need to be assured that you are coping on a personal and professional level with the effects of having to deal with an abusive situation.

Evidence in action (KS 1, 18, 21)

Ask your manager about the laws and guidelines that relate to protecting individuals from abuse in your workplace. Check with experienced colleagues about situations they have dealt with and ask them to tell you about what happened and the information they would have documented with regards to the situation.

Make notes for your portfolio, including the reasons why clear documentation is necessary.

Government policies and guidelines

The most important set of government guidelines, which lays down practices for co-operation between agencies, is *Working Together to Safeguard Children*. This was published in 1999 and forms the basis for child protection work. This set of guidelines ensures that information is shared between agencies and professionals, and that decisions in respect of children are not taken by just one person. Matters relating to abuse of children and adults now form part of mandatory training programmes.

Did you know?

Each week one child will be killed by their parent or carer in England and Wales. 16 per cent of children in England and Wales experience serious maltreatment by their parents (Source: www.nspcc.org.uk).

A government White Paper published in 2001, *Valuing People: A New Strategy for Learning Disability in the 21st Century*, sets out the ways in which services for people with a learning disability will be improved. *Valuing People* sets out four main principles for service provision for people with a learning disability:

- civil rights
- independence
- choice
- inclusion.

The White Paper also makes it clear that people with a learning disability are entitled to the full protection of the law.

Recent policy approaches to protecting children and vulnerable adults in care environments have concentrated on improving and monitoring the quality of the service provided to them. The principle behind this is that, if the overall quality of practice in care is constantly improved, well-trained staff working to high standards are less likely to abuse patients, and are more likely to identify and deal effectively with any abuse they find.

The law protecting children

The Children Act (1989) requires that local authority social services departments provide protection from abuse for children in their area. This Act gives powers to social services departments, following the procedures laid down by the Area Child Protection Committee, to take legal steps to ensure the safety of children.

The law protecting adults

The Care Standards Act (2000) made provision for the protection of adults by the use of the Provision of Vulnerable Adults (POVA) scheme. The scheme comprises of a list of care workers who have previously been convicted of harming vulnerable adults in their care. This list is checked when care providers wish to employ care workers to care positions working with vulnerable adults. This process is carried out by the Criminal Records Bureau (CRB) and since July 2004 there has been a statutory requirement on registered care providers to check with the CRB if a care worker they wish to employ is included on the

POVA list. Since 2002, people applying to work in health care services have had criminal record bureau checks in an attempt to identify and stop people who would be inappropriate to work in a care setting.

Information on ways to protect individuals

Safeguarding and protecting vulnerable adults and children is an area of work that has been in the public eye for many years. As a result of this, a great deal of research has been carried out, and plenty of information is available in order to develop and improve your understanding of this difficult subject.

Your manager will be able to advise you about the best way to find out information, and you should choose the way in which you find it easiest to learn – you may prefer to attend a training course, to read a book or to watch a training video. Ask your manager to find out what is available in your workplace.

Evidence in action (KS 1, 2, 3, 4, 5, 6, 7, 8, 11, 12, 17, 18, 19, 20)

Within your workplace you will have the opportunity to attend mandatory training sessions with regard to safeguarding children and vulnerable adults. If you have not attended this training, try to do this in the very near future. Make notes for your portfolio on how the knowledge you have gained can support your practice.

Further reading and research

Providing care for vulnerable people can be challenging and difficult, while at the same time rewarding. The more support you receive and information you gather, the better equipped you will be to cope with the demands and responsibility.

Websites

- www.dh.gov.uk (Department of Health: Health and Social Care related topics – Dignity in care, vulnerable adults, POVA, PoCA; No Secrets – guidance on Developing and Implementing Multi-Agency Policies and Procedures to Protect Vulnerable Adults from Abuse)
- www.gscc.org.uk (GSCC: General Social Care Council – Codes of Practice)
- www.crb.gov.uk (Criminal Records Bureau)
- www.pcaw.co.uk (PCaW: Public Concern at Work)
- www.nspcc.org.uk (NSPCC: National Society for the Prevention of Cruelty to Children)
- www.unison.org.uk (UNISON: Public services union – guides to POVA and PoCA including a leaflet called 'Reported')
- www.csci.org.uk (CSCI: Commission for Social Care Inspection – Care Provider – guidance related to the social care services you are researching)
- www.elderabuse.org.uk (Action on Elder Abuse)
- www.valuingpeople.gov.uk (Valuing People: A New Strategy for Learning Disability in the 21st Century)
- www.everychildmatters.gov.uk (Every Child Matters: Working Together to Safeguard Children)
- www.dca.gov.uk (DCA: Department for Constitutional Affairs)
- www.who.intsuggestions (World Health Organisation)

Publications

- Arroba T., Ball L. (2001) *Staying Sane: Managing the Stress of Caring*, Age Concern
- Maclean S., Maclean I. (2001) *Social Care and the Law*, Kirwin Maclean Associates
- Maclean S., Maclean I. (2005) *Supporting You, Supporting Others: Health and Social Care (Level 3)*, Kirwin Maclean Associates
- Moore R., Maclean I. (2004) *Cultural Sensitivity in Social and Health Care*, Kirwin Maclean Associates

Infection control

Introduction

The single most important thing you can do as a health care assistant is to help prevent the spread of health care infections in your clinical area.

Everyone working within a health care environment has a responsibility to protect themselves and others from the risk of infection. While it is generally accepted that not all infections can be prevented, it is believed that, by implementing strict infection control policies and guidelines, hospital-acquired infections could be reduced by 15 to 30 per cent (National Audit Office 2000).

As someone who has direct, day-to-day contact with patients, carers, relatives and other staff, you have a crucial part to play in infection control in your workplace. Identifying when a patient is at risk of acquiring an infection and knowing how to prevent it are key roles for you. To do this effectively, you need to have the necessary knowledge and skills concerning infection control and prevention and the competence to implement them in practice.

In this unit, we will discuss health care acquired infections, how they spread within the environment, who is at most risk, and what you can do to prevent such infections from spreading.

What you need to learn

- Infections in the health care setting
- The chain of infection
- Hospital staff involved in preventing the spread of infection
- Standard precautions
- Responsibilities of the health care assistant

Infections in the health care setting

As a health care assistant, it is vital that you understand how infections are caused, how they can spread between individuals and the actions you can take to prevent this happening. Applying standard precautions consistently in everyday practice is the single most important thing you can do.

The infections you will read about in this unit are put into particular categories in the health care setting.

- A **health care acquired infection** (HCAI) is any infection acquired as a result of contact with a health care system, either community- or hospital-based.
- A **hospital acquired infection** (HAI) generally means one that has arisen 48 hours after admission, which was not incubating on admission to hospital.

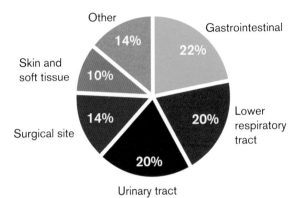

Major site of infection identified in the
Third Prevalence Survey of Healthcare-associated
Infections in England 2006

- Other 14%
- Gastrointestinal 22%
- Skin and soft tissue 10%
- Lower respiratory tract 20%
- Surgical site 14%
- Urinary tract 20%

Source: Pratt R J, Pellowe C M, Wilson J A, Loveday H P, Jones S R L J, McDougall C, Wilcox M H. epic2: National Evidence-Based Guidelines for Preventing Healthcare-Associated Infections in NHS Hospitals in England. *Journal of Hospital Infection*. February 2007; 65S: S1-S64

Main sites of health care infections.

Skin	*Staphyloccocus epidermis, Candida* species, *Streptococcus* species, *Corynebacterium* species
Throat	*Strep. viridans, Neisseria* species, diphtheroids
Mouth	*Strep. viridans, Moraxella catarrhalis,* spirocheates
Respiratory tract (upper)	*Strep. viridans, Neisseria* species, micrococci
Vagina	Lactobacilli, streptococci, yeasts
Intestines	*Bacteroides* species, anaerobic streptococci, *Escherichia coli, Proteus* species, *Strep. faecalis, Klebsiella* species, *Clostridium perfringens*

Common bacteria making up the body's normal flora. Adapted from Wilson (2001).

Reflect

Think about some of the patients you have nursed in your clinical area. What types of infection did they have? Make a list of the ones you can remember, e.g. wound infection.

What effect did the infection have on the patient? What impact do you think this would have socially and psychologically for the patient? Did the infection lead to a longer hospital stay?

Remember

It is the simple things you do on a day-to-day basis when caring for your patients – such as effective hand washing – that can have the biggest impact on the prevention and control of HAIs.

How infection happens and spreads

At any one time the human body is populated with a large number of **commensal** micro-organisms that live in harmony with the body (see the following table). These **micro-organisms**, also known as the body's **normal flora**, help to protect the body by occupying internal and external surfaces of the body, thereby reducing free surface space, which in turn prevents the multiplication of disease causing micro-organisms called **pathogens**.

Problems can occur, however, if the normal flora micro-organisms are transferred from one site on the body to a different site on the same body. At the new site, they are not recognised as normal flora and this can lead to infection. This is known as an **endogenous infection**. An example of this would be bowel flora entering the urethra while catheterising a patient, potentially leading to a urinary tract infection. This is why it is so important to apply a strict aseptic technique while undertaking this procedure (see aseptic technique on page 156 for more details).

If an individual becomes exposed to a micro-organism from another person or source, this is termed an **exogenous infection** (cross infection). Examples of this would be the injection of another person's blood through a needle stick injury, or the transfer of a micro-organism from a health care assistant's hand to a patient's wound.

The body's natural defences

As well as gaining some defence against infection from the normal flora, the body has other natural defence mechanisms. Examples of this include white blood cells and antibodies in the blood, the integrity of the skin and cilia in the upper respiratory tract.

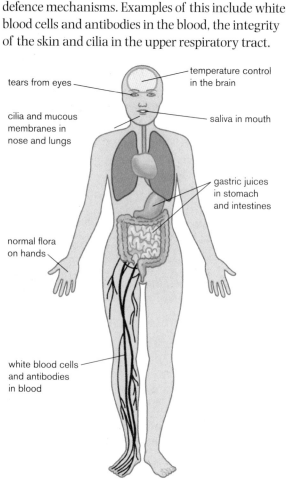

tears from eyes

temperature control in the brain

cilia and mucous membranes in nose and lungs

saliva in mouth

gastric juices in stomach and intestines

normal flora on hands

white blood cells and antibodies in blood

The body's defences against infection.

A patient in hospital is sometimes put in a situation where these natural defence mechanisms are breached. Examples of this include:

- a patient undergoing treatment that lowers his or her immunity by reducing their white blood cell count
- the insertion of a urinary catheter
- the insertion of an **invasive** device, such as a venous cannula.

All of these will put the individual more at risk of **infection** – and understanding this is a key learning outcome.

As a health care assistant, it is very important for you to understand that it is possible for micro-organisms to multiply in the tissues of an individual yet cause no outward signs or symptoms of disease. This is called **colonisation** and means that a person can be a **carrier** of a disease, yet have no knowledge of this. It is then possible for the pathogens to be transmitted to another person through contact, such as shaking their hand.

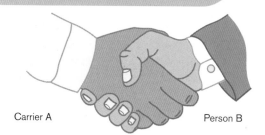

Carrier A

Person B

Carrier A shakes hands with non-carrier person B

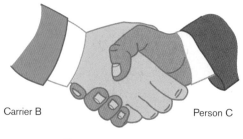

Carrier B

Person C

B, now a carrier, contaminates person C

Carriers carry pathogens without showing signs of illness. They are capable of transmitting pathogens to others who then become ill.

People and objects can become contaminated if they come into contact with a pathogen. If your hands become contaminated then you could pass the pathogen to another person if you were to touch them. This is why regular decontamination of your hands is so vitally important.

The risk to patients

Patients in hospital are at greater risk of infection: they already have a weakened immune system and will generally be exposed to a variety of invasive procedures during their stay. It is therefore extremely important that you have the knowledge and skills to identify those patients at risk of infection, as well as the signs and symptoms of infections, both local and systemic.

- A **localised infection** is an infection affecting one area of the body only, such as an elbow or toe – this could be due to a dog bite, insect sting or cut. The area becomes painful, red and inflamed, with the signs and symptoms remaining local to the injury.
- A **systemic infection** is an infection that enters the bloodstream and makes the patient feel very ill. The patient might complain of tiredness, headache, vomiting, aching limbs, nausea, flushing or a high temperature.

If you notice any of the above signs or symptoms when caring for your patient, you must report it immediately to the practitioner in charge and document your findings on the appropriate paperwork, such as the TPR chart or nursing care plan.

The chain of infection

The chain of infection is a series of six steps showing how infection can be spread.

This chain of infection will continue in a cyclic way, unless one of the links in the chain is broken. The easiest point at which to break this chain is generally considered to be at the means of transmission. One of the simplest ways to do this is by washing your hands, between every patient and before and after undertaking clinical tasks. By doing this, you can greatly reduce the likelihood of transmitting infection from one place to another.

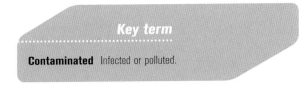

Infectious agent (pathogen)

Environment (reservoir)

Portal of exit (Excretion or secretion of body fluids)

Means of transmission (e.g. on hands)

Portal of entry (e.g. wound, catheter)

Susceptible host (e.g. elderly, very young)

The chain of infection.

Infectious agent

This is considered to be the first part of the chain. Infectious agents are disease-causing pathogens such as bacteria, virus, fungi and parasites. The table below shows some examples of diseases caused by these pathogens.

Environment

This is where the pathogen multiplies and survives. Certain conditions need to be met for the pathogen to grow, such as temperature, **humidity**, nutrients, **pH** and oxygen. The environment may not necessarily be in or on an individual, as pathogens have also been shown

to survive in places such as in water behind radiators, on food, on work surfaces and on equipment. This is why it is so important that you follow infection control precautions and ensure that work areas and equipment are kept clean and dry at all times.

> ### Key terms
>
> **Humidity** The amount of water vapour in the air.
>
> **pH** The percentage of hydrogen ions in a substance, which is a measure of the acidity or alkalinity of a solution.

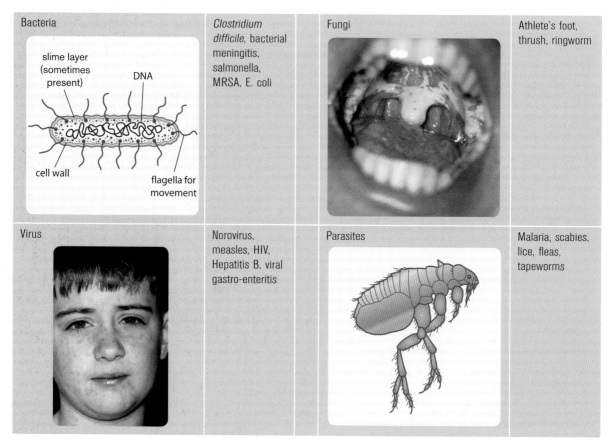

| Bacteria | *Clostridium difficile*, bacterial meningitis, salmonella, MRSA, E. coli | Fungi | Athlete's foot, thrush, ringworm |
| Virus | Norovirus, measles, HIV, Hepatitis B, viral gastro-enteritis | Parasites | Malaria, scabies, lice, fleas, tapeworms |

Examples of pathogens and the diseases they can cause.

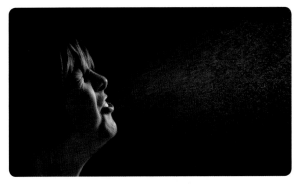

Pathogens can be transmitted through sneezing.

Portal of exit

If it is to spread, the pathogen needs a means of escaping the environment in which it is growing. This can be via the excretion or secretion of body fluids such as a bleeding wound, sneezing or productive cough or diarrhoea and vomiting. Other exits include the skin and placenta.

Means of transmission

This is the easiest link in the chain to break. Pathogens can be transmitted through a number of different routes.

- Direct contact – person to person contact, for example, during direct hands on patient care, sexual intercourse.
- Indirect contact – contact with a contaminated object, for example a surgical instrument, respiratory equipment
- Airborne – inhalation of pathogens carried on dust particles or skin scales
- Droplet – contact with contaminated respiratory secretions released through sneezing, coughing and talking or suctioning and bronchoscopy

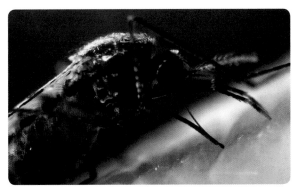

Mosquito sucking blood.

- Arthropods: flies, bugs, mites, etc. that transmit the pathogen by biting, sucking or via their droppings. Malaria is a disease caused by the mosquito sucking a human's blood and thereby transmitting the pathogen.

Portal of entry

The pathogen can gain entry through any of the body's **orifices**, e.g. mouth, vagina, rectum, nose and urethra.

> ### Key terms
>
> **In utero** In the womb.
> **Orifice** An opening, mouth of a cavity.

If the patient has an artificial orifice, such as a colostomy, jejunostomy or tracheostomy, they are equally at risk of infection if safe working practices are not followed during their care.

When a patient is at a critically ill stage, he or she may undergo the introduction of invasive devices to monitor their condition, such as urinary catheters, central venous catheters and intravenous cannulae. It is your joint responsibility to ensure that the patient's condition is not further compromised by acquiring a HAI.

Patients can also be at risk because they have a break in their skin. This could be due to a traumatic wound or surgical incision, or through an injection site.

With the patient at their most susceptible, it is imperative that you implement precisely your hospital's health and safety policies and guidelines. You must also ensure that you employ strict aseptic techniques when managing these devices (see Topic 2 Aseptic technique on page 156 and CHS 12 on wound care on page 256).

Susceptible host

The final link in the chain is the susceptibility of the host to acquiring an infection. You have already seen that patients undergoing procedures that include the introduction of an invasive device are more at risk of infection. However, there are other factors which can place the individual at risk, including:

MRSA	C. difficile
MRSA stands for methicillin resistant *Staphylococcus aureus*. MRSA is a variant of the *Staphylococcus aureus* bacterium which has become resistant to some commonly used antibiotics.	*C-difficile* is an abbreviation of *Clostridium difficile* which is a healthcare associated intestinal infection that mainly affects elderly patients with other debilitating illnesses.
• Transmitted mainly through contact with colonised skin or contaminated equipment. • Eliminated from hands by using alcohol handrub, and cleaning with most disinfectants. • Key risk of bloodstream infection is through piercing of skin (e.g. cannula or open wounds). • Survives less well in the environment. • Screening for colonised patients is simple (nose and skin swab), and colonisation known to increase risk of infection and transmission.	Present in 3% of healthy adults and is usually kept in check by the normal 'good' bacterial population of the gut. C-difficile can cause illness when certain antibiotics interfere with the balance of these 'good' bacteria. • Transmitted mainly through contact with spores from infected faeces, or contact with contaminated environment and equipment. • Reduced by washing hands with soap and water and cleaning with chlorine-based disinfectants. Alcohol hand gels are ineffective as spores are not killed by alcohol. • Key risk of infection is through ingesting spores, together with antibiotic treatment. • Spores survive very well in the environment. • Screening for colonised patients is inappropriate (most potential cases would not be identified and it requires a stool sample) and colonisation without symptoms is not considered to increase risk of transmission.

- the general health of the individual, e.g. if they are malnourished or oedematous
- having certain diseases, e.g. diabetes
- being very old
- being very young
- immunosuppression
- psychological illness
- poor general hygiene
- some drug therapies.

To demonstrate how the chain of infection is applied to common HAIs, read the sections above on MRSA and *Clostridium difficile*.

Hospital staff involved in preventing the spread of infection

Everyone working in a hospital or other health care environment has a responsibility to prevent the spread of infection. However, for certain key staff this responsibility is more evident in their day-to-day job roles.

Infection control team

This team includes the Director of Infection Prevention and Control, Infection Control Nurses, Audit nurses, surveillance staff and administrative staff.

The team's role is to support clinical staff in practice, undertake research, audit and surveillance, produce guidelines for practice, educate staff and advise on purchasing of products.

Microbiologists

Microbiologists working in hospitals assist the clinical team by using a range of scientific methods to isolate and identify organisms that cause infection, checking sensitivities to antibiotics and liaising with doctors and nursing staff about specific treatment options.

Matrons/lead nurses/senior nurses

All senior nurses, but matrons in particular, have a leadership role to play in infection prevention and control. They help to implement guidelines in practice, support staff with infection control issues, take part in audits and help to produce action plans, monitor cleanliness and review staff competence and personal development.

Managers

Managers liaise with the team to review the resources required, in terms of both staff and equipment, for infection control. They are also involved with policy development, specific infection control projects and the development of new services.

Nurses and health care assistants

The role of the nurse or health care assistant is to apply the principles of Standard Precautions, e.g. hand washing, aseptic technique, decontamination of equipment, appropriate disposal of waste and cleaning up of spillages. They also educate patients, undertake risk assessments and implement guidance laid down in the policies, such as isolation guidelines.

Cleaners/domestic staff

The role of cleaners and domestic staff is to maintain the general cleanliness of the ward environment, including patients' bed space, bathrooms and kitchen areas. They should work very closely with the ward sister and housekeeper (if appointed) to ensure that all areas of the ward are clean and dry, and that priority areas are addressed as required.

Housekeeper

Some hospitals have appointed staff called housekeepers. Their role varies from organisation to organisation, and even from ward to ward. However, most housekeepers have some responsibility for cleaning, catering and the patient environment. They tend to manage the laundry, maintain stock levels, liaise with the cleaning staff and ensure that sterile supplies are stored appropriately.

Clinical cleaning team

Not all hospitals will have a clinical cleaning team, but in those that do, the team is responsible for the various levels of cleaning required when patients with infections are transferred from side rooms or bays. This will include changing curtains, washing walls, possible steam cleaning of rooms and thorough cleaning of bed frame and mattress.

Doctors

Doctors also have a key role to play in both the prescribing and – just as important – the timely discontinuation of antibiotics. They also need to apply the principles of standard precautions when working in practice. Some doctors, particularly consultants, also take an active role in developing specific guidelines relating to their speciality and infection control.

Porter

Porters are key when it comes to preventing the spread of infection within an organisation. As their role requires them to move from ward to ward, transferring patients and equipment, they could easily spread infection if they did not follow infection control guidelines.

Chief Executive

The Chief Executive of an organisation is responsible for ensuring that there are effective plans and resources in place for the management of infection control, and for health and safety in general. Along with other members of the Trust Board, they should provide leadership and direction on all health and safety issues.

Activity: Following the chain

Think about the chain of infection and how infections can be transmitted within your clinical area. Make a list of all the day-to-day activities that help to reduce the spread of infection in your workplace, e.g. hand washing.

What policies and procedures are there in your organisation to support these activities? Who in your organisation can you contact if you need more information about an infection control matter?

Draw a spider diagram to illustrate all the people who could help you.

If you are working towards your NVQ you will gain evidence for: HSC 32 – K4 (b,c,d), K6, K11 (a,b,c), K12, K14.

Standard precautions

Standard precautions (previously called universal precautions) are designed to protect both patients and staff from infection. They should always be adopted wherever you work and applied to all patients at all times. As noted previously, it is impossible to identify all patients who are colonised or infected with disease-causing pathogens, therefore all blood and body fluids should be considered potentially dangerous at all times.

High risk	Low risk (if not visibly bloodstained)
blood	urine
body fluids – visibly bloodstained	faeces
CSF	vomit
semen	saliva – not dentistry related
vaginal fluid	
breast milk	
amniotic fluid	
pleural fluid	
peritoneal fluid	
pericardial fluid	
synovial fluid	
serous fluid	
saliva in dentistry	

Body fluids and level of risk.

Although the ultimate responsibility for the Health and Safety of staff rests with the Chief Executive of the organisation, you have a duty under the Health and Safety at Work Act (1974) to comply with all safety procedures and policies to ensure your actions will not harm the health and safety of yourself or others.

Memory jogger

What Acts and regulations are involved in preventing and dealing with infection? Look at pages 150–151.

Standard precautions cover the following safe working practices:

- hand washing
- personal protective equipment (PPE)
- safe use and disposal of sharps
- disposal of clinical waste
- spillages of blood and body fluids
- decontamination of equipment
- laundry management

Hand washing

It has been demonstrated that effective hand washing is the most valuable means of preventing cross-infection. Hand washing needs to become an unconscious habit – something that you do without thinking about it – and you need to ensure that you lead by example, acting as a good role model for other staff.

It is generally accepted that the major cause of the spread of infection from one person or source to another is via **transient micro-organisms** carried on the hands of health care workers. Your hands may appear visibly clean, but they can still be heavily colonised with a large number of disease-causing pathogens.

Key term

Transient micro-organisms Micro-organisms that lie on the surface of the skin and which can easily be transferred to another person or object by touching it. They can be removed by proper hand washing.

Did you know?

Cross infection via the hands of health care workers has been acknowledged as contributing to hospital outbreaks of methicillin-resistant staphylococcus aureus (MRSA).

Adequate and appropriately placed facilities for hand washing and hand drying should be available for you to use in the clinical area. These include automated, elbow- or wrist-controlled mixer taps, liquid soap dispensers, good quality hand towels and foot-operated waste bins.

Clear guidelines relating to hand hygiene should be accessible in your workplace, and can usually be found in the organisation's Infection Control Manual.

Activity

Have a look for your own organisation's policy on hand hygiene. Does it cover all the points mentioned in the best practice box?

Best practice: Hand washing

✔ Hands must be decontaminated immediately before each and every episode of direct patient contact or care, and after any activity or contact that potentially results in hands becoming contaminated.

✔ Hands that are visibly soiled or potentially grossly contaminated with dirt or organic material (i.e. following the removal of gloves) must be washed with liquid soap and water.

✔ An alcohol-based handrub should be used between caring for different patients or between different care activities for the same patient, unless visibly soiled. Hands should be washed with soap and water after several applications of alcohol handrub.

✔ All wrist jewellery and, ideally, hand jewellery should be removed.

✔ Cuts and abrasions must be covered with waterproof dressings.

✔ Fingernails should be kept short, clean and free from nail polish. False nails and nail extensions must not be worn by clinical staff.

✔ When decontaminating hands using an alcohol-based handrub, the solution must come into contact with all surfaces of the hand, just as if using soap and water.

✔ Staff should be encouraged to use an emollient hand cream regularly, for example after washing hands before a break or going off duty and also when off duty to maintain the integrity of the skin.

(Source: Pratt et al epic 2: *National Evidence-Based Guidelines for Preventing Healthcare-Associated Infections in NHS Hospitals in England*. Journal of Hospital Infection, February 2007)

An effective hand-washing technique involves three stages.

1 **Preparation:** This requires wetting your hands under tepid running water before applying the recommended amount of liquid soap or an antimicrobial preparation. The hand-wash solution must come into contact with all surfaces of your hand. You must rub your hands vigorously for a minimum of 10–15 seconds, paying particular attention to the tips of your fingers, your thumbs and the areas between your fingers.

2 **Hand washing and rinsing:** There are six steps to effective hand washing.

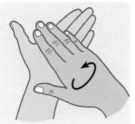

1 *Rub hands together palm to palm.*

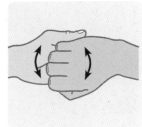

2 *Backs of fingers to opposite palms with fingers interlocked.*

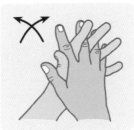

3 *Palm to palm with fingers interlocked.*

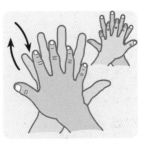

4 *Right palm over back of left hand with fingers interlocked and vice versa.*

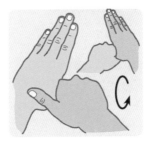

5 *Rotational rubbing of right thumb clasped in left palm.*

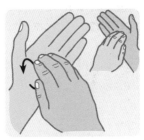

6 *Rotational rubbing backwards and forwards with clasped fingers of right hand in left palm and vice versa.*

You should rinse your hands thoroughly under running water. Use your elbow to turn off the tap.

3 **Drying:** Dry your hands thoroughly with good-quality paper towels.

If you do not do hand washing effectively, micro-organisms can be left on the surface of your hands which can be transferred to another person or piece of equipment at a later date.

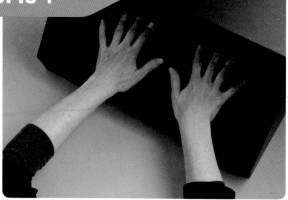

Areas commonly missed when washing hands.

As stated in Pratt et al (2007), 'Personal protective equipment should be based on an assessment of the level of risk associated with a specific patient care activity or intervention and take account of current health and safety legislation.'

Personal protective equipment

Personal protective equipment (PPE) includes items such as gloves, aprons, goggles, masks, visors, hats and footwear. It is used to protect both you and the patient from the risk of contamination and potential cross-infection.

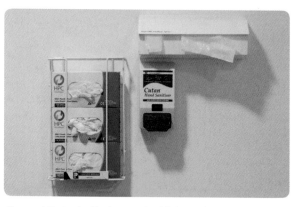

Personal Protective Equipment should always be easily accessible.

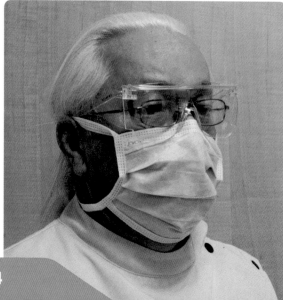

Some indications for wearing gloves

- Emptying a catheter bag
- Venepuncture
- Wound care
- Changing stoma bags
- Cleaning equipment – particularly if contaminated
- Cleaning up blood or body fluids.

Best practice Guidelines for Personal Protective Equipment

Gloves	Aprons/gowns	Face masks and eye protection
Gloves must be worn for all invasive procedures, contact with sterile sites, and non-intact skin or mucous membranes, and all activities that have been assessed as carrying a risk of exposure to blood, body fluids, secretions and excretions; and when handling sharp or contaminated instruments.	Disposable plastic aprons must be worn when in close contact with the patient or contaminated materials/equipment and when there is a risk that clothing may become contaminated with pathogens or blood, body fluids, secretions or excretions.	Face masks and eye protection must be worn where there is a risk of blood, body fluids, secretions or excretions splashing into the face and eyes.
Gloves must be worn as single use items. They are put on immediately before an episode of patient contact or treatment and removed as soon as the activity is completed.	Plastic aprons/gowns should be worn as single use items, for one procedure or episode of patient care, and then disposed of as clinical waste. Non-disposable protective clothing should be sent for laundering.	Respiratory protective equipment, e.g. a particulate filter mask, must be correctly fitted and used when recommended for the care of patients with respiratory infections transmitted by airborne particles.
Gloves are changed between caring for different patients or between different care/treatment for the same patient.	Full body fluid repellent gowns must be worn where there is a risk of extensive splashing of blood, body fluids, secretions or excretions, with the exception of perspiration, on to the skin or clothing of the health care worker.	
Gloves must be disposed of as clinical waste and hands decontaminated, ideally by washing with liquid soap and water after the gloves have been removed.		
Gloves that are acceptable to healthcare workers and European Community (CE) marked must be available in all clinical areas.		
Sensitivity to natural rubber latex in patients, carers and healthcare workers must be documented and alternatives must be available.		
Neither powdered nor polythene gloves should be used in health care activities.		

Evidence-based guidelines on the use of Personal Protective Equipment in NHS hospitals. Source: Pratt et al, epic 2: *National Evidence-Based Guidelines for Preventing Healthcare-Associated Infections in NHS Hospitals in England.* Journal of Hospital Infection, February 2007.

Safe handling and disposal of sharps

Sharps are items such as needles, stitch cutters, blades, glass ampoules and any other sharp instrument. Incorrect handing or disposal of sharps can lead to cross-infection of blood borne viruses such as Hepatitis B, Hepatitis C and HIV.

The safe handling and disposal of sharps is everyone's responsibility, and it is important that you are aware of your responsibilities in relation to this. Training should be available within your organisation and it is your responsibility to ensure that you attend the appropriate course and put into practice what you have learned.

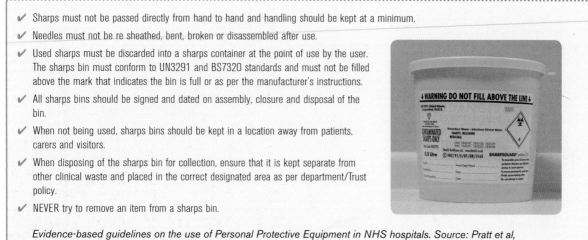

Best practice: Sharps

✔ Sharps must not be passed directly from hand to hand and handling should be kept at a minimum.

✔ Needles must not be re sheathed, bent, broken or disassembled after use.

✔ Used sharps must be discarded into a sharps container at the point of use by the user. The sharps bin must conform to UN3291 and BS7320 standards and must not be filled above the mark that indicates the bin is full or as per the manufacturer's instructions.

✔ All sharps bins should be signed and dated on assembly, closure and disposal of the bin.

✔ When not being used, sharps bins should be kept in a location away from patients, carers and visitors.

✔ When disposing of the sharps bin for collection, ensure that it is kept separate from other clinical waste and placed in the correct designated area as per department/Trust policy.

✔ NEVER try to remove an item from a sharps bin.

Evidence-based guidelines on the use of Personal Protective Equipment in NHS hospitals. Source: Pratt et al, epic 2: National Evidence-Based Guidelines for Preventing Healthcare-Associated Infections in NHS Hospitals in England. Journal of Hospital Infection February 2007.

If you see any of the above guidelines not being implemented, then it is your responsibility to report it promptly to the professional in charge of the clinical area or to act, if this is within your level of authority or competence. You must also be aware of your organisation's sharps injury and inoculation policy.

Waste disposal

Your employer has a duty under the Environmental Protection Act (1990) to ensure that safe working practices exist in relation to the disposal of all waste. It is your responsibility to know and implement the policies and guidelines as laid down by your organisation.

Waste can be divided into a number of sub-categories:

- **domestic** – this includes flowers, paper, packaging and food. Domestic waste can be placed in black bags (or clear in some organisations) and goes to landfill sites for disposal;

Procedure following contamination by bodily fluids

Needle stick injury, bite or scratch

ACTION

Encourage bleeding by squeezing

Wash thoroughly with soap and water

Cover with waterproof plaster

Splash to mouth or eyes

ACTION

EYE
Rinse eye thoroughly under running water

MOUTH
Rinse out mouth with water
DO NOT SWALLOW

Inform manager

Complete incident/accident form

Contact Occupational Health Department

If Occupational Health Department closed go to Accident and Emergency Department

Inform Occupational Health Department as soon as they are open again

An example of a sharps/splash injury pathway.

- **clinical** – any waste that is contaminated with potentially infectious material such as blood or body fluids. This waste is currently placed in yellow bags and goes for incineration;
- **sharps** – any devices that have the potential to pierce the skin, e.g. needles. These need to be placed in a sharps bin and are sent for incineration.
- **cytotoxic substances** – disposed of in purple waste bags/boxes.
- **glass** – the specific disposal of glass will depend on whether it has been contaminated or not. See your organisation's policy.

Memory jogger

Look back at the section on standard precautions when dealing with sharps, on page 145.

You must refer to your organisation's policy on waste disposal for the correct colour and type of waste receptacle in your particular work place. This is particularly important as, in 2005, the Hazardous Waste Regulations introduced a new classification system for healthcare waste along with a new colour coding system. This coding is not currently mandatory, so you will find that some organisations have already applied the new colour coding while others have not.

Ensure that waste is disposed of in the correct coloured waste bin for your organisation. In many organisations, this is still yellow for clinical waste and black for domestic waste.

Whichever colour coding system your organisation currently uses for its waste, there are other general rules which should be applied. All bags should be:

- filled to 2/3 full only and tied securely
- labelled with the address of the department and organisation
- kept segregated for collection.

Case study: Blood spill

A doctor working on your ward accidentally drops a glass bottle containing a blood sample. The glass bottle breaks into a number of pieces and the blood spills onto the ward floor.

1 What policies within your organisation could you access to help you deal with this situation?

2 What health and safety precautions would you consider prior to cleaning up the spillage?

3 How would you safely clean up and dispose of the glass?

4 How would you safely clean up the blood spillage from the floor? Where would you dispose the waste from this procedure?

5 What documentation would you complete concerning this incident?

If you are working towards your NVQ you may gain evidence for: HSC 32 K4 (a,b,c,d,e), K6, K11 (c), K12, K14, K16, K18.

Managing blood and body fluid spillages

Any spillage of blood or body fluids needs to be cleaned up immediately, to protect patients, carers and staff from potential contamination by harmful pathogens and/or a slipping hazard.

As discussed earlier, it is essential that you apply personal protective equipment of apron and gloves before cleaning any spillage, and that you follow local policies regarding the use of disinfectants to clean the area effectively.

Remember

If the floor is still wet, you must put out a warning sign.

Decontamination of equipment

Strict guidelines are in place regarding the decontamination of equipment used in clinical practice. The method of decontamination may be by cleaning, disinfection or sterilisation. Which method to use will depend on a risk assessment being undertaken to determine whether the piece of equipment is at low, intermediate or high risk of contamination.

Risk	Application of item	Recommendation
High	• In contact with an incision, wound or membrane • Introduced into sterile body areas	Sterilisation
Intermediate	• In contact with mucous membranes • Contaminated with particularly virulent or readily transmissible organisms • Before use on immunocompromised patients	Sterilisation or disinfection Cleaning may be acceptable in some agreed situations
Low	• In contact with healthy skin • Not in contact with the patient	Cleaning

Infection risk and recommended approaches to decontamination.
Source: *Gould D J (2005) Infection Control: the environment and service organisation.* Nursing Standard, *20, 5, 57–65.*

Cleaning

This is used for low-risk areas and equipment, using warm water and detergent to remove visible signs of contamination. It also removes a number of the micro-organisms present. Examples of things to be cleaned would include mattresses, drip poles and floors.

The National Patient Safety Agency has developed a national colour coding system for all hospital cleaning materials and equipment, e.g. mops, buckets and cloths.

Health care organisations also have different levels of cleaning, from standard cleaning through to deep cleaning. You will need to refer to you organisation's policies relating to the types available, the definitions

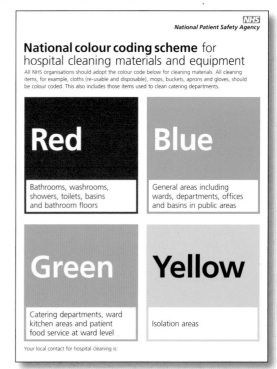

National Patient Safety Agency — NHS

National colour coding scheme for hospital cleaning materials and equipment

All NHS organisations should adopt the colour code below for cleaning materials. All cleaning items, for example, cloths (re-usable and disposable), mops, buckets, aprons and gloves, should be colour coded. This also includes those items used to clean catering departments.

Red — Bathrooms, washrooms, showers, toilets, basins and bathroom floors

Blue — General areas including wards, departments, offices and basins in public areas

Green — Catering departments, ward kitchen areas and patient food service at ward level

Yellow — Isolation areas

Your local contact for hospital cleaning is:

of each and when they are required. These policies should also state how each type of cleaning should be requested.

Disinfection

This is a deeper, more effective process than cleaning, which will reduce the number of micro-organisms, but does not eradicate all of them. Disinfection can be achieved using heat or chemicals. Before disinfection, the area or equipment in question must be cleaned of all visible signs of contamination.

When using chemicals, it is vital that you are aware of the hazards associated with certain chemicals and that you know the necessary precautions to take. Use of chemicals in the work area is covered by the Control of Substances Hazardous to Health (COSHH) Regulations (2002).

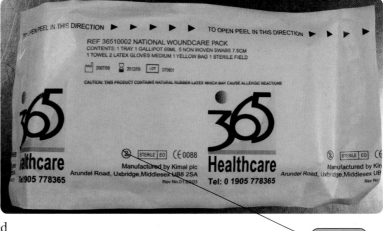

Symbol for single use only.

Test yourself

What should you do if you splash a hazardous chemical in your eye? What personal protective equipment should you use to prevent this?

Memory jogger

What do the COSHH regulations cover? Refer to the section on legislation, page 218.

Sterilisation

This process destroys all micro-organisms, including spores. It can be achieved through:

- heat – dry or moist heat under pressure (known as 'autoclaving')
- radiation – such as gamma rays and ultraviolet light
- chemicals – used for equipment that would disintegrate if exposed to high temperatures.

Prior to autoclaving equipment is packaged and sealed with autoclave indicator tape. This tape changes colour when the required temperature for sterilisation has occurred.

If the package is damaged or torn, it can no longer be considered sterile and must be withdrawn from use. Sterile packs should be stored in dry, clean environments prior to their use.

You should also be aware that an increasing number of pieces of equipment and medical devices are now single use only. You can recognise these because they carry the symbol shown in the image above.

It is extremely important that any equipment bearing this symbol is only used once. The reuse of single-use devices can affect their safety, performance and effectiveness, exposing patients and staff to unnecessary risk (MHRA DB 2006 (04) Oct 2006).

Laundry management

Once again, your hospital or workplace will have it's own policy relating to the safe management of used linen. Ensure that you know what the policy states, and make sure you follow it.

Soiled laundry needs to be kept separate from clean linen. Heavily soiled linen with blood, or body fluids, and infected linen needs to be placed in a red alginate bag and then placed into another bag depending on your organisation's policy. Other linen should be bagged as per policy.

Responsibilities of the health care assistant

Under the Health and Safety at Work Act 1974, you have a joint responsibility to protect yourself and others within your organisation from the risk of infection. In everyday practice, this would include:

- being aware of and implementing policies and procedures
- reporting hazards and potential risks
- maintaining a clean and safe working environment
- attending staff education sessions
- keeping up to date with necessary immunisation
- managing of your personal hygiene and dress.

Best practice: Training

Whenever you attend any training or education, where possible ask the person who has provided the training to give you a certificate of attendance or to sign a statement indicating that you have attended the session. On its own, this is not sufficient evidence for your portfolio, so you should always ensure that it is supported with a piece of reflection, considering:

✔ what you have learned

✔ whether your practice needs to change in light of this new information, and if so how

✔ whether you need to find out any more information

✔ how you can share this information with your work colleagues.

Professional dress

You should ensure that you present yourself professionally at all times at work. The way you look will be seen as a measure of your competence, by those who use the service and by your colleagues.

Your organisation will have its own uniform policy, which must be followed. The Department of Health (2007) recommends a number of general principles relating to uniforms and work wear.

- Wear a clean uniform each day. If your organisation does not launder your uniform, then you must wash it at, at least, 60°C in order to remove most micro-organisms.
- Change into and out of uniform at work.
- Change immediately if your uniform becomes visibly soiled.
- Tie long hair back off the collar.
- Keep your fingernails short and clean. Do not wear false fingernails for direct patient care.
- Do not go shopping or undertake similar activities in public in your uniform.
- Do not wear hand or wrist jewellery or wristwatches. A plain wedding ring may be acceptable.

- Never forget that you could be seen as a role model to others.

Memory jogger

What do you wear? Refer to the section on page 57.

Challenging bad practice

If you find yourself in a situation where you witness one of your health care colleagues behaving inappropriately or not following your organisation's policies and procedures, you can respond in a number of ways.

Depending on the severity of the problem and your competence/confidence to do so, you should:

- challenge the behaviour, or the source of the bad practice
- have a one-to-one discussion with the colleague in question
- act as a mentor with whom your colleague can share problems and difficulties
- act as a role model of good practice
- report the incident to the practitioner in charge.

Case study: Sarah

Sarah is a new health care assistant who has recently joined your team. You are both about to provide treatment to a patient who is being nursed in a side room. The sign on the door indicates that the patient is being nursed in 'Enteric Isolation'. When entering the room, you notice that Sarah does not put on an apron or any gloves.

- Describe what your actions would be on witnessing this.
- Would you inform anyone about this? If so, who would you inform and why?

If you are working towards your NVQ you may gain evidence for:
K3, K4d, K11a, K16, K18.

Health and safety legislation

There is a vast amount of legislation relating to infection control, some of which is specific to certain departments and practices. The diagram on the next page details some of the more commonly mentioned legislation. You should also refer to Unit HSC 35 page 131 for further details.

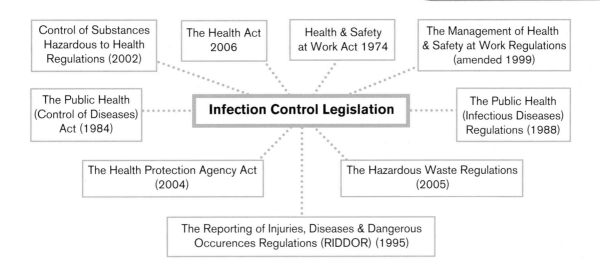

| Control of Substances Hazardous to Health Regulations (2002) | The Health Act 2006 | Health & Safety at Work Act 1974 | The Management of Health & Safety at Work Regulations (amended 1999) |

| The Public Health (Control of Diseases) Act (1984) | **Infection Control Legislation** | The Public Health (Infectious Diseases) Regulations (1988) |

| The Health Protection Agency Act (2004) | The Hazardous Waste Regulations (2005) |

The Reporting of Injuries, Diseases & Dangerous Occurences Regulations (RIDDOR) (1995)

Admission, transfer and discharge of patients

Admission

When patients are to be admitted to your clinical area, you need to know certain details about their current condition and their past medical history (if available) before they arrive. Depending on the details provided, patients will be allocated either to a side room or into a bay with other patients. If a side room needs to be prepared for a patient, the room and all equipment should be organised before the patient reaches the clinical area.

Some patients are isolated in side rooms until the results of certain investigations are known. You will need to know if the patient has had all the necessary investigations or whether more are required, e.g. MRSA swabs or a stool specimen. Certain risk assessments may also be undertaken when the patient reaches your clinical area, e.g. MRSA risk assessment. Following the outcome of the risk assessment, patients may be moved from an open bay into a side room until results of investigations are known.

The result of any risk assessment needs to be reported to the practitioner in charge of the patient's care, and then documented in the care plan.

When the patient reaches your area, you may be asked by his or her relatives or carers for information about the infection. Remember to work within the limits of your competence. You may need to refer any queries you cannot competently answer to the practitioner in charge.

If the patient is to be nursed in isolation, you need to place a sign on the door of the room indicating which type of isolation is required, and the door needs to remain closed.

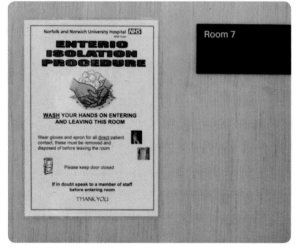

All patients in isolation need to have the appropriate signage on the door, indicating the type of barrier nursing to implement.

Types of isolation

Symptoms	Types of precautions required in addition to standard precautions
Diarrhoea/vomiting	enteric
TB (suspected/confirmed) Chickenpox, measles	airborne
Skin infection Infected/draining wounds Leaking skin rash	contact
Respiratory infection Rash indicative of mumps, rubella or meningococcal disease	droplet
Severely immunocompromised patient (must be requested by patient's clinician)	protective isolation

Please note that sometimes a combination of two categories may be needed: for example, when nursing a patient with oozing skin rash or lesions indicative of chickenpox, a combination of airborne and skin contact precautions will be needed.

Source isolation

This is undertaken to prevent the transfer of infection from the patient to others.

Types of source isolation include:

Contact isolation

This includes pathogens that are transmitted via hands or equipment. The source of the pathogen may be from wound secretions, fluid from skin lesions, pus or contaminated equipment and the environment. The patient may present with an infected or colonised skin lesion, a wound infection or an oozing skin rash.

Faecal/oral (enteric) isolation

This type of infection is spread from gastro-intestinal fluids or contaminated equipment and environment. The patient will present with diarrhoea and/or vomiting. The mode of transmission is via faecal/oral spread and viral causes can be airborne.

Case study: Mrs Betts

Mrs Betts is an 88-year-old lady who is being admitted to your ward with a two-day history of diarrhoea and vomiting. She is currently dehydrated and needs to be nursed in isolation on admission to your team.

- What type of isolation nursing do you think Mrs Betts requires? Explain you reason for choosing this type.
- Where on the ward do you think the practitioner in charge will allocate this patient and why?
- What equipment would you prepare before Mrs Betts' admission?
- What documentation do you think you might need to complete on admission?
- If you were unsure of any actions required, whom would you approach for advice?

If you are working towards your NVQ you may gain evidence for:
CHS32 K3, K4 (a,b,c,d), K6, K11, K12, K14.

Airborne isolation

As the name suggests, the mode of transmission is via the airborne route through breath, chest secretions or oral secretions. The patient presents with symptoms suggestive of an airborne infection, e.g. tuberculosis. The pathogens remain suspended in the air for prolonged periods. It is advisable to nurse these patients in a room with mechanical ventilation.

Droplet isolation

These infections are spread by droplets produced when patients sneeze, cough or talk, or during suctioning or bronchoscopy. Whooping cough is one example of a disease spread via droplet transmission. Special ventilation is not required for this type of isolation as the pathogenic particles are too large to remain suspended in the air, and fall to the ground close to the source.

Protective isolation

This type of isolation is required for patients who are at risk of acquiring infections from other people: for example, those who are immunocompromised, or burns patients.

Activity: isolation nursing

Identify your organisation's policies on isolation nursing. Make a list of all the things you need to think about before entering the side room of a patient with an infection.

- What risk assessments could you refer to in the patient's nursing notes?
- What special considerations do you need to think about when nursing a patient in isolation?

Consider both the patient and yourself.

If you are working towards your NVQ you may gain evidence for:

HSC32 – K2, K4(b,c,d), K6, K9(a), K14.

Notifiable diseases

Some infections must be notified to the local Consultant in Communicable Disease Control (CCDC). This notification is a legal requirement and is the responsibility of the doctor making the diagnosis. Most clinical areas have certificates that need to be completed and sent to the CCDC for their attention.

Although it is the doctor's responsibility to complete the certificate, the doctor may ask you to locate the certificate for him or her to complete.

You should make sure that you know where these certificates are kept, and make yourself aware of any other requirements under the Public Health (Infectious Diseases) Regulations 1988. This may contribute to evidence for CHS32 K4.

Current statutorily notifiable diseases and food poisoning under the Public Health (Control of Disease) Act 1984	
- Cholera	
- Plague	
- Relapsing fever	
- Smallpox	
- Typhus	
- Food poisoning	

Current statutorily notifiable diseases under the Public Health (Infectious Diseases) Regulations 1988	
- Acute encephalitis	- Mumps
- Acute poliomyelitis	- Opthalmia neonatorum
- Anthrax	- Paratyphoid fever
- Diphtheria	- Rabies
- Dysentery (amoebic or bacillary)	- Rubella
- Leprosy	- Scarlet fever
- Leptospirosis	- Tetanus
- Malaria	- Tuberculosis**
- Measles	- Typhoid fever
- Meningitis	- Viral haemorrhagic fever
- Meningococcal septicaemia (without meningitis)	- Viral hepatitis
	- Whooping cough
	- Yellow fever

Transfer

When transferring patients, either internally or externally, you must ensure that the receiving area has all the information necessary to nurse that patient safely.

The practitioner in charge of the patient's care is responsible for either completing a written transfer letter detailing all the necessary information, or contacting the new clinical area and giving this information verbally.

However, it may be your responsibility to physically transfer the patient to the new area. If you have been given any written or verbal information for the new clinical area, you must ensure that this is given to the appropriate member of staff. You should also make sure the patient is made comfortable in their new environment.

When the patient has been transferred, you should clear the room and ensure it is cleaned according to your organisation's policy.

Discharge

On discharge, it is crucial that the patient and his or her carers have all the information and equipment needed to safely care for the patient at home.

Written information of care needs, specifically concerning any infection still present, should be provided for any care agencies, such as community nurses, who will continue to care for the patient in the community.

Once the patient has been discharged, the room needs to be cleaned according to your organisation's policy. This may necessitate a standard clean, a clinical clean or a clinical clean with wall washing, depending on the infection present.

Documentation and record keeping

Documentation is an essential element in caring for a patient, and demonstrates both the care provided during his or her stay and the specific requirements on discharge. The most useful records are those that are interdisciplinary and involve the patient in the assessment, planning and evaluation of the care provided.

There are a number of factors that contribute to effective record keeping. Records should:

- be factual, consistent and accurate
- be recorded as soon as possible after the event has occurred
- be recorded clearly and in such a manner that the text cannot be erased or deleted without a record of change
- be accurately dated, timed and signed
- not include abbreviations, jargon, meaningless phrases, irrelevant speculation, offensive or subjective statements.

Source: NMC (2007) *Record Keeping Guidance*

To find out more about record keeping and your role in it, see Unit HSC 31 on page 36.

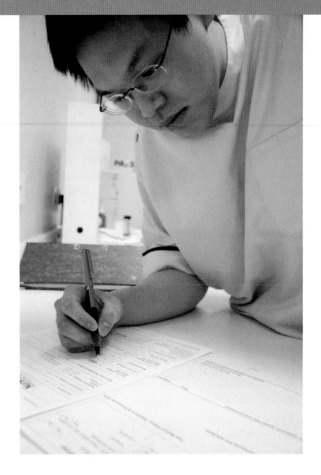

References

Department of Health (1984) *Public Health (Control of Diseases)* Act, London

Department of Health (1988) *Public Health (Infectious Diseases)* Regulations, London

Department of Health (2007) *Uniforms and Workwear. An evidence base for developing local policy*, London
http://www.dh.gov.uk/publications]

Emmerson A.M., Enstone J. E., Griffin M., Kelrey M.C., Smyth E.T. (1996) The Second National Prevalence Survey of infection in hospitals: overview of the results. *Journal of Hospital Infection*. 32, 3, 175 – 190

MDHA(2006) *Single Use Medical Devices. Implication and Consequences of Reuse*. DB 2006 (04) Oct.
http://www.mhra.gov.uk

National Audit Office (2000) *The Management and Control of Hospital Acquired Infection in Acute NHS Trusts in England*. The Stationery Office. London http://www.nao.org.uk/publications/nao_reports/9900230.pdf

National Patient Safety Agency (2007) *Colour Coding Hospital Cleaning materials and Equipment*, Safer Practice Notice 15, NPSA, London http://www.npsa.nhs.uk/patientsafety/alerts-and-directives/notices/cleaning-materials/

Nursing and Midwifery Council (2007) *NMC Record Keeping Guidance*, A-Z advice sheet, NMC, London http://www.nmc-uk.org.uk/aFrameDisplay.aspx?DocumentID=3170

Office of Public Sector Information (1988) *Public Health (Infectious Diseases) Regulations* 1988 London. HMSO. http://www.opsi.gov.uk/si/si1988/Uksi_19881546_en_1.htm

Pratt R.J., Pellowe C.M., Wilson J.A., Loveday H.P., Jones S.R.L.J., McDougall C., Wilcox M.H. (2007) epic2: National Evidence-Based Guidelines for Preventing Healthcare-Associated Infections in NHS Hospitals in England. *Journal of Hospital Infection*. February; 65S: S1-S64

Wilson J. (2001) *Infection Control in Clinical Practice*, 2nd Edition, Bailliere Tindall, London

Aseptic technique

Introduction

In its document *Winning Ways* (2004), The Department of Health stated that 'health care workers are a major route through which patients become infected'.

Two of their actions in this document stated that:

- clinical teams will demonstrate consistently high standards of aseptic technique

- induction programmes for all staff, including agency and locum staff, will include local guidance on infection control and the use of aseptic technique.

To support this, the Department of Health also published the Health Act (2006), which specifically addressed the aseptic technique. It stated that:

- clinical procedures should be carried out in a manner that maintains and promotes the principles of asepsis

- education, training and assessment in aseptic technique should be provided to all persons undertaking such procedures

- the technique should be standardised across the organisation

- audits should be undertaken to monitor compliance with aseptic technique.

With this in mind, it is vital that you are appropriately trained, assessed and deemed competent to undertake an aseptic technique in practice.

What you need to learn

- What is asepsis?
- Aseptic technique and aseptic non-touch technique
- Clean technique
- Standard precautions related to the aseptic technique
- How to apply sterile gloves
- Maintaining a sterile field
- Aseptic technique procedure
- Applying the technique to a simple wound dressing

What is asepsis?

Asepsis is defined as 'the state of being free from living pathogenic micro-organisms' (Hart, 2007). Antisepsis is a process or a treatment, which kills or inhibits micro-organisms. When related to hand washing, it is the process which removes transient micro-organisms from the skin and reduces the normal flora.

Sepsis, on the other hand, is the presence of pathogenic micro-organisms or their toxins in the blood or tissues.

Aseptic technique

An aseptic technique is the method used to prevent the introduction of harmful micro-organisms into wounds or susceptible sites when undertaking invasive procedures. If correctly implemented, the procedure also protects the health care assistant from becoming contaminated by the patient's body fluids.

> ### Checklist: Standard precautions
> - Hand washing
> - Personal protective equipment
> - Safe disposal of sharps
> - Safe disposal of clinical waste
> - Decontamination of equipment
>
> See also Unit HSC 32 page 60 and **Infection control** page 134.

An aseptic technique can be employed in a variety of different settings including the operating department, clinical areas such as the ward environment, clinic or GP surgery as well as the patient's own home. Depending on the environment and the procedure to be undertaken, the technique used will either be a surgical aseptic technique or an aseptic non-touch technique (ANTT) (Pratt et al 2007).

Using an aseptic technique helps to minimise the risk of exposure to potentially harmful micro-organisms and therefore reduces the incidence of Hospital Acquired Infections.

Surgical aseptic technique

The surgical aseptic technique is used primarily in the operating theatre where strict sterile procedures are required, due to the invasive nature of the surgery. However, the sterile aseptic technique can also be used in clinical areas for other highly invasive procedures, such as the insertion of central venous lines. Health care workers need to employ the same strict sterile procedures used in the operating theatre. This includes the use of drapes, sterile equipment, personal protective equipment and patient preparation.

Aseptic non-touch technique

The aseptic non-touch technique is still a fairly new concept. However, the epic2 guidelines recommended that ANTT should be the aseptic technique of choice (Pratt et al 2007). Because of this, there are now a growing number of health care organisations across the country implementing the aseptic non-touch technique for procedures such as urinary catheterisation, administration of intravenous drugs, wound care and venepuncture.

The key principle of the aseptic technique remains the same except that, when handling any sterile equipment, the key parts are not touched. The key parts are those parts of the equipment which are in direct contact either with the patient or, in the example of IV administration, with the infusion fluid, e.g. needle, syringe tip.

Activity

In relation to your clinical practice, choose an activity where you have used the aseptic non-touch technique. Make some notes that cover these areas.

- What sterile equipment did you need to prepare for the activity and why?
- Identify the key parts of the sterile equipment and write them down.
- What personal protective equipment did you wear and why?
- What documents did you complete following the procedure, and why is this an important part of the activity?

If you are working towards your NVQ you will gain evidence for: CHS 12 – KC 5, 15, 18a, c, K 26a, b.

A step-by-step guide for the aseptic technique is illustrated later in this topic on page 161.

Clean technique

A clean technique is a modified aseptic technique that can be used for certain wounds and procedures. The practitioner in charge of the patient's care must make the decision on which method is appropriate. This decision must also be documented in the patient's plan of care.

A clean technique can be used for a number of procedures including:
- chronic wounds healing by secondary intention, such as leg ulcers and pressure sores
- the removal of sutures

- endotracheal suctioning and tracheostomy dressings.

The main difference between an aseptic technique and a clean technique is that for a clean technique the following rules generally apply (Refer to your organisation's policy.).

- Clean gloves are used instead of sterile.
- Tap water suitable for drinking is used instead of sterile saline.
- A clean field is used, not a sterile one.

However, you should note that you should still use sterile equipment – such as dressings, stitch cutters and suction catheters – and implement a non-touch technique, so that no key parts are touched.

Who should undertake an aseptic technique?

Before undertaking any of the techniques described, you should ensure that the procedure is identified within your job description. If it is not documented as one of your specific job roles then you should not proceed to undertake it.

> ### Best practice: Undertaking aseptic technique
>
> Be sure that you are competent to carry out the procedure.
>
> Make sure that the task has been appropriately delegated to you. Only trained and competent staff should perform the aseptic non-touch technique or the clean technique.
>
> If you do not have the necessary skills or you do not feel confident to undertake the task, you should not proceed without direct supervision and support.

> ### Activity
>
> Imagine that you have been asked by a senior member of staff to undertake a procedure for which you have not been trained or assessed as competent for.
>
> 1 Explain what you would do, giving reasons for your actions.
>
> 2 What legislation, policies and practices relate to this issue?
>
> 3 Make some notes on this.
>
> *If you are working towards your NVQ you will gain evidence for: CHS 12 KC 1, 2, 3.*

Patient consent and preparation

As with any procedure involving the patient, it is important that you explain the reason why the procedure is necessary, giving the patient time to ask questions.

You will need to ensure that you have the patient's consent to undertake the required procedure. Do they have all the necessary information to make an informed decision?

> ### Memory jogger
>
> How do you make sure the patient has given their consent? Look back at Unit HSC 31, page 34.

At the beginning of your shift, you should make a list, with the assistance of the practitioner in charge, of the different dressings you need to

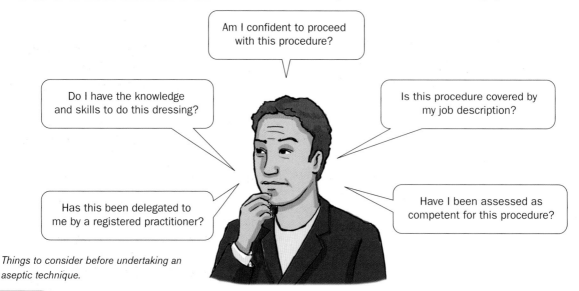

Am I confident to proceed with this procedure?

Do I have the knowledge and skills to do this dressing?

Is this procedure covered by my job description?

Has this been delegated to me by a registered practitioner?

Have I been assessed as competent for this procedure?

Things to consider before undertaking an aseptic technique.

undertake. Next, prioritise them depending on whether they are clean or contaminated dressings. You should always undertake clean dressings first and infected dressings last. This is to reduce the possibility of cross-infection from the infected dressing to the clean dressing. The same principle should apply when dressing wounds on the same patient. Always start with the cleanest wound first.

Depending on the required procedure, you may also need to position the patient in a specific way. Give the patient clear instructions and offer assistance if necessary.

Undertake a manual handling risk assessment to decide if you require help from a colleague or the use of a particular piece of equipment. See Unit HSC 32, page 58 on manual handling for more information.

Activity

Choose a patient you have cared for, who identified some worries and/or concerns about their wound care. Write a piece of self-reflection using the following questions as a guide.

- What was the procedure the patient required?
- What concerns or worries did the patient have?
- How did you deal with these concerns and worries?
- How did you feel about the patient raising their concerns?
- Did you need to seek support or advice from another member of staff?
- What information did you give to the patient?
- Would you do anything differently next time?

If you are working towards your NVQ you will gain evidence for: CHS 12 – pc 2; KC 3, 6, 7, 8, 25, 27

Standard precautions related to the aseptic technique

Hand washing

Hand washing is an essential part of any aseptic technique.

Hand washing has been identified as an effective measure in reducing the number of health care-acquired infections, and so should be undertaken before and after any patient contact, including an aseptic technique.

You should also wash your hands after removing your gloves, as it has been shown that hands can become contaminated through tears in the glove and because bacteria may increase under the gloves, due to the presence of moisture.

The use of alcohol hand gel during the procedure has now reduced the number of times that you need to leave the patient's bedside in order to wash your hands.

Remember, however, that alcohol hand gel should not be used on visibly soiled hands. If your hands are visibly soiled, you need to use soap and water to clean them.

Memory jogger

How should you wash your hands? Look again at the correct method, in Unit HSC 32, page 61.

Personal protective equipment

As discussed in Unit HSC 32 and Topic 1 *Infection control*, you should choose personal protective equipment (PPE) following an assessment of the risk associated with a particular care activity or intervention (Pratt et al 2007).

Some interventions or procedures will require the health care assistant to wear full PPE including gown, gloves, mask, goggles and specialised footwear; others will only require disposable plastic apron and gloves (either sterile or clean non-sterile).

It is generally accepted that a plastic apron should be worn during aseptic procedures for the following reasons:

- to protect the health care assistant's clothing from becoming contaminated with potential pathogens from the patient's body fluids
- to prevent the transfer of harmful pathogens to other patients or fellow workers
- to protect the patient from acquiring any harmful pathogens carried on the health care assistant's clothing

Source: Mallett & Bailey (1999)

All disposable personal protective equipment should be discarded between patients and procedures according to your organisation's policy, and all other equipment (e.g. goggles) should be thoroughly washed and dried.

How to apply sterile gloves

Sterile equipment will only remain sterile while it is in contact with other sterile products. It is therefore extremely important that you follow the correct procedure for applying sterile gloves, so that they do not become contaminated by your exposed hands or other contact.

Before applying the gloves, make sure that you have carried out the following points.

- Remove any rings or bracelets
- Cover any open cuts or abrasions on your hands
- Make certain that your nails are short
- Ensure that your hands are either washed with soap and water, or that you have used an alcohol hand gel.

The following six steps will illustrate how to apply a pair of sterile gloves so that at the end of the process they remain sterile.

Remove the gloves at the end of the procedure, using the checklist below. See also the illustrated steps in Unit HSC 32, page 60.

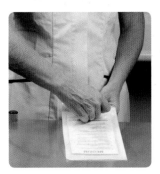

Open the packet by peeling apart the outer layer.

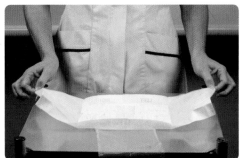

Open the inner packet by using the edges of the packaging to expose the sterile gloves within.

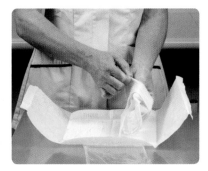

Take hold of the left glove with your right hand using only the exposed inside wrist section, as illustrated.

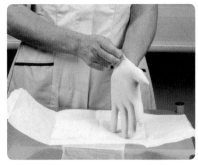

Insert your left hand into the glove, pulling on the glove with your right hand, **still holding only the inside wrist section**. Do not worry if all your fingers are not in the correct finger holes of the glove – this can be corrected later.

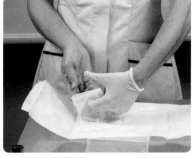

Insert your gloved left hand under the sterile cuff of the second glove, as illustrated. Pick up the second glove and insert your right hand into the glove.

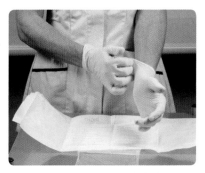

Now that you have both hands inside each glove, you can carefully rearrange the gloves so that they fit comfortably. **Ensure that you do not touch any exposed skin with a gloved hand while undertaking this part of the procedure.**

Checklist: Removing sterile gloves

- Remove left glove with gloved right hand, without touching exposed skin
- Hold left glove in palm of right hand
- Remove right glove, pulling it over the left glove, ensuring that it is still enclosed in your right palm.
- Dispose of gloves, holding only the inside of the glove, in a clinical waste bin.
- Wash hands and dry thoroughly after removal of gloves.

Maintaining a sterile field

A sterile field is created by the use of sterile drapes or sterile towels, and can be placed either around the site of the procedure or on a dressing trolley/stand. Only sterile equipment should be placed on the sterile field

Best practice: Sterile fields

Take care when opening packages to ensure that you do not touch the sterile contents with your exposed hands.

Do not allow any other person to place any un-sterile objects on the sterile field.

Do not allow any other person to touch the sterile equipment or lean across the sterile field.

Once a piece of equipment has become contaminated, you must dispose of it, if single use, and replace it if needed.

Keep contaminated reusable instruments separate from other sterile items until they can be placed in the used medical instruments box, usually kept in the dirty utility room.

Please refer to your own organisation's policy on cleaning medical instruments before returning them to the Sterile Services Department.

Aseptic technique procedure

The following step-by-step guide for undertaking an aseptic technique is based on a general sterile dressing pack. You may need to adapt this guide depending on the procedure you are undertaking and the content of the sterile packs held by your organisation.

Before you start

- Ensure that the procedure is within your job description and that you have the necessary skills and competence.
- Review the patient's care plan to ensure that you know what care is required: for example, does the patient have any allergies, is a wound swab needed or has the treatment been changed?
- Explain the procedure to the patient and gain their consent according to your organisation's policy.
- Ensure the procedure is undertaken in a clean

area – a clinical treatment room or 30 minutes after any cleaning activity has taken place, to allow airborne particles to settle.
- Do not undertake the procedure by an open window, as this will increase air movement and the potential for airborne contamination.
- Pull curtains around the bed space or close the door of the treatment room, and indicate that room is in use to maintain privacy.
- Ensure that there is alcohol hand gel by the patient's bed or easily accessible within the treatment room.
- Collect all the necessary equipment for the procedure, adhering to the details in the patient's care plan. Stopping and starting because you have forgotten vital equipment does not look professional, and the patient may lose confidence in your ability to undertake the task.
- Wash your hands – see page 143 for the step-by-step procedure – and apply plastic apron before proceeding.

Undertaking the procedure

1 Clean the trolley with detergent, water and paper towels or detergent wipes. Dry the trolley with clean paper towels.

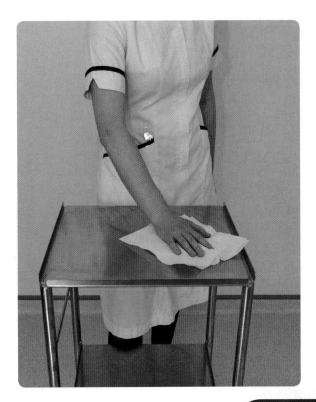

2 Check that all the packages are in date and undamaged.

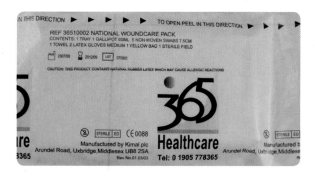

3 Place all the equipment on the bottom shelf of the trolley. Apply a disposable apron and/or other personal protective equipment. Take the trolley to the patient's bedside.

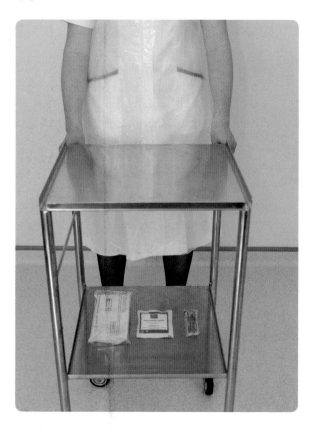

4 Make the patient comfortable and ensure privacy and modesty as much as possible.

If the procedure requires the removal of a soiled dressing, then at this point you will need to loosen the dressing using clean non-sterile gloves. Do not completely remove the dressing. Discard used gloves in clinical waste bin.

5 Decontaminate your hands using alcoholic hand gel. Take the dressing pack from the bottom shelf of the trolley. Hold it over the top shelf, open the pack and carefully drop the sterile contents onto the top shelf without touching it.

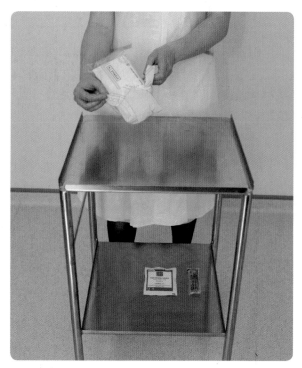

6 Open the sterile field using the corners only.

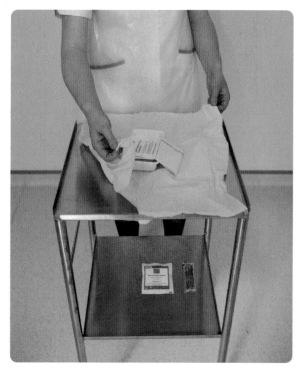

7 Open all the other sterile packs and drop them onto the sterile field. Place your hand in the yellow disposal bag and arrange the contents of the dressing pack on the sterile field.

If necessary, the bag may then be used to remove the soiled dressing. Invert the bag, ensuring that the dressing remains secure within the bag, and attach it to the side of the trolley.

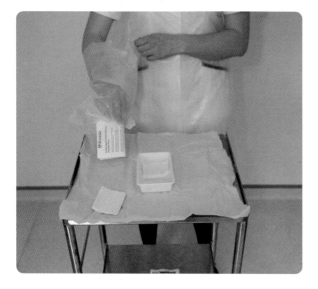

8 Decontaminante hands with alcohol gel. Open the lotion package carefully and pour it into appropriate container on the sterile field. Take care not to touch the sterile container with the lotion package. Decontaminate your hands with alcohol gel.

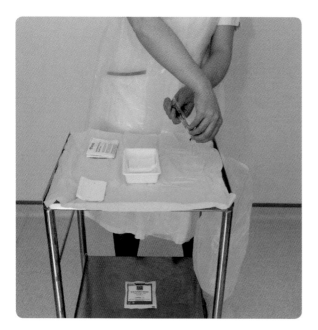

9 Apply sterile gloves, touching only the inside wrist section as described earlier in this topic, on page 160. Carry out the procedures.

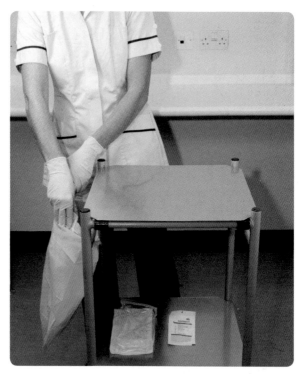

10 Once the procedure is complete, place all clinical waste including gloves and apron in the yellow bag and carefully seal. Decontaminate hands. Make sure the patient is comfortable before you leave.

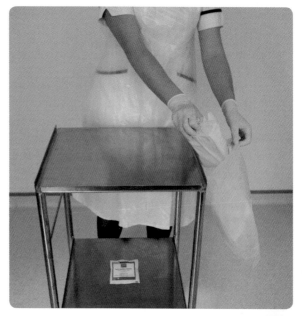

11 Dispose of clinical waste in yellow bin in dirty utility room or according to organisation's policy. Clean the trolley. Clean your hands with soap and water or alcohol hand gel. Document your actions in the patient's records and report to the practitioner in charge of the patient's care.

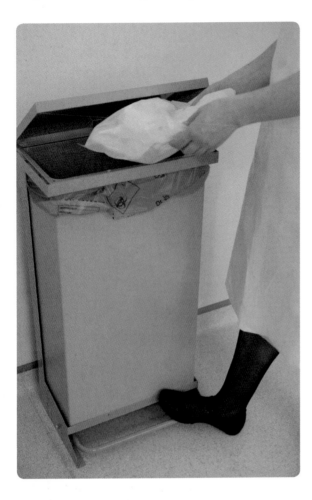

If during the procedure you are concerned about the patient's condition, or you notice something which you feel a registered member of the team needs to see, summon assistance using whichever method is appropriate to the concern. This may necessitate you pulling the emergency buzzer, calling for assistance or requesting the presence of the practitioner in charge of the patient's care.

Activity

Make notes on the following:

- While undertaking a wound dressing, you notice that the wound edges are red, inflamed and painful. What actions would you take and why?

  What might be the cause of the patient's signs and symptoms?

- The patient suddenly faints while you are undertaking their wound dressing. What actions would you take?

- After removing the patient's dressing, you notice blistering and they are complaining of pain and irritation. What actions would you take? What do you think may be the cause of this?

If you are working towards your NVQ you will gain evidence for: CHS 12 KC 3, 8, 9, 27

Applying the technique to a simple wound dressing

Please also refer to Unit CHS 12, page 256.

1 Check patient documentation to clarify the procedure required and to identify any allergies or potential adverse reactions.

2 Discuss the procedure with the patient and gain informed consent to undertake the procedure.

3 Wash your hands with soap and water and dry them thoroughly.

4 Clean the trolley with detergent and paper towels. Dry thoroughly.

5 Place all the equipment onto the lower shelf of the dressing trolley, checking contamination risks and expiry dates: dressing pack; sodium chloride sachet; new sterile dressing. Apply a disposable apron.

6 Take the trolley to the patient's bed space or escort the patient to the treatment room.

7 Position the patient comfortably, but in a position where you can access the wound.

8 Ensure privacy and dignity at all times.

9 Loosen the old dressing, but do not remove it totally. If the dressing is soiled, clean non-sterile gloves will be required. When loosened, dispose of the gloves in the clinical waste bin.

10 Decontaminate your hands with alcohol gel and open the dressing pack, sliding the contents onto the top shelf of the dressing trolley. Open the dressing pack using corners only to create a sterile field. Open the new sterile dressing and tip it onto the sterile field.

11 Place your hand inside the sterile disposable bag in order to arrange contents of dressing pack. Then use the disposable bag to completely remove the old dressing, invert the bag to ensure the contents remain inside, then attach it to the side of trolley using adhesive strip. Decontaminate your hands with alcohol gel.

12 Assess the wound for signs of infection (red, inflamed or oozing) and to see whether there has been any improvement or deterioration. Depending on your findings, you may immediately need to inform the practitioner in charge or after completion of the dressing. A wound swab may be required.

13 Open the sterile sodium chloride sachet and pour the contents into the container on the sterile field.

14 Decontaminate your hands with alcohol gel and apply sterile gloves – see page 160 for instructions.

15 If the wound is visibly dirty or there is heavy exudates, you will need to clean it – see the principles of wound cleaning in Unit CHS12, page 259. The procedure may vary depending on the wound type and depth. Wound irrigation is preferable as it causes less wound trauma, but it may not be appropriate for some surgical incisions.

16 Apply the clean sterile dressing aseptically using a non-touch technique and following the manufacturer's instructions. Again, depending on the exudate, you may require just a primary dressing (one that is in contact with the wound) or a primary and a secondary dressing (a dressing which covers the primary).

17 Remove your gloves and apron, place them in a yellow disposable bag and seal.

18 Make the patient comfortable before leaving.

19 Dispose of the clinical waste in the clinical waste bin in the dirty utility room.

20 Clean down the trolley.

21 Wash your hands thoroughly with soap and water and dry them.

22 Report the procedure to the practitioner in charge and record your actions on the appropriate nursing/medical documentation.

References

Department of Health (2003) *Winning Ways. Working Together to Reduce Healthcare Associated Infection in England, London*
http://www.dh.gov.uk/en/
Publicationsandstatistics/Publications/
PublicationsPolicyAndGuidance/DH_4064682

Department of Health (2006) *The Health Act. Code of Practice for the Prevention and Control of Health Care Associated Infections*, London
http://www.dh.gov.uk/en/
Publicationsandstatistics/Publications/
PublicationsPolicyAndGuidance/DH_4139336

Hart S. (2007) Using an aseptic technique to reduce the risk of infection. *Nursing Standard.* 21, 47, 43-48

Mallett J. & Bailey C. (1999) *The Royal Marsden NHS Trust Manual of Clinical Nursing Procedures*, 4th Ed. Blackwell Science, Oxford.

Pratt R.J., Pellowe C.M., Wilson J.A., Loveday H.P., Jones S.R.L.J., McDougall C., Wilcox M.H. (2007) epic 2: National Evidence-Based Guidelines for Preventing Healthcare-Associated Infections in NHS Hospitals in England. *Journal of Hospital Infection.* February; 65S: S1-S64

Further reading

Information on aseptic non-touch technique can be found at http://www.antt.co.uk

Anatomy and physiology

Introduction

Have you ever thought about how your body works? Think about a simple action such as catching a ball. You need to use your senses to locate the ball, and follow its movement through the air, and your brain to maintain balance, coordinate and produce movement of your limbs. Nerves and various chemicals allow the passage of information to and from the brain. Nutrients from digested food and oxygen are required to produce the energy needed by all parts of the body to work, grow and repair.

As a health care assistant, you have to understand how all of these systems work. To do this, you need to know some anatomy – what the different parts

of the body are like – and some physiology – what functions these parts perform.

As you study each section related to a different part of the body, you will see that there are direct links to your practice at work. You will discover what happens when people become unwell and what the body requires in order to remain healthy. So, for example, learning about the types of cells and tissues will help you to understand what happens when wounds become infected with organisms and why good hygiene is necessary. You may be required to teach patients and carers how to promote health and avoid illness and you will need to understand how the body works in order to do this.

What you need to learn

- What are anatomy and physiology?
- Cells and tissues
- Skin, hair and nails – the integumentary system
- Skeleton, joints, muscles, bones and cartilage – the locomotor system
- The nervous system
- The endocrine system
- The digestive system
- Homeostasis
- The blood and circulatory system
- The lymphatic system
- The respiratory system
- Chemical aspects

What are anatomy and physiology?

To understand how a body works and does the things it can do, you need to look at the smallest parts of the body and understand their structure, how they link together and how they are controlled.

Anatomy literally means 'a cutting up' – and dissection is the way in which scientists study the body. It allows them to discover where each part is located, its size, shape and how it is formed.

Physiology is the study of the functions of living

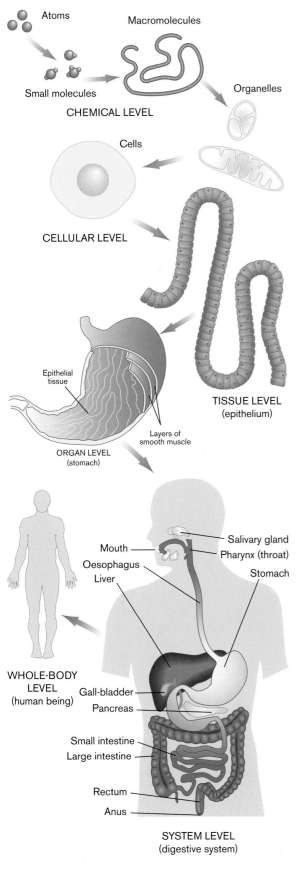

CHEMICAL LEVEL

Atoms
Macromolecules
Small molecules
Organelles

CELLULAR LEVEL

Cells

TISSUE LEVEL
(epithelium)

Epithelial
tissue

Layers of
smooth muscle

ORGAN LEVEL
(stomach)

WHOLE-BODY
LEVEL
(human being)

Mouth
Oesophagus
Liver
Salivary gland
Pharynx (throat)
Stomach
Gall-bladder
Pancreas
Small intestine
Large intestine
Rectum
Anus

SYSTEM LEVEL
(digestive system)

Levels of biological organisation.

organisms and their parts. Scientists experiment in order to investigate why each part is of a particular size and shape and in a particular position. They have been able to discover how this enables unique and specialised activity when the smallest units link together. In this section of the book you will learn about how the body is organised from the smallest part (the cell), to the largest part (the whole body).

Cells and tissues
Cells

Cells are the smallest independent units of life and are the basic living units of all organisms. They are so small that, until microscopes were available about 300 years ago, they could not be seen at all. Now, with the aid of **electron microscopes**, we are able to see the parts of the cell, which allow it to function. Cell size varies in the human being, the largest is the ovum (female sex cell) and the smallest is the sperm (male sex cell).

As shown in the flow chart, some cells combine to form larger units and so the whole body is made up of 50 million, million cells.

Key term

Electron microscope A microscope that uses small particles – electrons – and electromagnets to magnify up to half a million times.

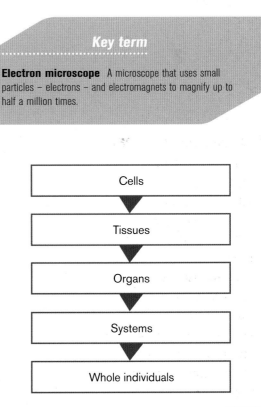

Cells

Tissues

Organs

Systems

Whole individuals

Cell	Smallest biological structure which is able to exist independently
Tissue	Groups of cells with a shared structure and function
Organ	Specialised structure which consists of different types of tissues organised in a specific way
System	Group of organs which work together
Organism	The whole being – human, animal or plant

- **excretion:** removal of waste through the cell membrane
- **growth:** grow to a set size
- **reproduction:** division of cells to produce daughter cells
- **irritability:** ability to respond to external factors.

Human cells are made up of three main parts: plasma membrane, cytoplasm – containing smaller structures (**organelles**) and nucleus. They have the following properties of life:

- **movement:** activity or movement within the cell (or, as with muscle, more general movement)
- **respiration:** use of oxygen to produce energy and by-products
- **metabolism:** use of energy and production of waste

Key terms

Organelle A minute structure within a eukaryotic cell that has a particular function. Examples of organelles include the nucleus, mitochondria and lysosomes.

ATP Adenosine Triphosphate, the chemical that provides energy for all cellular material.

Cytoskeleton Filaments forming the supportive scaffolding of the cell.

DNA Deoxyribonucleic Acid, the genetic material that provides the blueprint for all cell types.

Structure and function of different parts of a cell

Cell part	Structure	Function
Cell membrane	Double layer of phospholipid and protein molecules. Some proteins form pores or gaps	Separates cell from its environment, and controls the passage of many substances in and out of the cell
Cytoplasm	A gel-like material made up of 80 per cent water	Maintains shape of cell. Contains nutrients and gases that pass in and out as the cell functions. Supports smaller structures, organelles
Ribosomes	Tiny particles, constructed mainly of Ribosomal Ribonucleic acid (RNA). Some are temporarily attached to endoplasmic reticulum	Make enzymes and other protein compounds – hence they are known as 'protein factories'
Endoplasmic reticulum (ER)	Complex network of membranes connecting sacs and canals. Two types: rough and smooth	Rough ER receives and transports newly made proteins; smooth ER makes the new membrane
Golgi apparatus	Series of flattened cavities packed tightly on top of one another. Constantly added to from the ER as proteins are made.	Chemically processes the molecules from the ER, packages them into vesicles and slowly moves them out to the cell membrane for release
Mitochondria	Elongated, sausage-shaped organelles	Form **ATP** during aerobic respiration
Lysosomes	Small vesicles containing digestive enzymes	When released, digestive enzymes remove dead or foreign material
Centrioles	Rod-shaped pairs formed of fine tubules. Found in area of cytoplasm known as centrosomes	Important in cell division – form the **cytoskeleton** of the cell and organise spindle
Cilia	Tiny, hair-like projections made of microtubules	Allow movement e.g. lining upper respiratory tract, which moves mucus upwards
Flagella	Single extensions of cells, larger than cilia	Propel cells forward e.g. tail of sperm
Nucleus	Small sphere in centre of cell, inside double membrane containing nucleoplasm. Contains nucleolus and chromatin granules, made of proteins and chromosomes containing **DNA**. These are constantly added to from ER as protein is made	Controls all organelles in cytoplasm, particularly important role in cell reproduction. Nucleolus programmes formation of ribosomes, chromatin, chromosomes – vital in inheritance.

Tissues

Tissues are collections of similar, specialised cells that work together to carry out particular functions. Getting familiar with tissue types and recognising what is normal and abnormal is important: many diseases affect specific tissues, so your knowledge of tissues can be the difference between life and death.

There are several different types of tissue, including:

- epithelial tissue
- connective tissue
- muscle tissue
- nervous tissue.

Tissues are also classified as **simple** (with one layer of cells) and **stratified** (with several layers of cells).

Functions, type and structure of tissue cells

Epithelial tissue

Function	Type	Structure	Illustration
Lining and covering	Simple	Single row of cells	
	Stratified	Several layers of cells	
Glands	Exocrine glands	Ducts carry the secretions from the gland, e.g. sebaceous glands	
	Exocrine glands	Do not have ducts but secrete the substance directly into the blood supply, e.g. the hormone thyroxine from the thyroid gland.	

Connective tissue

Function	Type	Structure	Illustration
Joins other tissues together	Loose (areolar) connective tissue	Collagen and elastin fibres	Elastic fibre / Connective tissue cell / Fat cells / Collagenous fibres
	Adipose (fatty) tissue	Fat filled cells	Collagenous fibres / Elastic fibres / Fat cells
	Fibrous (dense connective) tissue • collagen fibres • reticular fibres • elastic fibres	Very strong fibres; tendons and ligaments	Fibroblast nuclei / Collagen bundles
	Cartilage: • hylaline • fibrocartilage • elastic	Fibrous and hard connective tissues	Pure cartilage / Cartilage cell
	Bone: • compact • cancellous	Collagen impregnated with minerals, mostly calcium	Channel (for nerves and blood vessels) / Bone cells
	Blood	Corpuscles and plasma	Red blood cell – seen from the side / Red blood cells / Platelets / Nucleus / Cytoplasm / Cytoplasm containing granules / Nucleus / Lymphocytes / Phagocytes

Muscle tissue

Function	Type	Structure	Illustration
Contracts and can produce movement	Skeletal	Striped or striated fibre	
	Smooth	Smooth fibres	
	Cardiac	The heart muscle	

Nervous tissue

Function	Type	Structure	Illustration
Receives stimuli and conveys impulses	The brain, spinal cord and nerves	Single row of cells	

Membranes

Function	Type	Structure
Covering, lining, dividing, anchoring	Serous	Lines body cavities and outer layer of organs
	Mucous	Lines tubes which lead to the outside of the body; secrets mucus
	Cutaneous	The skin; consists of an outer layer of epithelium
	Synovial – a connective tissue membrane	Lines the joint cavity; produces synovial fluid to allow for ease of movement

Epithelial tissue

This provides the covering of the body and many organs, and also forms linings. The cells in this sort of tissue are packed closely together, giving a smooth surface. The cells do not have blood vessels or supporting tissue, and often form sheets. Types of epithelial tissue are grouped according to the shape of their cells and the way in which they are arranged (squamous, cuboidal, columnar and transitional).

Connective tissue

There are several types of connective tissue.

Areolar and adipose

Areolar connective tissue is formed of delicate webs of fibres in a loose base of sticky gel, containing a variety of cells. It is the most common of the tissues, as it surrounds all organs.

Adipose connective tissue is a storage point for lipids or fat. Fat accumulates in the large spaces found inside cells.

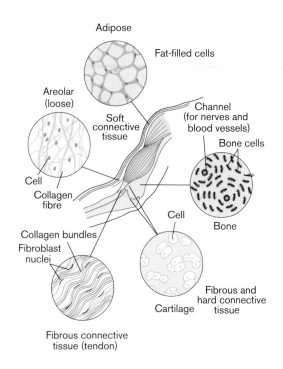

Types of connective tissue.

Types of epithelial tissue

Type of epitelial tissue	Illustration
Simple squamous • Lines the blood vessels and air sacs (alveoli) in the lungs • Allows for the exchange of nutrients, gases and waste products	Squamous epithelium
Simple cuboidal • Lines the tubules of the kidneys and some glands • Secretes and absorbs water and small molecules	Cuboidal epithelium
Simple columnar • Lines most of the organs of digestion • Absorbs nutrients and produces mucus	Ciliated columnar epithelium
Stratified squamous • Found in the epidermis and the mouth • Protects against friction, dehydration and bacterial invasion	Squamous cells
Stratified cuboidal • Lines the ducts of sweat glands • Secretes water and mineral salts	
Stratified culumnar • Lines the mammary glands and the larynx • Secretes mucus	Basement membrane Columnar basal cells

Fibrous connective tissue

This is made up of white collagen fibres, in parallel rows. It provides strength and flexibility, but does not stretch and so is the ideal material for tendons, which attach muscle to bone.

Cartilage and bone

Cartilage is what you see covering the ends of animal bones. It appears shiny and is often referred to as 'gristle'. It has a firm basis with a consistency of a plastic gel.

Bone is complex connective tissue. It develops from cartilage when specialised cells called osteoblasts lay down bone tissue, which becomes impregnated with calcium. If you look at bone under a microscope, the **matrix** appears as a series of hard circular structures or osteons. Bones give structure and support to the body, store minerals and form blood cells.

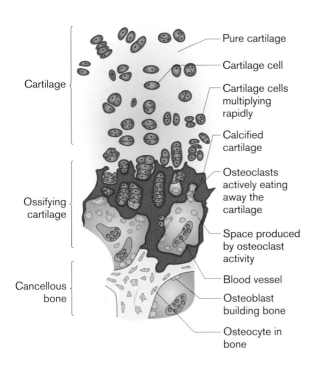

The ossification and growth of bone.

Blood and haemopoietic tissue

Blood may not seem like a tissue, but it is just an unusual type of tissue, as it has a liquid matrix. Blood provides a transport medium for a variety of cells and other materials that are needed by cells throughout the body. It is vital in protecting the body when injury occurs by allowing clotting.

> **Key term**
>
> **Matrix** Base material forming a framework for other cells or substances.

Haemopoietic tissue is found in the centre of bone cavities and in lymphoid tissue in organs, such as spleen and tonsils. It is the centre for blood and lymphoid cell production.

See also Blood on page 200.

Muscle tissue

The cells in muscle tissue have the ability to contract and to stretch, and are the specialist cells for movement. They are frequently slow to heal if damaged, often being replaced by scar tissue, which allows only restricted movement.

There are three types of muscle: skeletal, smooth and cardiac.

Voluntary or skeletal muscle

When viewed under a microscope, this tissue has a striped appearance, with cells that are long and threadlike. Many of these cells together form the muscles, which attach to bones and joints. When your skeletal muscle tissue is stimulated, it produces movements that you can control – when you walk, for example.

Voluntary muscle is there to:

- allow movement – at joints
- maintain posture – muscles always have some degree of contraction to keep the body upright
- maintain body temperature – shivering will increase heat production
- aid venous return and lymph flow – blood and lymph vessels are squeezed as they pass between muscles, so blood is encouraged to flow back towards the heart.

Involuntary or smooth muscle

This type of tissue consists of narrow, spindle-shaped cells, which have one nucleus per fibre. Smooth muscle has no stripes or 'striations' – hence the name. It is found in the walls of blood vessels and hollow organs, such as the stomach and intestines. Contractions in the muscle layers of the digestive tract move food along and expel the waste. Unlike skeletal muscle, this sort of muscle is not under voluntary control. Instead, it is controlled by the autonomic nervous system (ANS – see page 190). *See also* The digestive system *on page 194.*

Activity

Find out about the muscle in the bronchioles of the respiratory system. Explain how contractions here may lead to difficulty in breathing in some of the patients you may look after.

Cardiac muscle

This type of tissue is found only in the heart. It is formed of highly specialised cells, which, under the light microscope, appear striped with darker bands and interlocking branches. These cells have the unique ability to produce contractions when there is no other stimulation. In the heart, this causes the regular, involuntary contractions that you feel and hear as your heartbeat. *See also* The circulatory system *on page 207.*

Nervous tissue

This tissue allows rapid communication between body structures and controls the actions of all cells tissues and organs. There are two main types of cells:

- **neurones** or **nerve cells**, which are the conducting units,
- **glia** or **neuroglia**, which provide support for neurones.

Neurones consist of a cell body and processes. The axon transmits impulses away from the cell body; dendrites carry impulses towards the cell body.

See also The nervous system *on page 185.*

Pathogens

We have considered human cells and tissues, but our bodies can be also affected by other organisms made up of cells, known as pathogens.

Pathogens are disease-causing organisms such as bacteria, viruses, fungi and protozoa. These organisms can infect any part of our bodies, leading to symptoms such as high temperature, pain and swelling. Usually, human beings can fight infection as we have specialised cells – antibodies and enzymes – which are part of our immune system. *See* Infection control *on page 134.*

If bacteria cannot be destroyed by our immune systems, antibiotics may be used as a treatment. Frequent and inappropriate use of antibiotics has resulted in bacteria which are unaffected by many **antibiotics** e.g. Methacylin resistant staphylococcus aureus (MRSA).

Key terms

Antibiotics Chemicals that attach to particular parts of bacteria and either destroy them or prevent them multiplying.

Skin, hair and nails – the integumentary system

Skin

The skin is a sheet-like structure covering the outer surface of the body. The skin has a number of important functions:

- protection
- temperature regulation
- excretion
- absorption
- making vitamin D.

The condition of your skin also reflects your general state of health and your emotions.

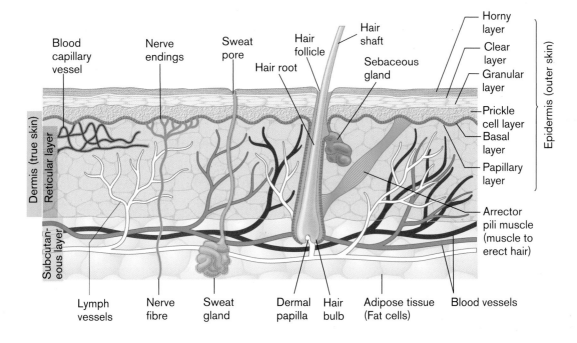

The structure of skin.

It is divided into three layers: the outer layer or epidermis; the true skin or dermis; and the bottom, protective layer, called the subcutaneous layer.

Epidermis
The epidermis is made up of five layers or strata:

- basal layer (*stratum germinitavum*)
- prickle cell layer (*stratum spinosum*)
- granular layer (*stratum granulosum*)
- clear layer (*stratum lucidum*)
- horny layer (*stratum corneum*).

Basal cell layer
This is the deepest of the layers, formed of tightly packed epithelial cells, which are constantly dividing in a process called mitosis. As they move towards the surface, the cells become hardened, providing a protective, waterproof layer. As cells are replaced, they are rubbed off at the surface into the atmosphere. Much of the house dust we clean away consists of skin cells.

Within this layer are cells called melanocytes. These cells provide our skin colour and protect us against **ultraviolet (UV) light**.

If the basal cell layer is damaged, cells will not regenerate (re-grow). It may grow in from the edges but, depending on the extent of damage, this could be a lengthy process. Skin may be grafted from another site to speed up the process and prevent wound contamination and infection.

Prickle cell and granular layers

As they move up, the basal cells change in structure, developing spindles or prickles – hence the name prickle cell layer. As they move up further, they start to die, and by the time they reach the granular layer, mitosis – or cell division – has stopped. The cells in this layer contain a granular protein called keratin.

Clear and horny layers

In some areas of the body, a thicker covering is required e.g. points of 'wear and tear' such as soles of feet. Here the granular layer becomes clear (stratum lucidum). By the time the cells reach the top, horny layer at the surface, they are flat, hard and slough off easily, in a process called **desquamation**.

> **Key term**
>
> **Desquamation** The natural process where surface dead cells rub off as they are replaced by new cells from the germinative layer.

The dermis

Made up of mainly connective tissue with collagen and elastic fibres, the dermis is much thicker than the epidermis, but is more loosely packed.

The upper layer of the dermis is thrown into bumps – the ridges and dips form our fingerprints. At a junction, this arrangement helps bind the skin layers together.

The deeper layers have more tough, elastic fibres, which give it the ability to spring back into shape when pinched or stretched. These fibres, plus the subcutaneous fat, decrease with age – that is why your skin loses its elasticity and becomes less springy as you get older. A similar effect is seen in dehydration where water is lost from cells; for example, when you lose large volumes of fluid or fail to replace it by drinking.

Blood vessels run at the base of the dermis and capillaries branch into the higher layers but do not penetrate the epidermis.

In the dermis, different nerve endings respond to different sensations:

- pain – free nerve ending
- pressure – Pacinian corpuscle
- touch – Meissner's corpuscle
- temperature – free nerve ending.

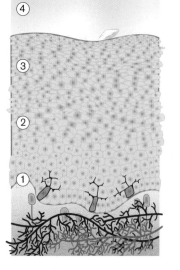

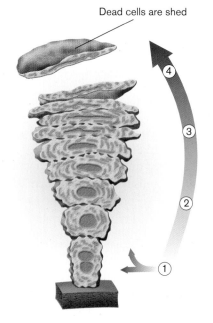

Dead cells are shed

The process of desquamation.

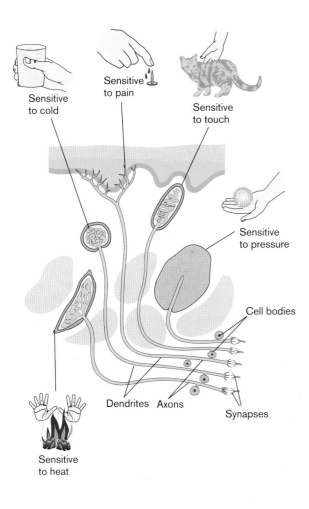

Nerve receptors in the skin.

At various levels of the skin

A number of features can be found at different levels, not just in one specific layer of the skin:

- **hair follicles** from which hair grows. A fine growth is present all over the body but it is profuse in the axilla, head, pubis and eyebrows
- **muscle fibres** that attach to hair follicles and, when stimulated, make the hair rise, trapping air – this helps to insulate your body when it is cold
- **sebaceous glands** which secrete oil at the base of hair follicles, acting as 'nature's skin cream'
- **sweat glands** of two types: eccrine (found all over body) and apocrine (armpits, pubic areas). These help with the removal of waste, and are critical in helping to maintain body temperature.

Subcutaneous layer

At the deepest level, below the dermis, is a layer of subcutaneous tissue (also called the hypodermis). Fat cells form layers here, to insulate the body and provide a storage area for energy. This layer provides protective padding, acting as a shock-absorbing layer to protect the underlying organs from trauma.

Nails

Nails are technically classed as accessory organs of the skin, which protect the tips of fingers and toes. They are produced by the cells of the epidermis. The cells in the nail bed are supplied with abundant blood vessels – hence this area normally appears pink. When levels of oxygen in the blood drop, the nail bed develops a blue tinge (cyanosis). For this reason, when you are preparing a patient for surgery, you should make sure their nail polish is removed to allow for accurate observation. When a patient has a circulatory disease or diabetes, you should be especially careful that you do not damage tissue when caring for their nails – especially their toenails. You should usually refer them to a podiatrist, who specialises in care of the feet.

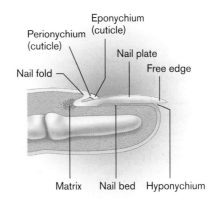

Cross-section of the nail in its nail bed.

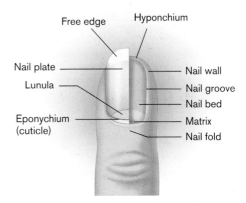

The structure of the nail.

Activity

Find out what the effects of burns might be to skin layers. How could you assess the size and severity of the damage?

Why do pressure sores or decubitus ulcers occur? How might these be prevented?

Healing

When skin is damaged there is a natural sequence of events, which results in repair. The process differs slightly depending on the depth of the damage.

If the damage is epidermal (for example, following minor burns and abrasions), the epidermal cells migrate across the wound, then the relocated cells build new layers.

If the damage is deeper, multiple tissue layers need to repair so there is a more complex healing process, potentially resulting in scar tissue formation and the loss of normal function. If large areas of deep tissue are lost, grafting of tissue from another site on the body will be required.

The phases of healing

Inflammatory phase – blood clot forms in the wound, uniting the edges. Increased blood flow to the damaged area. Phagocytes destroy organisms and remove dead matter

↓

Migratory phase – clot reorganised into a scab. Epithelial cells to bridge the gap, fibroblasts make scar tissue, damaged blood vessels re-grow.

↓

Proliferative stage – a continuation of the migratory phase. Extensive growth of epithelial cells and blood vessels. Fibroblasts make lots of scar tissue

↓

Maturation phase – Epithelial tissue is restored, scab sloughs off and tissues below return to normal.

Did you know?

The tissue filling the space is now known as **granulation** tissue and has a rich pink colour.

Scar tissue

Scar formation is known as **fibrosis**. Scar tissue contains more densely arranged collagen fibres, but has fewer blood vessels, elastic tissue and accessory organs such as hairs and glands.

Did you know?

If there is so much scar tissue that it goes above the normal epidermal surface, it is called **hypertrophic scarring**; if it is extensive, it is called **keloid scarring**.

See also Dressing wounds *on page 277.*

Activity

Find out why epidermal wound healing does not result in scar formation.

Skeleton, joints, muscles, cartilage, ligaments and tendons – the locomotor system

The locomotor system is made up of the skeleton, joints, muscles, tendons and cartilage.

The skeleton

The skeleton forms the main framework of your body, protecting your inner organs. Because of associated tissues – muscle, tendon and cartilage – movement occurs at the joints in the skeleton. Blood cells are formed in the skeleton, and it also provides storage for minerals.

The bones forming the skeleton are light but, in a healthy body, very strong. The whole system is very flexible, although it deteriorates with age, illness, certain treatments and a poor diet.

The skeleton can be divided into two parts: the axial skeleton and the appendicular skeleton.

The skeleton

The structure of the skeleton

The human skeleton consists of 206 individual bones which can be divided into different parts.

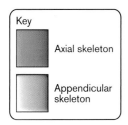

Key
- Axial skeleton
- Appendicular skeleton

- The **axial skeleton** consists of 80 bones and incorporates:
  – the skull (cranium and facial bones)
  – the vertebral column
  – the thorax.

- The **appendicular skeleton** consists of 126 bones and incorporates:
  – the shoulder girdle
  – the upper limbs
  – the pelvis
  – two lower limbs.

The axial skeleton

The skull

Frontal × 1	Nasal × 4
Parietal × 2	Vomer × 1
Temporal × 1	Maxilla × 1
Occipital × 1	Mandible × 1
Ethmoid × 1	Zygomatic × 2
Sphenoid × 1	Palatine × 2
Lacrimal × 2	Hyoid × 1

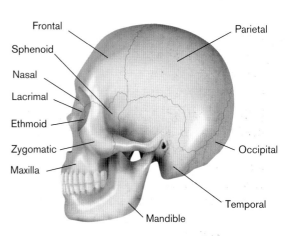

Frontal
Sphenoid
Nasal
Lacrimal
Ethmoid
Zygomatic
Maxilla
Parietal
Occipital
Temporal
Mandible

▲ *The bones of the skull.*

The vertebral column

Cervical vertebrae × 7	Coccyx × 4 fused vertebrae
Sacrum × 5 fused vertebrae	Lumbar vertebrae × 5
Thoracic vertebrae × 1	

▼ *The bones of the vertebral column*

The thorax

Ribs × 12 pairs
Sternum × 1

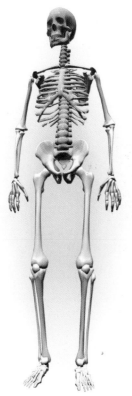

▲ *The axial and appendicular skeletons.*

▼ *The bones of the thorax.*

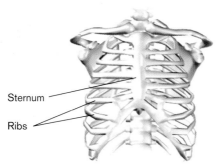

Sternum
Ribs

Cervical vertebrae (seven)

Thoracic vertebrae (twelve)

Intervertebral discs

Lumbar vertebrae (five fused)

Sacral vertebrae (five)

Coccygeal vertebrae (four fused)

The appendicular skeleton

The shoulder girdle

Scapula × 2	
Clavicle × 2	

▼ The bones of the shoulder girdle.

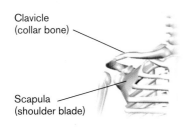

Clavicle
(collar bone)

Scapula
(shoulder blade)

The pelvis

Pelvic bone × 2:
each pelvic bone is a fusion of 3 individual bones: ilium, ischium and pubis

▼ The bones of the shoulder pelvis.

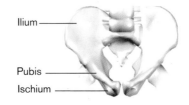

Ilium

Pubis

Ischium

The upper limbs

Two upper limbs, each with:	
Humerus × 2	Metacarpals × 5
Carpals × 8	Ulna × 1
Radius × 1	Phalanges × 14

▼ The bones of the upper limbs.

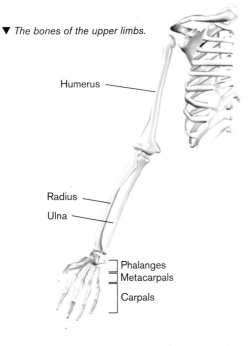

Humerus

Radius

Ulna

Phalanges
Metacarpals

Carpals

The lower limbs

Two lower limbs, each with:	
Femur × 1	Tibia × 5
Tarsals × 7	Phalanges × 14
Patella × 1	Fibula × 1
Metatarsals × 5	

▼ The bones of the lower limbs

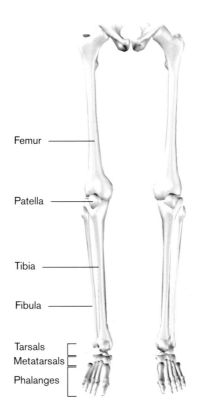

Femur

Patella

Tibia

Fibula

Tarsals

Metatarsals

Phalanges

Fascinating fact

The human body has more bones at birth than as an adult. This is because some bones become fused together, such as the sacrum, coccyx and pelvis.

Development of bone

During the early stages of a foetus' development, rods and plates of cartilage (and, in one case, connective tissue) are laid down as a 'blueprint', to be replaced in the seventh week by bone. This process is called ossification.

Ossification

Osteoblasts form new bone in the cartilage rods or plates. They secrete collagen, which forms a strong framework. Minerals, mainly calcium salts, are then deposited there.

Osteoblasts become trapped in the framework and form mature cells called osteocytes. These can release further calcium ions that become part of the bone tissue. Osteoclasts break down the minerals and protein in old bone tissue by releasing **enzymes**. This allows bone to be remoulded. The balance between the work of the osteoblasts and osteoclasts helps to maintain the skeleton and keep it light.

Key term

Enzymes Complex chemicals that control reactions in living cells and speed up changes.

Bone continues to develop into early adult life, until the age of 25 or so. Some tissues, such as cartilage of the nose and ears, will continue to grow very slowly.

For bones to remain healthy, there is some growth, repair and destruction of bone throughout your life. Healthy bone growth needs a nutritious diet, with calcium, phosphorus, vitamins A, D, C and B12, protein, a good blood supply, physical exercise and hormones, such as thyroxin.

There are five shapes of bones within skeleton.

Type	Description	Examples
Long	The typical 'bone' shape.	femur, humerus (see diagram)
Short	Usually box shaped. Outer shell of compact bone with centre of cancellous bone. Often articulates with other bones, for range of movement.	carpals (wrist bones)
Flat	Often thin and curved to fit area, made up of cancellous bone sandwiched between outer compact bone.	skull bones
Irregular	Similar to short bones but of varying shapes.	vertebrae
Sesamoid	Only found in certain tendons. Provides protection in areas of stress and load, reduces friction at joint.	patella (knee cap)

Bones of all shapes share similar characteristics, so by studying a typical bone, you will learn about the whole group.

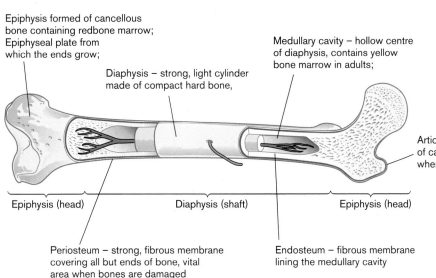

Epiphysis formed of cancellous bone containing redbone marrow; Epiphyseal plate from which the ends grow;

Diaphysis – strong, light cylinder made of compact hard bone,

Medullary cavity – hollow centre of diaphysis, contains yellow bone marrow in adults;

Articular cartilage – thin layer of cartilage, smoothing movement where joints meet

Epiphysis (head)   Diaphysis (shaft)   Epiphysis (head)

Periosteum – strong, fibrous membrane covering all but ends of bone, vital area when bones are damaged

Endosteum – fibrous membrane lining the medullary cavity

Structure of a long bone.

Activity

Investigate some of the following disorders and identify why and how they occur: osteoporosis, arthritis, tendonitis, bursitis.

How could your knowledge of anatomy and physiology improve the care you give?

Joints

Joints are formed where two or more bones meet, allowing movement. They are classified as fibrous, cartilaginous or synovial.

Fibrous joints

Also known as fixed or immovable joints, these are held together with fibrous connective tissue rich in collagen. No movement occurs when ossified. An example is the skull, where movement or 'moulding' is required during the birth process.

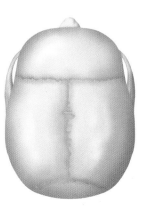
Fibrous joint in the cranium.

Cartilaginous joints

Articulating bones are connected by hyaline or fibrocartilage. They allow only slight movement, for example at the joint where the pubic bones meet – the symphasis pubis and vertebral bodies.

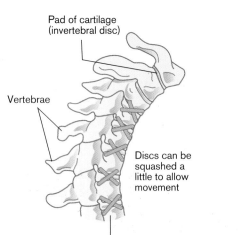

Cartilaginous joint in the vertebral column.

Pad of cartilage (invertebral disc)

Vertebrae

Discs can be squashed a little to allow movement

Ligaments hold the bones together

Synovial

Bone ends are covered with articular cartilage and contained within a cavity containing synovial fluid which enables free movement and provides nutrients to underlying cartilage. The fluid is produced by the synovial membrane, which lines the cavity. The joint is surrounded by a fibrous capsule.

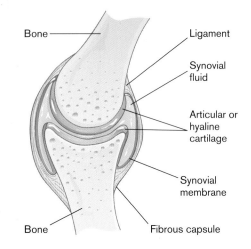

Bone

Ligament

Synovial fluid

Articular or hyaline cartilage

Synovial membrane

Bone

Fibrous capsule

The structure of a synovial joint.

There are five types of synovial joints, each with a different structure and function.

Type of synovial joint	Example	Movement
Gliding	Clavicle/scapula	Small, versatile gliding movements
Hinge	Phalanges	Flexion, extension; in one plane only
Pivot	Radius and ulna	Rotation including pronation and supination
Ball and socket	Pelvis/femur	The widest range of movement: flexion, extension, adduction, abduction, circumduction and rotation (including pronation and supination)
Condyloid	Carpals	Movement in two planes; adduction, abduction, flexion, extension, limited circumduction

Different sorts of movement are possible at synovial joints, as this illustration shows.

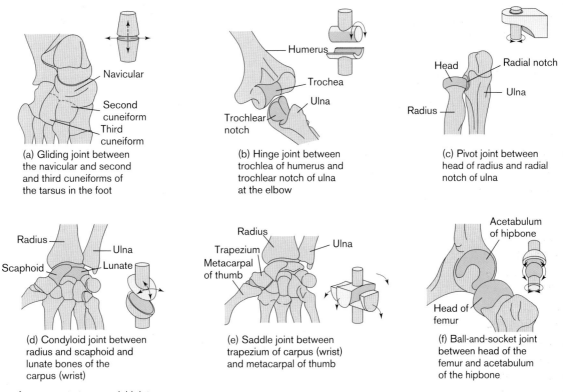

(a) Gliding joint between the navicular and second and third cuneiforms of the tarsus in the foot

(b) Hinge joint between trochlea of humerus and trochlear notch of ulna at the elbow

(c) Pivot joint between head of radius and radial notch of ulna

(d) Condyloid joint between radius and scaphoid and lunate bones of the carpus (wrist)

(e) Saddle joint between trapezium of carpus (wrist) and metacarpal of thumb

(f) Ball-and-socket joint between head of the femur and acetabulum of the hipbone

Types of movement at a synovial joint.

Cartilage

Cartilage is a type of firm connective tissue with a dense network of collagen and elastin. Unusually, cartilage contains no blood or nerve vessels. There are two main types of cartilage.

- **Hyaline cartilage** covers bone ends and forms the larynx, tip of the nose and rings within the trachea and bronchi.
- **Fibrocartilage** provides strength and rigidity: for example, as pads between the vertebrae of the spine.

Ligaments

Ligaments are bands of strong, fibrous connective tissue that hold bones together across joints. Ligaments have little elasticity, as they are there to stabilise the joint when the muscle contracts to allow movement.

Tendons

Like ligaments, tendons are strong, fibrous bands of connective tissue, but tendons attach muscle to bone, rather than bone to bone. It is the contraction of a muscle through a tendon which causes the movement of a bone at a joint.

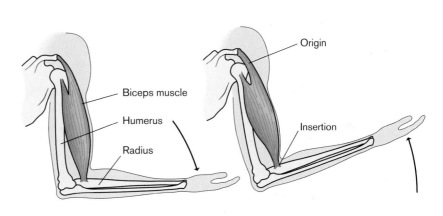

Muscle attaches to bone to facilitate movement.

Muscle

You have already been introduced to the three types of muscle, their structures and functions on page 173. Look back now and refresh your memory before reading on.

Memory jogger

Can you remember the three types of muscle, and the differences between them? Look back at page 173 to check.

The only type of muscle directly involved in the locomotor system is voluntary or skeletal muscle. This is the type of muscle that most people recognise, as it provides shape to the body. Voluntary muscles become more developed with exercise – as you can see in athletes and bodybuilders – but they can also waste away when activity is reduced.

Voluntary muscles are attached to bones by tendons, at points known as the origin and the insertion. Groups of muscles work together to allow movement, and maintain stability and muscle tone.

Structure of voluntary muscle

If you looked at individual muscle cells under an electron microscope, you would see threadlike filaments. Some are thin and formed of a protein called myosin; some are thick and formed of a protein called actin. Many of these filaments are grouped together and arranged so that they appear to have light and dark bands. These units are known as sarcomeres, and are separated from one another by Z lines.

How a voluntary muscle works

To start a contraction, skeletal muscle cells have to be activated. A motor neurone rests on each muscle fibre, forming a junction. Chemicals released here make the impulse carry on to further muscle cells.

During contraction, the thin filaments are pulled towards the centre of each sarcomere, shortening the whole muscle.

When the muscle relaxes, the filaments return to their normal state. The whole muscle contracts by means of this sliding system: the filaments attach to one another, forming bridges, which then work as levers and ratchets, pulling the fibres past one another.

This activity requires energy, which is supplied by Adenosine Triphosphate (ATP) molecules. Carbohydrates are broken down to form glucose which can be stored in muscle as glycogen. When this interacts with oxygen, ATP is formed. When ATP is broken down to form energy, the by-products are water, carbon dioxide and pyruvic acid. If there is insufficient oxygen, pyruvic acid is converted to lactic acid, which builds up causing muscle fatigue – felt as soreness and cramps.

As muscles shorten, the bones into which they are inserted move towards the origin.

Muscles work in teams to ensure smooth movement: one set of muscles contracts, while the opposing muscles relax.

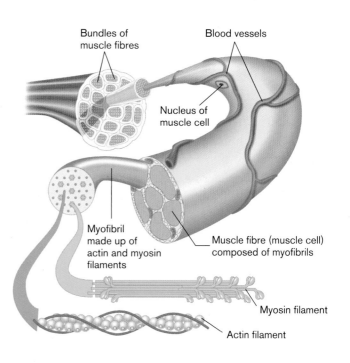

The internal structure of skeletal muscle.

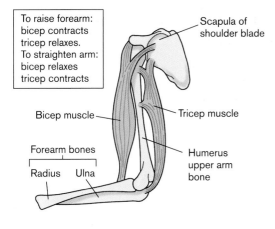

To raise forearm:
bicep contracts
tricep relaxes.
To straighten arm:
bicep relaxes
tricep contracts

Scapula of shoulder blade

Bicep muscle

Tricep muscle

Forearm bones

Humerus upper arm bone

Radius   Ulna

Movement at the forearm.

Characteristic	Endocrine system	Nervous system
Time of signal	Hormones circulated in blood (chemical signal)	Electrical impulses along nerve fibres; chemicals released at synapses aid movement
Size of signal	Depends on the amount of hormone	Depends on the number of fibres stimulated and frequency of impulses
Site affected	May have widespread effect on cells in different parts of the body but may also be specific	Generally localised; each neurone links with only one or two cells but fibres may be very long
Speed	Usually slower – seconds, hours or days	Rapid – within a thousandth of a second
Control	Overall via a feedback system to producing gland	Via brain

Activity

Identify which muscles may be used as injection sites and when this route might be used to administer medication.

Activity

Look up information on the causes of tenosynovitis and carpel tunnel syndrome. Think of ways of avoiding these problems.

Key term

Synapse   The minute gap between neurones, across which impulses pass.

The nervous system

Your nervous and endocrine systems are the main controllers of the activities which the cells of your body carry out. The endocrine system produces chemicals that are passed directly into your blood and circulated round your body. The nervous system, on the other hand, works by means of nerve cells and fibres, which connect with one another and all organs of the body.

Both systems transmit information, but in different ways.

The nervous system can be split up into two divisions:

- **the central nervous system (CNS)** – the brain and spinal cord, which are the central control of nervous functions
- **the peripheral nervous system (PNS)** – the nerves which extend to outlying areas, subdivided into autonomic and somatic.

The basic units of this system are the **glia** or supporting nervous tissue, and the **neurones** or nerve cells, which conduct impulses. These units vary in shape, size and function.

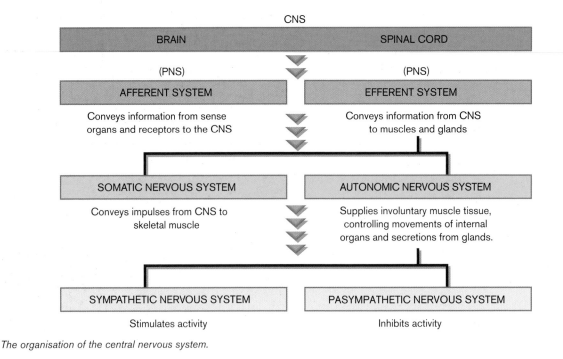

CNS

BRAIN	SPINAL CORD

(PNS)	(PNS)
AFFERENT SYSTEM	**EFFERENT SYSTEM**

Conveys information from sense organs and receptors to the CNS	Conveys information from CNS to muscles and glands

SOMATIC NERVOUS SYSTEM	**AUTONOMIC NERVOUS SYSTEM**

Conveys impulses from CNS to skeletal muscle	Supplies involuntary muscle tissue, controlling movements of internal organs and secretions from glands.

SYMPATHETIC NERVOUS SYSTEM	**PASYMPATHETIC NERVOUS SYSTEM**

Stimulates activity	Inhibits activity

The organisation of the central nervous system.

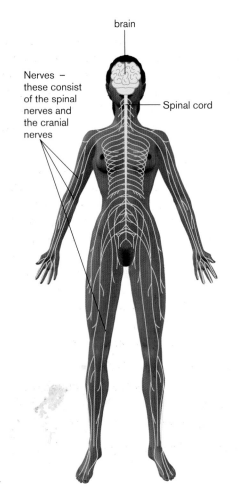

brain

Nerves – these consist of the spinal nerves and the cranial nerves

Spinal cord

The nervous system.

Neurones

Each neurone consists of three parts: the dendrite, the axon and the myelin sheath.

Dendrites are projections (one or more) that pass impulses to the cell body. The axon is a projection which passes impulses away from the cell body. The myelin sheath insulates the nerve, to stop the impulses spreading to neighbouring neurones.

There are three types of neurones, classified according to the direction in which they transmit impulses.

- **sensory neurones (afferent)** – these transmit impulses to the spinal cord and brain from all areas
- **motor neurones (efferent)** – these transmit impulses away from the brain

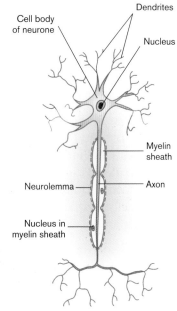

Cell body of neurone

Dendrites

Nucleus

Myelin sheath

Neurolemma

Axon

Nucleus in myelin sheath

The structure of a neurone.

and spinal cord, and cause movement. The impulses go only to muscle and glandular tissue

- **interneurones (central or conducting neurones)** – these conduct impulses from sensory to motor neurones.

Myelin is formed from protein and lipids (fat). In cells that are outside the central nervous system, this is produced by Schwann cells, which surround the axon. Schwann cells have segments, and the areas between the segments are known as Nodes of Ranvier. This area, with the myelin, allows the impulse to move rapidly movement along the fibre. The outer cell membrane of the Schwann cell – the neurolemma – is essential for cut or injured axons to grow back again. As axons in the central nervous system have no neurolemma, their potential for regrowth is limited.

Reflect

Think of any patients in your care who have injuries to their CNS. How has this affected them? What are the implications of having injuries that cannot heal, for them and their carers?

Voluntary muscle is there to:

- allow movement – at joints
- maintain posture – muscles always have some degree of contraction to keep the body upright
- maintain body temperature – shivering will increase heat production
- aid venous return and lymph flow – blood and lymph vessels are squeezed as they pass between muscles, so blood is encouraged to flow back towards the heart.

Nerve impulse or action potential

A nerve impulse or action potential is a wave of electrical disturbance along the surface of neuronal membranes. It is set off in sensory nerves by a change in the environment, such as pressure, pain, temperature or a chemical change.

When the impulse reaches another neurone, chemicals called neurotransmitters are released at the junction, and the impulse passes across the gap or synapse.

There are at least 30 different neurotransmitters specific to different sites, including:

- **acetylcholine** – at synapses in the spinal cord and neuromuscular junctions, sometimes referred to as cholinergics
- **monoamines** – noradrenalin (adrenergic), dopamine, serotonin, which are involved in sleep, mood and motor function
- **neuropeptides** – endorphins and enkephalins, natural painkillers that are released in the brain and spinal cord at a point called the pain conduction pathway.

Activity

Find out why Multiple Sclerosis occurs and why the symptoms may vary.

What are Muscular dystrophy and Parkinson's disease? What are their symptoms?

Nerves are collections of peripheral nerve fibres bundled together. They form the white matter in the brain and spinal cord – 'white' because they usually have myelin sheaths. Tissue composed of cell bodies and unmyelinated axons and dendrites forms the grey coloured tissue in the brain and spinal cord.

Nerve impulses run in neurone pathways. One form of neurone pathway is the reflex arc. The simplest versions of this are two- and three-neurone arcs. They work like one-way streets, where impulses pass in one direction only. One simple example is the 'knee jerk' reflex arc, where, if you tap the area under the patella, the stretch receptors are stimulated, resulting in a rapid response which initially bypasses the route up to the brain. Testing the knee jerk reflex assists diagnosis of an area of damage or disease.

Two other important reflexes are:

- the withdrawal reflex, when something hot is touched
- the reflex of swallowing or sneezing.

An example of a reflex response controlled by the ANS is micturition.

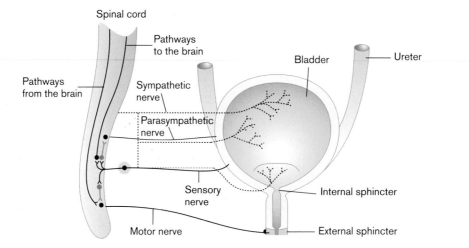

Control of the urinary bladder is a reflex action controlled by the autonomic nervous system.

The central nervous system (CNS)

The two major parts of the CNS are the centrally-placed brain and spinal cord. The skull protects the brain, and the central canal of the vertebral bodies protects the spinal cord. Both brain and spinal cord also have a continuous protective membrane covering them, called the meninges. A layer of fluid known as cerebro-spinal fluid (CSF) circulates between the CNS and the meninges, acting as a cushion and providing nutrients. CSF is filtered from blood vessels in the ventricles (cavities) of the brain, and is eventually returned to the circulating blood.

Activity

A lumbar puncture is a procedure where CSF is sampled. Find out about the conditions in which a lumbar puncture might be used.

Activity

What is meningitis? Investigate what it is, what the symptoms are and what treatment you might be involved in.

The brain

The brain is one of our largest organs. it is responsible for receiving, analysing and storing information, and for initiating responses and actions. It acts as a computer; the spinal cord is the route by which all information passes in and out of the computer.

The brain is divided into sections with different functions.

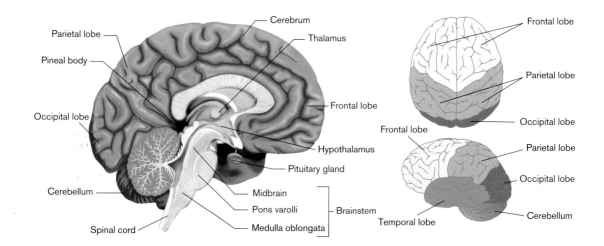

The brain. Each cerebral hemisphere is divided into four lobes.

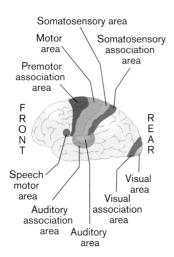

The functional area of the left cerebral hemisphere.

Area of the brain	Function
Left hemisphere	Language, rational, logical, analytical
Right hemisphere	Visuo-spatial, artistic, emotional, intuition, creativity
Motor cortex in frontal lobe	Fine movement
Pre-frontal cortex	Planning, working memory, goal-oriented behaviour
Limbic system	Emotions
Hypothalmus	Regulates ANS and endocrine system

Summary of the functional areas of the brain.

The meninges – the coverings of the brain – continue down to cover the spinal cord in three layers, with circulating CSF between them.

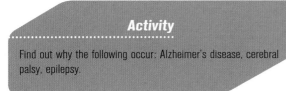

Activity

Find out why the following occur: Alzheimer's disease, cerebral palsy, epilepsy.

Activity

Find out how surgeons might use the spinal nerves and their coverings to control pain and operate without a general anaesthetic. What do they use?

The spinal cord

The spinal cord is about 45 cm long, stretching from the base of the skull to the level of 1st lumber vertebrae (if you put your hands on your hips, this is roughly the level at which your spinal cord ends). It provides a pathway between the brain and the rest of the body. The tracts in the spinal cord serve individual functions: for example, sensory (touch, temperature).

The spinal cord has been compared with a telephone switchboard system, which allows incoming and outgoing messages to be passed to the correct rooms. Sensory impulses travel up to the brain; motor impulses travel down and out towards the organs and muscles.

There are 31 pairs of nerves leaving each side of the cord:

- 8 cervical
- 12 thoracic
- 5 lumbar
- 5 sacral
- 1 coccygeal.

Where these nerves form a network, they are called nerve plexuses.

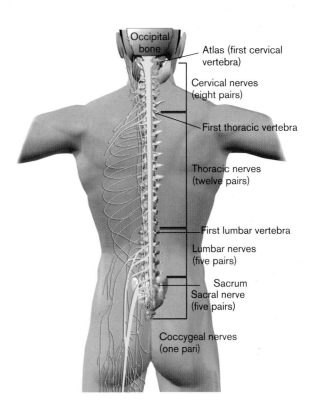

The spinal cord and spinal nerves.

The peripheral nervous system (PNS)

These are the nerves connecting the CNS to the body. The PNS includes the nerves affecting voluntary control (for example, skeletal muscle) and involuntary control (for example, glands, heart muscle and abdominal organs).

Areas not supplied by the spinal nerves are controlled by the 12 pairs of cranial nerves attached to the underside of the brain. The fibres mainly supply organs in the head and neck, the thoracic and abdominal cavities.

Sensory system

This system carries information from organs within the body, the skin and special senses (ears, eyes, tongue and nose) to centres in the cerebral hemispheres (see the summary of the functional areas of the brain, on page 189). Here the information is interpreted, and you become aware of particular sensations – pain, touch, sound or external or internal **stimuli**.

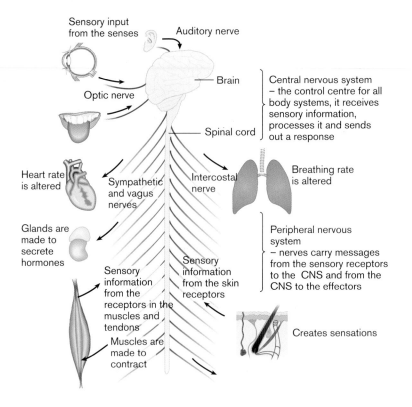

The peripheral nervous system.

> ### Key term
> **Stimuli** Physical event causing a change we are able to detect, for example, heat, cold, etc.

The nature of the sensation and the type of reaction depends on the CNS and the final destination of the nerve impulses. This is important in helping to protect against injury, since we can respond by reducing the damage or avoiding the danger.

Impulses reaching the lower brain stem have more complex reflexes, such as changes to breathing and heart rate.

The autonomic nervous system (ANS)

The ANS consists of types of motor neurones, conducting impulses from the spinal cord or brainstem to:

- cardiac muscle
- smooth muscle
- glandular epithelial tissue.

It tends to regulate functions e.g. heart rate, contractions of stomach and glandular secretions.

The autonomic system has two divisions: the **sympathetic** and parasympathetic systems. The sympathetic system functions as an emergency system when you exercise and when you have strong emotional arousal. It is vital when you are trying to cope with stress.

Autonomic functions

Organs affected	Sympathetic control	Parasympathetic Control
Heart muscle	Increased heart rate	Slows heart rate
Smooth/involuntary muscle In most blood vessels Blood vessels in: • skeletal muscle • digestive tract • anal sphincter • urinary bladder • urinary sphincter • muscles • iris of eye • ciliary muscle of eye • hairs	 Constricts Dilates Slows gut movement, reduces defecation Closes sphincter Relaxes bladder Closes sphincter Dilates pupil Flattens lens Pulls hairs upright on skin	 No change No change Increases gut movement Opens sphincter Contracts bladder Opens sphincter Contracts pupil Allows lens to bulge No parasympathetic fibres
Glands Adrenal medulla Sweat glands Digestive glands	 Increases secretion of adrenalin Increases secretion Decreases secretion of digestive enzymes	 None None Increases secretions

Consider how you might feel while watching a very frightening film. The sympathetic system comes into operation, preparing your body for 'fight or flight'. Blood flow increases to skeletal muscle to enable you to run; blood vessels to the gut are constricted so digestion is reduced; sphincter muscles close so you will not pass urine or defecate; the pupils of your eyes dilate to allow more light onto the retina, and the lens alters in order to focus accurately; you sweat, which will allow increased cooling; and adrenalin secretion is increased. Adrenalin and other hormones will support and maintain the stress response – and as it is released as a neurotransmitter, adrenalin will speed up impulse transmission too.

The autonomic nervous system is there to maintain or restore your normal, balanced body activity, known as homeostasis. Many organs have fibres from both sympathetic and parasympathetic divisions, and they work in an opposite or 'antagonistic' way. For example, this ensures that the heart beats at a regular rate, but responds to changing body needs. You can reduce the effects of sympathetic activity by meditating and relaxing.

The endocrine system

The endocrine system consists of a series of glands. These glands produce chemicals called hormones in varying quantities, depending on the body's needs. These hormones pass or 'diffuse' directly into the bloodstream.

The endocrine and nervous systems work together to co-ordinate and maintain body functions (homeostasis). However, their mechanisms are different. The nervous system operates by means of impulses triggered by a mediator, a neurotransmitter; the endocrine system works via hormones (see the table on page 193).

Did you know?

The word hormone comes from the Greek *hormon* meaning to excite or get moving.

The glands which produce hormones are spread widely throughout the body, and the hormones are transmitted round all the cells and tissues of the body.

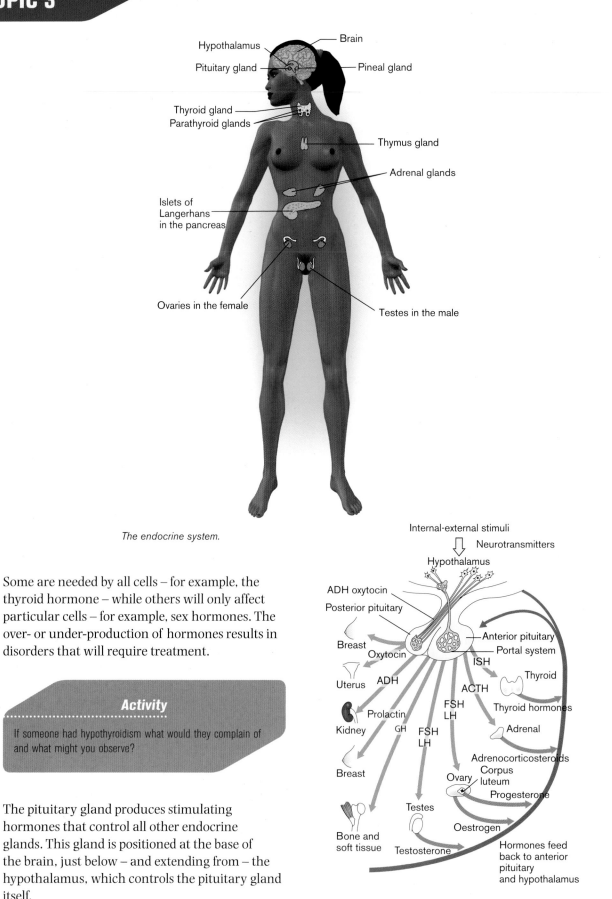

The endocrine system.

Some are needed by all cells – for example, the thyroid hormone – while others will only affect particular cells – for example, sex hormones. The over- or under-production of hormones results in disorders that will require treatment.

Activity

If someone had hypothyroidism what would they complain of and what might you observe?

The pituitary gland produces stimulating hormones that control all other endocrine glands. This gland is positioned at the base of the brain, just below – and extending from – the hypothalamus, which controls the pituitary gland itself.

The hormones secreted by the pituitary gland.

Summary of the endocrine glands and their functions

Gland	Hormones	Function	Disorders
Anterior lobe of pituitary	Growth hormone (GH)	To regulate growth of all body tissues	Giantism; dwarfism; acromegaly
	Adrenocorticotrophic hormone (ACTH)	To regulate the production of steroids; to regulate the ovarian follicle and the production of progesterone; to stimulate milk production in the breast	
	Gonadtrophins	To regulate the function of the ovaries and testes	
Posterior lobe of pituitary (these hormones are merely stored in the pituitary gland until needed. They are secreted by the hypothalamus)	Anti-diuretic hormone (ADH)	To regulate the absorption of water in the kidney, thus regulating urine output	Diabetes insipidus
	Oxytocin	To control milk production during breastfeeding; to promote the contraction of the smooth muscles of the uterus during childbirth	
Thyroid	Thyroxin	To regulate the metabolic rate; influences mental and physical activities	Hypothyroidism; hyperthyroidism
	Calcitonin	To regulate calcium levels in the bloodstream	
Parathyroid	Parathyroid hormone	Promotes the absorption of calcium which is needed for muscle contraction	Tetany
Pineal gland	Melatonin	To regulate the sleep–wake cycle; it is produced at night	Affected by flying from west to east (jet lag)
Thymus	Thymosin	To assist the production of T-lymphocytes	
Adrenal medulla	Adrenalin	To raise blood pressure and pulse as part of the 'fight or flight' response	Stress-related symptoms
Adrenal cortex	Steroids	To assist in the metabolism of carbohydrates, fats and proteins; to regulate the water balance in the body	Cushing's syndrome; Addison's disease
Pancreas	Insulin and glucagon	To regulate blood glucose	Diabetes mellitus (Types 1 and 2)
Ovaries	Oestrogen and progesterone	To regulate menstruation and secondary sexual characteristics in women; to prepare for and maintain pregnancy	Hirsutism; precocious puberty (early onset)
Testes	Testosterone	To regulate sperm production and secondary sexual characteristics in men	Low levels may cause delayed puberty

There are two major classes of hormones:

- water-soluble – such as adrenalin, noradrenalin, dopamine, antidiuretic hormone, oxytocin, growth hormone, insulin, thyroid stimulating hormone, prostaglandins, serotonin, melatonin
- lipid soluble – such as steroids, thyroid hormones, nitric oxide

Water-soluble hormones work as first messengers. They arrive at the target cell and link with the receptor on the cell – a bit like a lock and key mechanism. A second messenger is then activated from inside the cell, and this messenger then controls the cell activity.

Lipid soluble hormones can connect with the target receptor, pass into the nucleus of the cell and act on DNA, leading to specific effects in the cell. An example of this would be oestrogen leading to breast development in the female adolescent.

Hormone levels are regulated by specialised homeostatic mechanisms called feedback. This can be either positive or negative.

Negative feedback can be illustrated by looking at the hormone, insulin. The mechanism is 'negative' because it reverses the change in blood sugar.

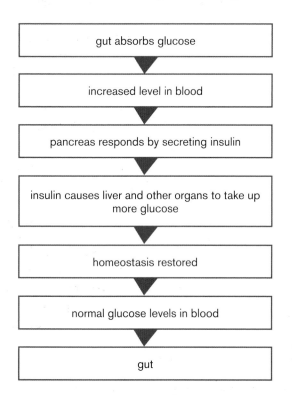

gut absorbs glucose

↓

increased level in blood

↓

pancreas responds by secreting insulin

↓

insulin causes liver and other organs to take up more glucose

↓

homeostasis restored

↓

normal glucose levels in blood

↓

gut

Positive feedback systems are rare, but they are 'positive' because they increase the changes, rather than reversing them. An example would be the control of oxytocin during labour, when contractions need to increase in order to push the baby out.

The digestive system

This is the system that takes in food and breaks it down into tiny **molecules**, which can then pass into the blood and on to all cells of the body. The cells can then generate energy, which enables our bodies to work (*see also* Cells and tissues, *page 167*). Waste is produced which is then passed out of the body – a process called elimination.

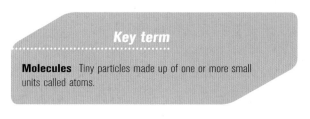

The digestive system consists of a series of hollow tubes, stretching from the mouth to the anus. There are associated organs *en route*, which either mechanically break food down or produce secretions to help with the chemical breakdown and absorption of the nutrients.

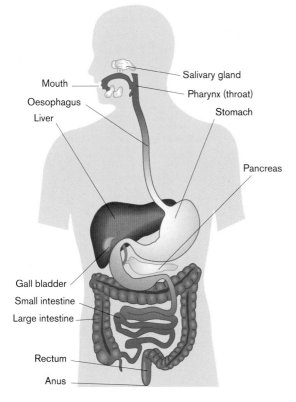

The digestive system.

Structure of the intestine

The structure of the different parts of the intestine varies slightly but in general it contains:

- **peritoneal covering (serous membrane)** single layer of squamous epithelium with underlying areolar connective tissue

- **muscle layers** (varies from one to three layers) – skeletal muscle in mouth, pharynx and upper part of oesophagus

- **submucosal layer** – areolar connective tissue

- **mucosa** – mucus membrane (epithelial), areolar connective tissue, thin layer of smooth muscle.

See also Cells and tissues, *page 167.*

Three kinds of processing occur within the system: digestion, absorption and metabolism.

Key term

Enzymes A chemical which controls reactions in cells, frequently speeding them up.

- **Digestion** of foodstuff is both mechanical (such as chewing and gut movement) and chemical, through the action of **enzymes** (chemicals which change and increase reactions).
- **Absorption** is the movement of the molecules through the wall of the tract and into the surrounding blood vessels.
- **Metabolism** is the cellular activity where food molecules are used to produce energy for cellular activity.

The digestive process

Food is taken in at the mouth, where teeth break it into smaller portions before it is swallowed. When food enters the oral cavity, saliva is produced by three pairs of glands in the oral cavity. The saliva, which contains the digestive enzyme **ptyalin**, mixes with the masticated food and chemical digestion starts, converting starch to maltose. The mixture then passes down the oesophagus into the stomach.

The stomach is situated just under the diaphragm; it is an expanded area of the tube, which acts as a reservoir for food. Hydrochloric acid produced by the cells in stomach mucosa converts the enzyme **pepsinogen** to **pepsin**, which can partially digest proteins. The acid also kills any ingested bacteria. The stomach muscle has three layers so it can mix and churn the contents, now known as chyme, to digest them further. A thick fluid called mucus lines the stomach, protecting it from the acid and mechanical damage.

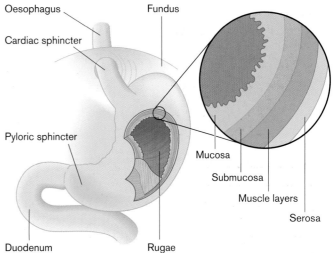

The stomach, showing the structure of the walls and lining.

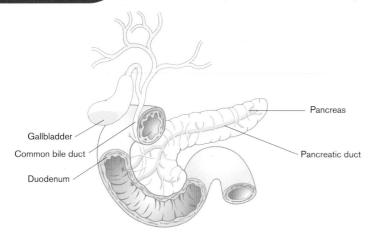

The pancreas, gall bladder, duodenum and liver.

The stomach produces a protein called the intrinsic factor, which enables the absorption of vitamin B12 – an essential vitamin for red cell production. A lack of vitamin B12 causes a particular type of **anaemia**.

> ### Key term
>
> **Anaemia** A condition when there is lack of red cells or haemoglobin, the substance that carries oxygen round the body.

Bile enters the duodenum at the common bile duct and breaks fats into smaller droplets (or 'emulsifies' them).

The pancreatic duct enters at the same point and delivers pancreatic juice. This juice contains the following types of enzyme, which digest proteins, carbohydrates and fats.

- **Three protease enzymes:** When activated from **trypsin**, these complete the digestion of proteins. They are converted into amino acids, which can then be absorbed into the blood. Further enzymes in intestinal juice will continue to digest any remaining undigested proteins.

- **Lipases:** These then digest the emulsified fats, converting them to fatty acids and glycerol. Fatty acids and glycerol can diffuse into the cells of the intestine, and are secreted into the vessels of the lymphatic system (see page 211), eventually joining the blood as it circulates to all tissues.
- **Amylase:** This converts carbohydrates into maltose. Maltose is digested further along the intestine.

The intestinal mucosa produce the last secretions to complete digestion:

- **peptidases** which convert peptides to amino acids
- **sucrase** which works on sucrose, converting it to the simple sugars, glucose and galactose
- **maltase** which converts maltose to glucose.

The activation of enzymes depends on the acid/alkaline levels (pH) of the body fluids and cells.

Mechanical digestion in the small intestine helps to mix the enzymes and the chyme together. Circular and longitudinal muscle fibres contract alternately, squeezing the chyme along the tract in a regular, continuous way (this process is known as segmentation and peristalsis).

Absorption

The table below shows you where in the digestive tract different substances are absorbed.

The two main organs associated with absorption are the pancreas and the liver.

The **pancreas** is both an endocrine and an exocrine gland. Pancreatic enzymes are produced in small clusters of cells called acini, which make up 99 per cent of the glandular tissue. The remaining cells produce insulin and glucagons,

Mouth	Stomach	Small intestine	Large intestine
	Water	Water	Water
		Amino acids	
Simple sugars	Simple sugars	Monosacharides (Simple sugars)	
	Minerals	Minerals	Small amounts minerals
	Water-soluble vitamins	Vitamins	Some vitamins
	Drugs e.g. aspirin and alcohol	Drugs and alcohol	Some drugs
		Lipids (fatty acids and glycerol)	

which are absorbed straight into the bloodstream (endocrine) (*see* The endocrine system, *on page 191*). Insulin plays a vital role in the use and storage of glucose.

Pancreatic juice is slightly alkaline and buffers the acid in chyme, stopping the pepsin from the stomach from working.

The liver is a large gland to the right of the stomach. As blood flows through it, the cells take up oxygen, nutrients and toxins, and produce bile. The sodium and potassium salts that form a major part of bile play a key role in emulsifying fats. The pigments which give bile its colour are formed from the broken-down red cell component, haemoglobin. It is one of the pigments, stercobilin, which gives faeces their normal brown colour.

As well as excreting bilirubin, the liver also:
- helps to maintain blood glucose levels
- breaks down some fats
- converts excess protein to amino acids and urea
- makes plasma proteins
- processes drugs and hormones
- stores glycogen, vitamins A, B12, D, E and K, as well as the minerals, iron and copper
- breaks down some bacteria, and aged red and white cells
- activates Vitamin D.

All this activity means the liver produces a great deal of heat, which contributes to maintaining body core temperature.

Some people may produce an excess of cholesterol – too much for the bile salts to cope with. In these instances, the salts may crystallise, creating gallstones which can obstruct the bile duct. Having gallstones is often debilitating, and may require surgery.

Did you know?

Damage to the liver can make it harden and fail to work. This is known as cirrhosis – a condition that is often caused by drinking too much alcohol.

Activity

Find out what the signs and symptoms are when someone is suffering from gallstones.

At the end of the gastro-intestinal tract, the waste is expelled as faeces, which consists of mainly undigested materials – cellulose, pigments, water, inorganic salts, dead epithelial cells and bacteria. The consistency depends on the type of foods in the diet, the intake of fluids and the **motility** of the gut. Constipation is a common problem as people age and fail to eat a diet high in fibre. As practitioners you may be required to observe the consistency of patients' faeces (stools).

Key term

Motility How well something can move and be active.

Bristol Stool Chart				
Type 1	Separate hard lumps. like nuts (hard to pass)		Type 5	Soft blobs with clear-cut edges (passed easily)
Type 2	Sausage-shaped but lumpy		Type 6	Fluffy pieces with ragged edges, a mushy stool
Type 3	Like a sausage but with cracks on its surface		Type 7	Watery, no solid pieces Entirely liquid.
Type 4	Like a sausage or snake, smooth and soft			

The Bristol Stool Chart helps you to report accurately on the texture of faeces.

Homeostasis

Homeostasis means 'steady body state', and it is essential in all systems of the body for survival. Conditions must be constant – and this includes concentrations of water and salts, fluid volumes, temperature, acid/alkaline levels (pH), cell numbers, hormone and enzyme levels.

Much of the control happens by way of feedback mechanisms and an example has been given in the control of hormones within the endocrine system (see page 191).

The excretory system

In order to function all the body cells use nutrients taken in as food and oxygen. The result will provide energy and waste products e.g. carbon dioxide, some electrolytes, excess water, by products of digestion. These need to be expelled from the body otherwise toxins would build up impairing body functions.

A number of systems work together in order to maintain the balance required (homeostasis). Two of these systems have already been mentioned.

- The digestive system – (see page 194)
- The skin or integumentory system – (see page 174)
- Respiratory system – (see page 213)
- The urinary system

The urinary system

The functions of the urinary system are as follows.

- Filters blood and excrete wastes, such as urea and drugs.
- Regulates blood volume by preserving or secreting water.
- Regulates composition of blood by preserving or excreting substances like sodium, potassium, calcium, phosphate and chloride.
- Regulates blood pressure.
- Produces hormones – Calcitrol (an active form of Vitamin D, and erythropoietin (stimulates red cell production).
- Regulates blood glucose levels – uses amino acids to synthesise glucose molecules.
- Regulates blood pH – excretes hydrogen ions and conserves bicarbonate ions.
- Excretes waste substances.

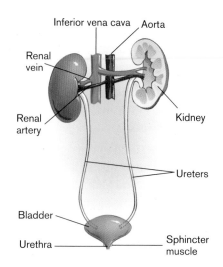

The renal system.

The primary organs of this system are the kidneys. They are positioned behind the peritoneum on either side of the spine and are protected by lower ribs and muscle.

Key term

Peritoneum A serous membrane which covers the digestive organs and the upper surface of the female uterus and is reflected back to line the wall of the abdominal cavity. This forms a double layer with a small amount of fluid between the layers allowing easy movement.

The functioning units of the kidney are microscopic structures called nephrons, of which there are more than a million in each one. It appears like a tiny funnel with a long twisted tube.

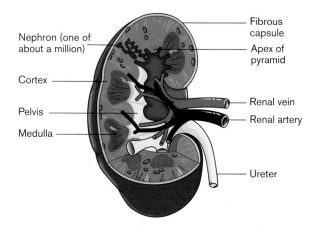

Cross-section of a kidney.

Blood enters the expanded portion of the Bowman's Capsule via a branch of the renal artery. This structure enables filtration under pressure.

The arterial capillaries form a network within the capsule, and then unite to leave the capsule and wind around the tubule loops. The capillary is termed the afferent vessel as it enters, and the efferent as it leaves. Blood enters under pressure and results in waste being filtered from the blood. The fluid is referred to as glomerular filtrate and the process, **filtration**.

Glomerular filtrate passes into the first part of the tubule, the proximal convoluted tubule and here reabsorption of water, glucose, various ions and amino acids take place. This means these molecules move from the tubule back into the surrounding capillaries and ensures that in healthy individuals, essential substances are not lost. The process is known as **selective reabsorption**.

Fluid then moves into a loop of the tubule which dips down into the medulla (deep tissue of the kidney) and is known as the loop of Henle. Because of the structure and length of the tubule at this point, the concentration of the urine is controlled by selective reabsorption which

continues in the collecting duct. Only those substances which are needed by the body are absorbed.

When kidney filtration is severely impaired, it is possible to use a machine or 'artificial kidney' to do this job. Its correct name is renal dialysis or haemodialysis.

The end product is urine which then passes into the pelvis of the kidney, flows down the ureters and into the bladder where it is stored until convenient to expel.

Urine will vary in acidity, concentration and content depending on the needs of the body, the state of health, diet and any medications taken.

All patients will have their urine tested at some point in their treatment. You will be able to monitor the amount of water and other substances in solution and this may allow ill health to be recognised and treated.

Urine moves into the bladder via the ureters. Movement is assisted by waves of muscular contraction. Urine is prevented from passing back up the ureters because they enter at an angle and as the bladder stretches the muscular wall blocks the exit.

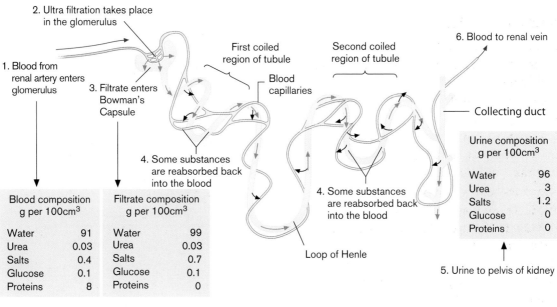

2. Ultra filtration takes place in the glomerulus

1. Blood from renal artery enters glomerulus

3. Filtrate enters Bowman's Capsule

First coiled region of tubule

Second coiled region of tubule

6. Blood to renal vein

Blood capillaries

Collecting duct

4. Some substances are reabsorbed back into the blood

4. Some substances are reabsorbed back into the blood

Loop of Henle

5. Urine to pelvis of kidney

Blood composition g per 100cm^3	
Water	91
Urea	0.03
Salts	0.4
Glucose	0.1
Proteins	8

Filtrate composition g per 100cm^3	
Water	99
Urea	0.03
Salts	0.7
Glucose	0.1
Proteins	0

Urine composition g per 100cm^3	
Water	96
Urea	3
Salts	1.2
Glucose	0
Proteins	0

Filtration under pressure.   *Selective reabsorption.*   *Active secretion.*

The bladder is a muscular bag, which can hold up to 500 ml of urine. The base is fixed behind the symphysis pubis (front of the hip bone) but as it fills with urine it expands up into the abdominal cavity.

In males, the urethra is also involved in the reproductive system. The urethra passes through the prostate gland and finally through the penis – a distance of 15-20 cm. The prostate and several other glands deliver secretions into the urethra during sexual arousal, but sphincter muscles around the bladder neck close at this time so that urination does not occur.

Activity

Explain the tests you might routinely carry out on a urine specimen and say what they mean. Find out how the urinary tract is affected by ageing. Why are urinary infections more common as we grow older? Why might stones form in the kidneys? Find out how dialysis works and relate it to natural kidney functioning.

Blood and the cardiovascular system

In this section, you will look at how materials are transported around the body, the composition of those materials and their functions.

Blood and lymph are the fluids that do two jobs: they carry the materials cells need if they are to work, and they carry away the wastes the cells produce.

When circulating, blood is contained in a series of vessels. A pump – the heart – provides the power to move the fluid round the body.

Blood

Blood is a connective tissue (*see also* Cells and tissues *on page 167*), composed of a liquid matrix, plasma which contains a variety of cells, nutrients and gases.

All cells and tissues are bathed in a fluid called interstitial fluid (or tissue fluid). Everything needed for cellular activity diffuses out of the blood and into interstitial fluid and then into the cells. Similarly, the waste materials produced by the cells are able to diffuse in the opposite direction into the blood. These waste products can then be transported to organs which will remove them from the body (*see also* Excretory systems *on page 198 and* The respiratory system *on page 213*).

Functions of blood

Regulation	Transportation	Protection
Maintains water balance	Transports oxygen and carbon dioxide	Various blood elements interact to allow clotting which protects against loss of blood (Haemorrhage) following injury
Regulates acid/base balance (pH)	Carries nutrients from GI tract to cells	White cells protect against disease by phagocytosis (engulfing foreign cells and breaking them down)
Assists in temperature regulation	Carries hormones and enzymes to cells to regulate function	Various types of blood proteins and antibodies also protect against disease
	Transports heat and waste products to lungs, kidneys and skin for elimination	

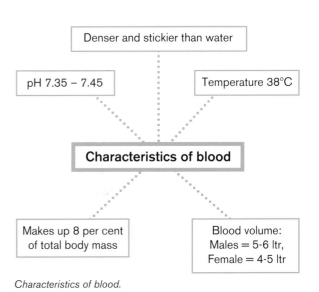

Characteristics of blood.

Structure of blood

Plasma 55%		Functions
Water	91.5%	
Proteins	7% = Albumins 54% Globulins 38% Fibrinogen 7% All others 1%	Maintain osmotic pressure
Other solutes	Electrolytes	Maintain cell function and fluid compartment integrity.
	Nutrients	Cell growth and function.
	Gases	As above
	Regulatory substances (hormones, enzymes)	Cell activity
	Waste products	Allows removal and reduce toxicity
Cells 45%		
Red cells or erythrocytes		
White cells or leukocytes		
Platelets		

55%
Plasma

45%
Blood cells

The structure of blood.

Patients will frequently need to have their blood tested to ensure that all cells and fluids are at normal working levels.

Formed elements in blood

Erythrocytes or red blood cells (RBCs)
All blood cells are produced in red bone marrow in the centre of long and flat bones from stem cells.

Erythrocytes, or red blood cells, are shaped rather like doughnuts with a thin central area and contain a protein called haemoglobin. This gives the cell its red colour. The function of this protein is to carry oxygen and, to a lesser extent CO_2. Oxygen is transported by red cells from the lungs to all tissues and CO_2 from tissues to lungs for excretion. The shape provides a huge surface area for the exchange of gases between blood and body cells. It has no nucleus and therefore is unable to repair or divide to form more cells. The lifespan is about 120 days but they are replaced constantly. Worn-out or damaged cells are removed from circulation and broken down by specialised cells in the spleen and liver. Breakdown products are recycled to form more cells and haemoglobin. The waste materials are excreted in urine and faeces.

Reduced oxygen carriage is referred to as anaemia and may be due to lack of either haemoglobin or red cells.

Activity
Find out and document how anaemia might occur and what treatment may be given. Why might Sickle Cell anaemia lead to symptoms in those who are affected by the disease?

Leucocytes or white blood cells (WBCs)
These vary in shape, size and function, but they all have a nucleus and are produced in red bone marrow. They are divided into two groups: granular leucocytes and agranular leucocytes. Leucopoenia is the correct term for an abnormally low WBC count.

Activity
What diseases might cause leucopaenia and what effects might this have on a patient? Are there conditions that might result in an increase in WBCs?

Classification of granulocytes

Granulocytes		Function
Neutrophils	Neutrophill	Neutrophils in the blood squeeze through the capillary walls and move into infected tissue. They kill invaders such as bacteria; they then eat the remnants.
Basophils	Basophill	The number of basophils increases during times of infection in the body. Basophils leave the blood and accumulate at the site of infection or where they are needed. They release substances such as **histamine**, which increases the blood flow to the area.
Eosinophils	Eosinophill	The number of eosinophils in the blood is normally quite low. However, numbers increase sharply if certain diseases are present, such as asthma, eczema or parasitic infections. Eosinophils are toxic to cells (cytotooxic); they release substances to attack invader cells.

Classification of agranular leucocytes

Agranular leucocytes		Function
Lymphocytes	Lymphocyte	There are several kinds of lymphocytes, each with different functions to perform. The most common types of lymphocytes are: • *B-cells*: these are responsible for making antibodies • *T-cells*: these are concerned with defending the body from viruses and other types of infection.

Classification of granulocytes and agranular leucocytes.

Thrombocytes or platelets

These third type of formed elements are tiny cell fragments, which contain many vesicles and do not have a nucleus. They are essential in clotting: the vesicles contain clotting factors and enzymes that make the platelets stick together.

These platelets start the clotting process, which is continued through a chain of clotting factors in plasma, labelled using a roman numeral. When the smooth muscle in the blood vessels contracts and the vessel narrows (a process called vasoconstriction), a clot can form.

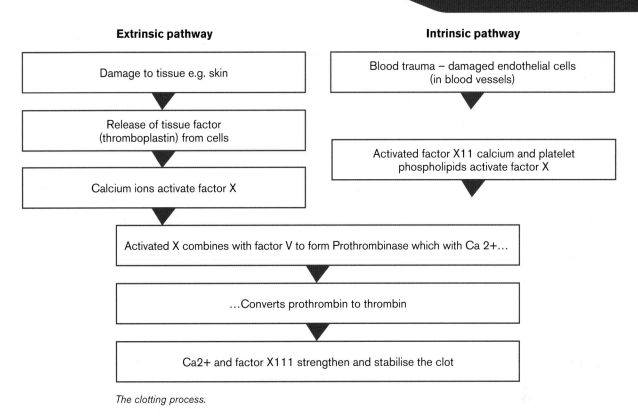

The clotting process.

The clotting process

There are two ways in which the clotting process starts, but they share a common pathway at the end.

From this flow chart, you can see that each of the substances affects another factor – like a 'domino effect' – eventually resulting in a clot to prevent further blood loss. Some people may be missing one or more of the factors involved which will result in an increased tendency to bleed (haemophilia).

On completion of the process, clot retraction occurs, where there is tightening of the fibrin threads. In time the healing process repairs the vessel lining or the tissue which has been damaged. *See also* Wound healing *on page 259*.

Normal clotting is dependent on adequate Vitamin K, as it is required for synthesis of four clotting factors by liver cells. Vitamin K is normally produced by the action of bacteria in the large intestine and is absorbed with lipids (fat soluble). *See also* The digestive system *on page 194*.

Activity

Why might inadequate release of bile result in problems with clotting?

Why does clotting not occur in blood vessels in a healthy body?

What might be prescribed to slow the clotting process in patients who have suffered a stroke or heart attack? Document how the medication you identify works.

Blood types

A blood transfusion can be a life-saving intervention. However, there are major factors to consider to ensure the transfusion is as safe as possible.

Remember: when you are putting in materials, primarily proteins, which are not the individual's own, it is a transplant. This means there is always a risk of a major reaction, which can be fatal. To make sure the patient is receiving blood from their own blood group, you must take a blood sample, which is used to identify the specific blood type.

Antigens

Blood types are identified by **antigens**, which may be situated on the outside of the RBC membrane. They are primarily protein compounds, which have an area on their membranes which will allow specific antibodies to attach.

> ### Key term
>
> **Antigen** A molecule, or part of a molecule, that is detected by the body immune system as 'foreign'. An antibody is produced in response, which will react with that antigen.

There are many different sorts of antigen, but a small number are very reactive and must be identified. An antigen can trigger the immune system to respond in a variety of ways, one of which is to produce antibodies. Many antibodies react with a specific antigen to cause 'agglutination': they attach to the foreign antigen, and stick together in clusters, which are then broken down.

We use the ABO system to group individuals' blood. The antigens are A and B, and this illustration shows how they may be present.

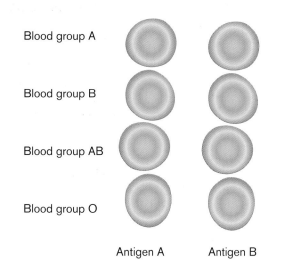

Blood group A

Blood group B

Blood group AB

Blood group O

Antigen A   Antigen B

Antigens in blood groups.

The rhesus factor

There may be one other antigen present on the red cell that can cause major reactions. This is D, or the rhesus factor. If it is present, you are identified as 'rhesus positive'; if it is not, you are 'rhesus negative'.

Plasma never naturally contains anti-rhesus antibodies, but if rhesus positive cells are introduced into a rhesus negative person's circulation, rhesus antibodies will develop. If positive cells continue to be transfused, at this time or in the future, the antibodies will react with the rhesus antigens, will agglutinate the incoming cells and cause a major reaction.

Women are most at risk, as if a mother is rhesus negative and has a rhesus positive partner, their child could inherit the positive antigen. If the woman bleeds from the placenta at any point in the pregnancy, red cells can pass back into the mother – which is just like transfusing her with rhesus positive cells. The woman will develop antibodies that could, in a future pregnancy, pass into the foetus' circulation. If the new foetus is rhesus positive the mother's rhesus D antibodies will start to break down the foetus' red cells. The foetus will be badly affected, and may die before birth or be born severely damaged. This is why a woman's blood group and rhesus antibodies are monitored carefully throughout her pregnancy.

In an emergency, where the blood group is unknown, O rhesus negative blood is used: because it lacks antigens on the cell membrane, it can only cause limited reactions. However, it is always best to provide blood of the patient's own group which has been screened for antibodies and infectious organisms.

> ### Activity
>
> Find out how women may be protected from reactions occurring as a result of RhD antibody formation.

Blood group	Antigens present	Antibodies present in plasma	Can donate to	Can receive from	Proportion in UK population
A	A	Anti-B	A, AB	A, O	Rh + ve = 85%
B	B	Anti-A	B, AB	B, O	
AB	AB	None	AB	A, B, AB, O	Rh − ve = 15%
O	None	Anti-A and B	A, B, AB, O	O	

The cardiovascular system

The heart and the blood vessels together are called the cardiovascular system.

Blood vessels

Blood is pumped from the heart through a series of tubes known as arteries. The larger ones close to the heart are elastic, to enable them to stretch when pressure is great. These larger arteries divide into medium-sized, muscular arteries, which continue to branch into small arteries, and then arterioles and finally capillaries. The capillaries gradually unite to form larger vessels, known as venules and veins, which convey blood back to the heart. Blood is then pumped to the lungs, where exchange of gases takes place.

All blood vessels are similar in structure, but have certain differences – these can be seen in the diagram below.

Arteries

Elastic arteries have a high proportion of elastic fibres in their walls, which are relatively thin. The heart contracts and, as the blood passes into the arteries, they stretch. The heart then relaxes, and the arteries recoil. This action propels the blood forward, even though the heart is resting.

Blood then moves on into smaller arteries and arterioles, which contain increasingly large proportions of muscle (rather than elastic fibre) in their walls. This muscle is well supplied with sympathetic nerve fibres (*see* The nervous system *on page 185*), which enables the artery to constrict (a process called vasoconstriction).

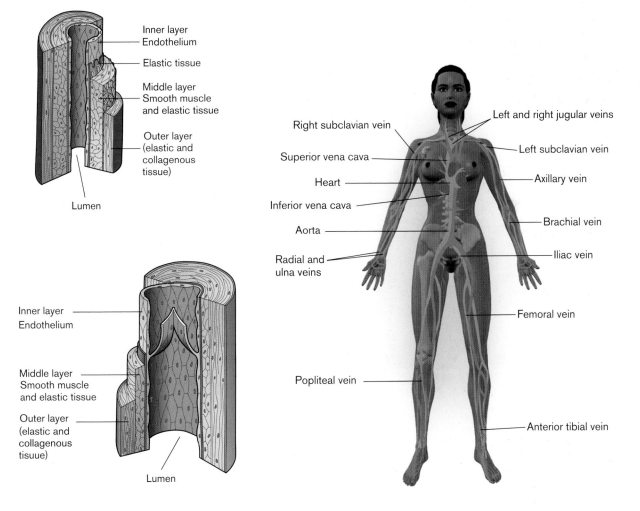

Arteries and veins have both similarities and differences.

The major arteries of the body.

Arterioles

Arterioles deliver blood to the capillaries. As the arterioles branch and get closer to the capillaries, all their layers get thinner, although some muscle fibres are always present. Arterioles are key in regulating blood flow into the capillaries. They do this by narrowing or widening, depending on the needs of various tissues. This is what you can observe when a patient's blood pressure changes.

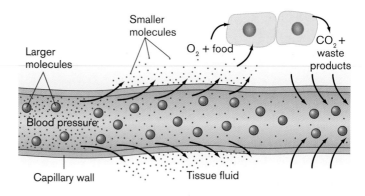

Capillary exchange.

Capillaries

Capillaries are found close to all tissues but the numbers making up the network varies, depending on how active the tissue is. So there are large networks in muscle, liver, kidney and the nervous system.

Some tissues lack blood vessels e.g. cornea and lens of the eye.

They are just one cell thick and are semi-permeable. This allows fluid, salts, gases and nutrients to pass through into cells and waste from the cell to pass back into the capillary. Some fluids, white cells and waste do remain in the tissue fluid surrounding all cells and if there is excess this will drain into lymphatic capillaries and eventually be returned to the blood.

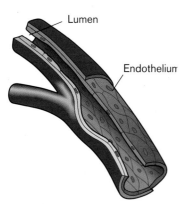

The structure of a capillary.

Here are some factors that affect the movement of substances through the capillary wall.

- **Diffusion** When substances such as oxygen and nutrients are present in high concentrations in blood, they can diffuse through the capillary wall to an area of lower concentration. So when O_2 concentration is lower in the tissues and higher in the capillary, it passes into the tissues; when CO_2 is higher in the tissues and lower in the capillary, it moves into the capillary.

- **Hydrostatic pressure** This is the pressure of the water in blood pushing against the vessel wall. Pressure is higher at the arterial end of the vessels, and this enables fluid to be 'pushed' into **interstitial** fluid.

> ### Key term
> **Interstitial** Similar to plasma but lacking large proteins.

- **Osmotic pressure** Plasma proteins in the blood also exert pressure. This is what 'pulls' fluid from the interstitial fluid back into the capillaries.

The circulatory system

The heart is the body's pump, providing the power to circulate blood to all its cells of the body. It is a cone-shaped, hollow organ, roughly the size of a closed fist. It is located near the midline of the chest (thoracic cavity), in the cavity between the lungs (the mediastinum): the sternum is in front, the vertebral bodies behind. The heart lies on its side, resting on the diaphragm (see The respiratory system on page 213).

The heart pumps blood through a 'double circulatory system'. One part of this is the system supplying the body, and the other part is the lungs.

The pericardium is the tissue which covers, protects and anchors the heart. It is formed of two main parts: the fibrous and the serous pericardium.

- **Fibrous pericardium** This is a tough, inelastic bag, the open end being fused to the outer connective tissue of the blood vessels leaving the heart. It prevents over-distension of the heart.
- **Serous pericardium** This is a thinner, more delicate double membrane. The outer layer is fused to the fibrous layer, while the inner layer sticks closely to the heart. Between the layers is a thin film of serous fluid, which reduces friction between the membranes as the heart moves.

The wall of the heart is composed of three layers.

- The **epicardium** is the inner layer of the pericardium, with a thin, transparent, smooth surface.

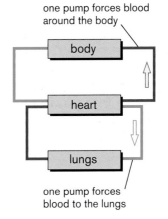

one pump forces blood around the body

body

heart

lungs

one pump forces blood to the lungs

The double circulatory system.

- The **myocardium** is the cardiac muscle tissue that makes up most of the heart, and is is specially adapted to contract independently.
- The **endocardium** is the innermost tissue, and consists of endothelial cells. It provides a smooth lining, continuous with the lining of the blood vessels, and forms the valves.

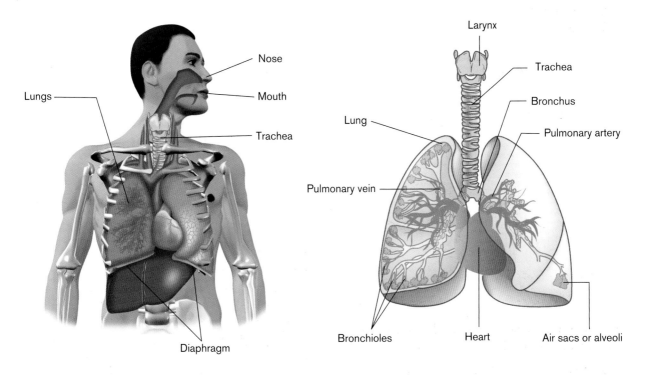

The respiratory system.

Lungs — Nose — Mouth — Trachea — Diaphragm

Larynx — Trachea — Bronchus — Pulmonary artery — Lung — Pulmonary vein — Bronchioles — Heart — Air sacs or alveoli

The cavity of the heart has four chambers. wA central septum divides the left from the right, and each side is divided in two. The upper two chambers are the atria and the lower the ventricles. The upper chambers contract together, followed by the lower ones. Valves control the flow of blood between the upper and lower chambers and also from the main vessels, supplying blood to the lungs and the body.

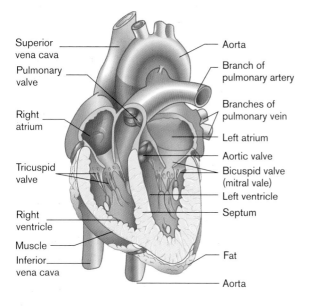

The structure of the heart.

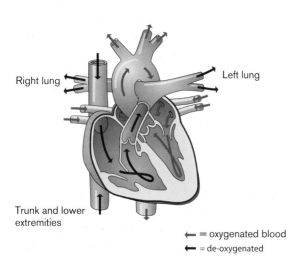

← = oxygenated blood
← = de-oxygenated

The cardiac cycle.

How circulation works

This is the sequence of events when blood is pumped round the body.

1. Blood from the lower body and the head and neck, enters the right side of the heart via the superior and inferior vena cava. This blood has low levels of O_2 and high levels of CO_2.

2. As the right side of the heart fills and the pressure rises, the atrioventricular valves open, the atria contract, and blood is pumped into the ventricles.

3. The ventricles contract, and blood is forced out into the pulmonary arteries and on into the lungs, where gases are exchanged. *See also* The respiratory system *on page 213*.

4. Blood returns from the lungs, via the pulmonary veins, and enters the left atrium. It is now high in O_2.

5. As pressure rises, the bicuspid valve opens, the atria contract and blood is pumped into the aorta, which branches to supply all body tissues.

Note: the atria fill at the same time and then contract, followed by the ventricles so that the pulmonary and systemic circulations work simultaneously.

How the heart works

The heart has a specialised network of cardiac fibres originating from two sites, which are the source of electrical stimulation for the cardiac muscle. They can generate the impulses that cause contraction themselves.

The sinoatrial (SA) node is situated in the wall of the right atrium, below the opening of the superior vena cava; the atrioventricular (AV) node is located in the septum between the two atria.

When the atrioventricular node fires, an impulse or 'action potential' moves across the heart muscle, causing the atria to contract, then the ventricles.

Did you know?

The contracting of the atria is what you can see happening on an electrocardigram. An ECG can be used to assist in diagnosing damage or disease in the heart.

When the heart rate is 75 beats minute, a cardiac cycle lasts 0.8 seconds.

When the atria and ventricles contract, it is called a systole; when they relax, it is called a diastole. Relaxation lasts about 0.4 seconds but, as the heart rate increases, the relaxation period gets shorter.

As the heart beats and blood is pumped into the arteries, there is a regular wave of contraction followed by a wave of relaxation. This can be felt at points where an artery comes close to the surface, usually over a bony prominence. This pulse is strongest nearer to the heart.

Remember

Recording the pulse rate is one of the ways you can assess normal cardiovascular functioning. A patient's heart rate varies depending on their age, level of activity, anxiety, and state of heath.

The heart muscle is supplied with blood from vessels that are the first branches of the main artery – the aorta. If these become narrowed or blocked, the myocardium is deprived of oxygen and nutrients, and this causes pain. The affected myocardium dies and it cannot regenerate, so the functioning of the heart is permanently affected. This is called a heart attack or myocardial infarction.

Activity

Take your own pulse. Now run up a flight of stairs or perform ten jumping jacks. Take your pulse again. What changes do you notice?

Control of cardiac output

As you've seen, the heart generates its own impulse. To maintain body function, this impulse must be regular, yet it must also respond according to increased demand – for example, when you run.

The heart rate is maintained and regulated by both the nervous system and chemicals in the body. In the brain stem, there is an area called the medulla oblongata. This area holds the cardiovascular centre, which can increase or decrease the frequency of impulses in the sympathetic and parasympathetic branches of the ANS.

Blood pressure

As a health care assistant, you will have to monitor your patients' blood pressure often: blood pressure can tell you a lot about the patients' health, the amount of exercise they are doing and the levels of stress they are experiencing.

Blood pressure is the pressure exerted by the blood as it flows through the vessels. Pressure is higher in arteries, and lower in veins. In the arteries, the pressure reaches its maximum when the heart contracts (systole), and drops to a minimum when it is relaxing (diastole).

The pressures are then expressed as one recording – the systolic over the diastolic: for example 120/80, or 'one-twenty over eighty'. *See also* Physiological measurements *on page 291.*

Factors affecting blood pressure

The levels of someone's blood pressure depend on a number of factors.

- **The blood volume** The greater the volume, the higher the pressure. When someone has a haemorrhage, the volume drops and so does pressure. The volume of blood in the arteries is determined by the amount of blood pumped into the arteries, and how much is then drained into the arterioles.
- **The strength of heart contractions** The strength and rate of the heartbeat affects cardiac output, and therefore blood pressure. The amount of blood pushed out on each ventricular contraction is called the stroke volume. The stronger the contraction, the greater the stroke volume (blood pressure is greater); the weaker the contraction, the smaller the stroke volume (blood pressure is lower).
- **Peripheral resistance** Blood flow – and therefore blood pressure – is maintained because the capillaries are so tiny. The diameter of the arterioles is a key factor in determining how much blood drains from these two types of vessels.
- **Blood vessel lumen (diameter of the tube)** If the tubes are large, the pressure falls.

Think about what happens when you squeeze a hosepipe that is turned on. The force with which the water flows out is increased. So for example, the aorta stretches as pressure rises, and then recoils, making the blood move on continuously. This elasticity is an important factor in maintaining homeostasis.

- **Heart rate** As the heart rate increases, the amount of blood entering the aorta increases, as does the arterial blood volume – and the blood pressure. This is only true as long as the stroke volume does not decrease sharply, which it may do if there is insufficient time for ventricular filling.
- **Blood viscosity (stickiness or thickness of the blood)** If a patient has a haemorrhage, fluid from the interstitial spaces moves into the blood and it becomes diluted. As the blood is less viscous (thinner) the blood pressure falls. If there is an increase in red cell numbers (polycythemia), the blood becomes thicker, and blood pressure increases.

To respond to changing circumstances, blood flow is shunted from one area to another, so your blood pressure is changing constantly. It increases to transport more O_2 and nutrients to tissues which are increasing in activity – for example, your muscles when you exercise.

- Blood pressure also varies according to:
  - your state of health
  - your level of activity
  - your age
  - your body size
  - alcohol and drugs used
  - your stress levels
  - the time of day (diurnal variation)
  - when you have eaten.

Range of blood pressure

The range of blood pressure	Measurement
Low	90/60 or less
Normal	120/80 or less
Mild	140/90 or less
Moderate	160/100 or higher up to
Severe	180/110 or higher up to
Crisis	210/120 or higher

Pressure in the venous system is low in the large vessels, and falls to almost nil by the time blood returns to the heart from the cells of the body. When it enters the right atrium it is termed the central venous pressure and is important because it affects the pressure in the large peripheral veins. If the heart fails, central venous pressure rises and flow into the right atrium is slowed.

A number of mechanisms help to keep venous blood moving back to the right side of the heart:

- the continuous heartbeat
- adequate arterial pressure, which moves blood on into the venous system
- contraction of skeletal muscle, which squeezes the veins running through them and so moves blood forward
- valves within the veins that prevent backflow
- changes of pressure in the thoracic cavity when breathing occurs: this causes a further pumping action, which encourages the movement of venous blood back towards the heart.

Activity

Why does blood pressure increase in the condition of arteriosclerosis? Why might someone suffer from angina? What symptoms might the patient complain of if they had heart failure?

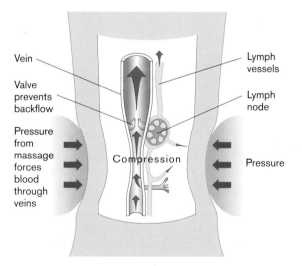

Massage assists blood flow back to the heart (venous return), helping with the removal of waste products from the body.

The lymphatic and immune system

The lymphatic system drains and recycles excess fluid, protein and fat, removes waste, and helps to protect the body from infection. It works with the cardiovascular system so that fluids from the tissue spaces are returned to the blood (*see* The circulatory system *on the previous pages*).
The lymphatic system consists of:

- fluid – lymph
- capillaries
- vessels
- tissues
- nodes.

The lymphatic system is different from the circulatory system in a number of ways. This table summarises the differences and similarities.

Circulatory system	Lymphatic system
Continuous series of tubes which branch into small vessels, and then unite to form a circular system	Blind-ended tubes in tissue spaces, uniting to form larger vessels but not forming a circular pathway
Has a pump, the heart, which drives fluid round the system, but relies also on pressure within body to aid venous return	Has no pump. Flow relies on pressure within the body cavities (breathing and blood pressure)
Contains blood	Contains lymph
Smallest vessels are microscopic, formed of squamous epithelium, the cells of which fit tightly together.	Similar microscopic vessels of squamous epithelium, but cells are a looser fit so that larger molecules can move into them from tissue spaces. Special vessels in large intestine allow movement of molecules of fat onto the lymph for transportation
	Contains lymphatic tissue-forming organs through which lymph is filtered – nodes, thymus, spleen, tonsils
White cells contained in blood play a protective roll	Lymphoid tissue plays a protective role as lymph is filtered. Lymphoid tissue contains phagocytic white cells
Veins contain valves to prevent backflow	Lymphatic vessels also contain valves

Lymph

Lymph is usually a clear or milky colour, depending on which areas of the body it has drained from.
It contains:

- water
- protein
- white cells, such as lymphocytes
- waste materials.

It may also contain:

- foreign bodies
- bacteria and viruses
- fat molecules.

Its main purpose is to act as a transport medium and to defend the body against infection. The white cells carried in lymph produce **antibodies** that destroy foreign cells, and also engulf dangerous organisms (phagocytes) and allow them to be removed from the body.

> ### Key term
>
> **Antibodies** Particular proteins that can lock on to foreign or diseased molecules and make them harmless or enable them to be destroyed by white cells in the body.

> ### Did you know?
>
> It is possible to give someone antibodies that will protect them from a particular infection. This is known as passive immunity.

Lymphatic capillaries

These are blind ended minute tubes, similar to blood capillaries but they are formed of overlapping cells which allow larger molecules to pass through from the tissue spaces. They are said to be more permeable.

Lymph vessels

The lymphatic capillaries unite to form vessels that are similar to veins but wider, with many more valves. The vessels flow through specialised lymphatic tissue called nodes. They eventually unite to form two final vessels: the right lymphatic and the thoracic duct.

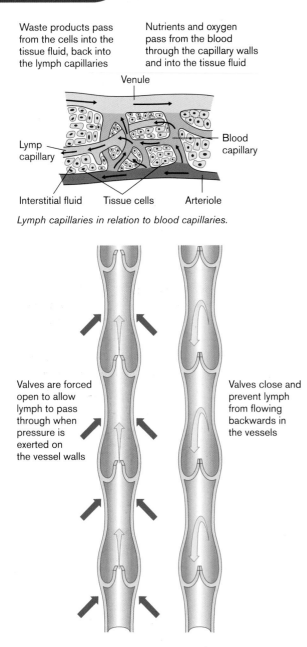

Waste products pass from the cells into the tissue fluid, back into the lymph capillaries

Nutrients and oxygen pass from the blood through the capillary walls and into the tissue fluid

Venule

Blood capillary

Lymp capillary

Interstitial fluid   Tissue cells   Arteriole

Lymph capillaries in relation to blood capillaries.

Valves are forced open to allow lymph to pass through when pressure is exerted on the vessel walls

Valves close and prevent lymph from flowing backwards in the vessels

The flow of lymph fluid through lymph vessels. When pressure is exerted on the vessel walls, valves are forced open to allow lymph to pass through. The valves close to prevent the backflow of lymph in the vessels.

Lymphatic tissue

This is a framework of epithelial tissue containing large numbers of lymphocytes that form chains along the route of lymph vessels. Larger lymph organs are commonly found in areas where infection is more likely to occur. These include:

- lymph nodes: clusters are found in the intestinal tract, in the central thorax, the axilla, and the groin and around the knees.

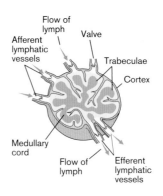

Flow of lymph

Afferent lymphatic vessels

Valve

Trabeculae

Cortex

Medullary cord

Flow of lymph

Efferent lymphatic vessels

The structure of a lymph node.

- tonsils: these form a protective ring round the oral and nasal cavities. Sometimes they swell and interfere with breathing. If this continues, the oral and nasal tonsils (adenoids) may be surgically removed.
- thymus: this is positioned behind the sternum. It is important before birth and in early childhood as it forms lymphocytes.
- spleen: as with other lymphoid tissue, the spleen filters and removes bacteria and foreign material, but it also destroys worn-out red blood cells and acts as a reservoir for blood.

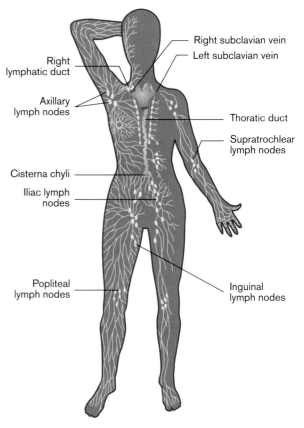

Right lymphatic duct

Axillary lymph nodes

Cisterna chyli

Iliac lymph nodes

Popliteal lymph nodes

Right subclavian vein

Left subclavian vein

Thoratic duct

Supratrochlear lymph nodes

Inguinal lymph nodes

The position of lymph nodes in the body.

Lymphatic ducts

There are two lymphatic ducts: the right and the left. Lymph passes through a number of lymph nodes where it is filtered, and then forms large lymphatic vessels or trunks. Lymph from the lower part of the body, the left side of the head and neck, left arm and left side of the chest enters the thoracic duct. It then passes into the left subclavian vein.

Lymph from the right side of the head and neck and the right arm and shoulder passes its contents into the right lymphatic duct, and then returns to the blood by means of the right subclavian vein.

You need to know about this drainage because accumulation of tissue fluid in particular areas often indicates disease, such as infection or cancer. Cancer cells may be drained from the sites where they have developed and, if the system is overwhelmed, cells travel in blood to distant sites where they may proliferate, forming secondary growths. *See also* The circulatory system *on page 207.* Blockage of the system may result in oedema – an excessive collection of tissue fluid.

See also The circulatory system on page 207.

Activity

Why might people who have had a breast and lymph nodes removed suffer from problems with oedema in the arm on the affected side?

Is there anything you can do to assist with drainage in affected areas?

Find out what Hodgkin's disease is.

Why might you get swollen sore lumps under your chin when you have mouth ulcers?

The respiratory system

The main function of the respiratory system is to allow the exchange of O_2 and CO_2 between the lungs and the atmosphere. The system works in combination with the circulatory system to transfer a continuous supply of these gases to the cells of the body. O_2 is required for **metabolism**, which results in the production of energy. CO_2 and water are by-products and will be excreted.

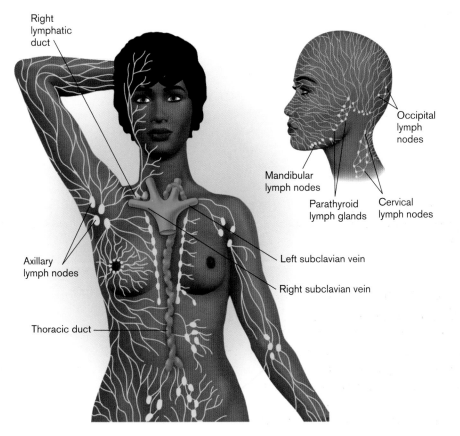

Right lymphatic duct

Occipital lymph nodes

Mandibular lymph nodes

Parathyroid lymph glands

Cervical lymph nodes

Axillary lymph nodes

Left subclavian vein

Right subclavian vein

Thoracic duct

The thoracic duct and right lymphatic duct.

To function normally, all cells need a constant supply of O_2 and rapid removal of CO_2. You can survive for days or weeks without water or food, but your brain cells will die after a matter of minutes if deprived of O_2.

There are two main processes involved in the respiratory system:

- breathing – the exchange between the lungs and the atmosphere, when the lungs inflate and recoil
- respiration – the exchange of gases between the blood and alveoli, and between the blood and the cells throughout the body.

Organs involved in respiration

You can take in air through your mouth or your nose. As the air moves through the nasal cavity, it is warmed and filtered before moving into the lungs: at the entrance to the nose, there are tiny hairs which catch any particles of dust.

The nose is divided into two cavities by the nasal septum. It is well supplied with blood vessels, and lined with mucus membrane. On each side of the cavity are three bony 'shelves' that project into the centre (nasal conchae). This arrangement increases the surface area that warms and moistens the air.

The olfactory end organs are situated close to the nasal conchae and are stimulated by droplets entering with air.

The pharynx

The pharynx is a funnel-shaped tube reaching from the internal nares (nostrils) and extending to the cricoid cartilage. This area, common to the respiratory and digestive tracts, provides a resonating chamber for the production of sound and contains the tonsils (*see* The lymphatic system *on page 211*). The pharynx consists of two layers of muscle. The upper portion is lined with pseudo stratified epithelium, while the lower portion is lined with squamous epithelium. Tiny projections on the epithelium waft any dust-laden material to a position where it can be expelled by coughing.

The larynx (glottis)

The larynx connects the pharynx to the trachea; it is composed of cartilage, the most prominent

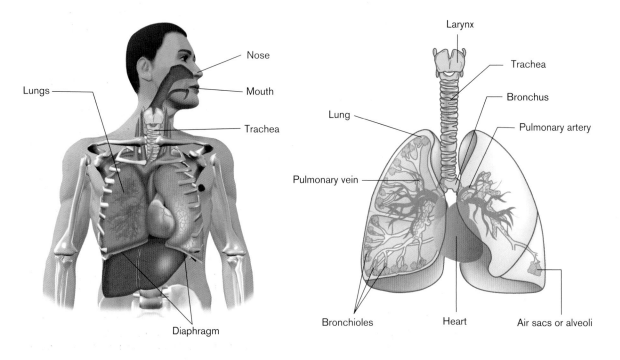

The respiratory system.

being the thyroid cartilage or Adam's apple. The larynx contains the vocal cords, which vibrate as air passes over them, resulting in sound. A leaf-shaped section of cartilage – the epiglottis – acts like a trap door: when you swallow, it drops down to cover the larynx, and prevents food from entering the trachea.

The trachea

The trachea is about 12 cm long, stretching from the larynx to level of the fifth thoracic vertebra where it divides into the right and left bronchi. It is formed of C-shaped rings of cartilage that keep the lumen open while allowing the passage of masticated food down the oesophagus, which passes behind the trachea.

When there is serious obstruction to breathing, it may be necessary to make an artificial opening into the trachea to allow air to enter the lungs. This is known as a tracheostomy.

Lungs and pleura

The lungs consist of the bronchi, bronchioles, alveolar ducts and alveoli, all supported by elastic connective tissue. There are two lungs – the right and the left lungs – which occupy most of the thoracic cavity. Lung tissue is naturally pink and spongy in appearance. The heart is situated between them in the mediastinum; the large blood vessels, nerves, lymph vessels and oesophagus pass between them. *See also* The circulatory system *on page 207.*

Each lung is divided into two lobes on the left, and three on the right. Each has its own secondary bronchus, dividing into further bronchi supplying the lobes and smaller sections known as lobules. The lobules each have a lymphatic vessel, arteriole and venule. The lobules are made up of alveoli, which are described later.

The lung is covered by a double layer of serous membrane, rather like a double bag, which lines the diaphragm below and fuses with the large vessels above. The visceral pleural layer adheres to the lung tissue, and the outer layer parietal is attached to the rib cage. Between the two layers there is a minute amount of serous fluid, which causes the layers to adhere to one another just as fluid would cause two layers of glass to stick together (*see* Pericardial layers *on page 207*). These tissues are vital for breathing.

The bronchi

The structure of the bronchi is similar to that of the trachea, both being lined with pseudo stratified epithelium. As the bronchi enter the right and left lungs, they divide into smaller tubes called bronchioles.

The bronchioles

The bronchioles branch into increasingly smaller tubes and, as they decrease in size, the amount of cartilage reduces and is replaced by smooth muscle. The muscle is controlled by the autonomic nervous system. When this is stimulated, the bronchioles dilate, enabling more air to pass into the lungs. These tiny tubes end in expanded air sacs called alveoli.

The alveolar ducts and alveoli

The bronchioles divide into tiny stems called alveolar ducts, which end in alveolar sacs. The walls of these sacs are made up of many alveoli, resembling individual grapes clustered together in a bunch. There are networks of blood vessels around and in close contact with the alveoli, rather like a hairnet.

The alveoli walls are one cell thick (epithelial cells) and the capillaries surrounding them are also formed of a single layer. The inner surface of the alveoli is covered with a substance called surfactant, which reduces surface tension and prevents the alveoli from collapsing as air moves in and out as you breathe. Premature babies often lack surfactant and may need machine assistance with their breathing (ventilation) while their lungs mature.

Pulmonary ventilation and the exchange of gases in the body

This process can be divided into three steps.

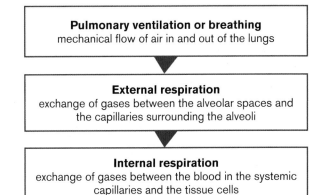

Pulmonary ventilation or breathing
mechanical flow of air in and out of the lungs

External respiration
exchange of gases between the alveolar spaces and the capillaries surrounding the alveoli

Internal respiration
exchange of gases between the blood in the systemic capillaries and the tissue cells

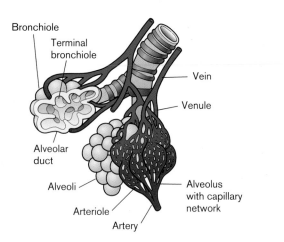

Gaseous exchange takes place in the alveoli.

When the air pressure inside the lungs drops below the pressure of the atmosphere, air moves into the lungs; when the pressure in the lungs rises above the pressure in the atmosphere, air moves out.

For breathing to occur, the lungs must expand: this increases the lung volume and decreases the pressure in the lungs, to below that of the atmosphere.

The main respiration muscles contract to increase the size of the chest, and the diaphragm, which forms the floor of the thoracic cavity, flattens out. At the same time, the external **intercostal** muscles (muscles between the ribs) contract, raising the rib cage. The double layer of pleural tissue is pulled outwards with the rib cage because:

- one layer adheres to the rib cage and one layer to the lung tissue
- the pressure between the pleural layers is below that of the atmosphere.

Because of the reduction in pressure inside the lung tissue, air moves in. This is known as inspiration. The pressure in the lungs then exceeds that of the atmosphere. As the lung tissue is elastic, it recoils or springs back, forcing air out of the lungs. This is known as expiration.

As you breathe in, air enters your lungs, passes to the alveoli, where it rapidly diffuses through the cell walls and into the circulating blood in capillaries surrounding the alveoli. Most of the O_2 attaches to haemoglobin in the red cells and is transported round the body. At the same time, CO_2 diffuses out of the blood into the alveoli and is exhaled.

Breathing is primarily involuntary, but we are able to change the movements consciously too (*see* Physiological measurements *on page 306*).

The processes involved in breathing are controlled by a centre in the brain stem called the respiratory centre (*see* The nervous system *page 185*). Information is passed via nerve pathways in the spinal cord. Some nerves leave the cord high up at about the 3rd-5th cervical vertebrae, to supply the diaphragm; others leave at 3rd-6th thoracic level, to supply the intercostal muscles. Other nerves supply muscles used in laboured breathing: for example, the muscles of the clavicle.

Factors affecting the control of respiration

Changes within the body are monitored by specialised receptors, which transmit information to the respiratory centre. Impulses can then be sent out to adjust respiration to meet the needs of the body.

Chemoreceptors

Chemoreceptors are receptor cells in the walls of the aorta at the point where it leaves the heart (aortic arch). These cells are sensitive to changes in the circulating blood – changes of levels of carbon dioxide and, to a lesser degree, oxygen. The impulses from the chemoreceptors are relayed to the respiratory centre, resulting in the passage of nerve impulses to the muscles of respiration. This alters the rate and depth of breathing.

A number of other receptors also relay information to the brain to enable adjustments to breathing. These are the stretch receptors in the lungs, diaphragm and chest wall, and the muscle and joint receptors. All these are stimulated when exercise is increased.

There is some voluntary control from higher centres in the brain. We can, for example, alter breathing movements when we sing, yawn, laugh or speak.

The respiratory system is affected by ageing, since the airways and tissues such as the alveoli become less elastic and more rigid. The chest wall also becomes more rigid, so the **vital capacity** decreases. By the age of 70, it may have dropped by 35 per cent, which explains why older people are more likely to develop disorders such as pneumonia, bronchitis and emphysema.

Activity

Using a range of resources, find out how the following affect respiration:

- pollution
- climbing above sea level
- being 8 months pregnant.

Key term

Vital capacity the largest amount of air we can breathe out in one expiration

Resources

Thibodeau G.A., and Patton K.T. (2007) *Structure and Function of the Body*, Mosby, London.

James J, Baker C and Swain H (2002) *Principles of Science for Nurses*, Blackwell Scientific, Oxford.

Tortora G.J. and Grabowski S.R (2007) *Introduction to the Human Body: The Essentials of Anatomy and Physiology*. John Wiley, Oxford.

Nicpon E.M. (2007) *Essentials of human physiology*, Pearson.

Benjamin Commins (CD Rom).

Relevant legislation and organisational policy and procedures

Laws, in their simplest form, can be defined as society's behavioural rules on how people can live orderly, safe and peaceful lives. The process of making these formal rules is usually through primary legislation – the passing of laws by Act of Parliament. These Acts, or Statutes, come into force when a majority of Members of both Houses of Parliament vote them in.

The original idea for a law can come from one of several sources. These include the Government, advisory agencies (such as the Commissions for Equal Opportunities or Human Rights), pressure groups and charities supporting a particular cause or interest (like Age Concern) or individual Members of Parliament (MPs) who promote certain issues (such as the quality of care in nursing homes or whether young people should be prosecuted for carrying knives).

Ideas for new laws are first aired in an open-ended discussion document entitled a Green Paper. If it is decided to take them further, the discussion produces a set of proposals which is published in a White Paper, as a Bill. The Bill is discussed, voted on, amended and consolidated during three separate debates in Parliament, and then passed to the House of Lords for final approval. When everyone agrees that it says what's needed, it goes to the Queen for Royal Assent. At this stage it passes from a Bill to an Act, and becomes law.

Within Europe the European Union adopts legislation in the form of Directives and Regulations. These Directives and Regulations must then be adopted by European member states within their own domestic legislation.

In Scotland health (and social care) are the responsibility of the Scottish Parliament so legislation and policy differ from England, Northern Ireland and Wales. These variations are shown in blue below.

Legislation policy procedure	Website	Relevant content	EU directive implemented by the Act
Data Protection Act (1998)	www.dh.gov.uk	The protection of the individuals' personal data with regard to processing and safe storage: • storing confidential information • protection of paper based information • protection of information stored on computer • accurate and appropriate record keeping.	95/46/EC
Access to Medical Records 1988			
Freedom of Information Act (2000)	www.dh.gov.uk	Introduced to promote a culture of openness within public bodies. Allows anyone the right of access to a wide range of information held by a public authority. Access to information is subject to certain limited exemptions, such as information about an individual. It is under this Act that individuals can access their health records.	95/46/EC
Freedom of Information (Scotland) Act 2002		In Scotland this Act established the office of Scottish Information Commissioner who is responsible for ensuring public authorities maximise access to information.	
Health and Safety at Work Act (1974)	www.hse.gov.uk	• Ensuring the environment is safe and free from hazards. • Assessing risks before carrying out tasks. • Checking equipment for faults before use. • Use of appropriate personal protective clothing. • Handling hazardous/contaminated waste correctly. • Disposal of sharp implements appropriately. • Shared responsibilities – employers/employees.	89/391/EEC

Legislation	Website	Details	Directive
Manual Handling Regulations (1992)	www.hse.gov.uk	• Preparing the environment before moving or handling anything. • Checking equipment is safe before use. • Safe moving and handling of patients. • Safe moving of equipment/loads.	90/269/EEC
Control of Substances Hazardous to Health (2002) (COSHH)	www.hse.gov.uk	• Storing cleansing materials correctly. • Labelling of hazardous substances correctly. • Appropriate handling of bodily fluids such as blood and urine. • Appropriate handling of flammable liquids/gases. • Appropriate handling of toxic/corrosive substances/liquids.	67/548/EEC
Reporting of Injuries, Diseases and Dangerous Occurrences Regulations (1995) RIDDOR	www.hse.gov.uk	• Reporting accidents and injuries objectively and accurately. • Reporting diseases to the appropriate bodies. • Reporting dangerous occurrences to the appropriate bodies. • Completion of relevant paperwork.	89/391/EEC
Lifting Operations and Lifting Equipment Regulations (1998)	www.hse.gov.uk	The Lifting Operations and Lifting Equipment Regulations aim to reduce risks to people's health and safety from lifting equipment provided for use at work by ensuring it is: • strong and stable enough for the particular use and marked to indicate safe working loads • positioned and installed to minimise any risks • used safely, that is the work is planned, organised and performed by competent people • subject to ongoing thorough examination and, where appropriate, inspection by competent people.	89/655/EEC amended 95/63/EC
Environmental Protection Act (1990, section 34) and the Environmental Protection (Duty of Care) Regulations (1991)	www.dh.gov.uk	Section 34 of the Environmental Protection Act (1990) imposes a duty of care on persons concerned with control of waste. It places a duty on anyone who in any way has a responsibility for control of waste to ensure that it is managed properly and recovered or disposed of safely.	2006/12/EC

Legislation	Website	Relevant content	European or UK Legislation
Human Rights Act (1998)	www.dh.gov.uk	The European Convention on Human Rights was passed by the Council of Europe in 1950 in response to the Universal Declaration of Human Rights which was drawn up by the United Nations (UN) in 1948. The Human Rights Act is the UK's response to this European Law. It includes: • involvement of the individual and informed consent • individual treatment and respect • appropriate response to patient need • ensuring individuals exercise their rights and can make choices • ensuring individuals privacy and dignity.	The European Convention on Human Rights (1950)
Mental Capacity Act (2005)	www.dh.gov.uk www.bma.org.uk	Provides a legal framework for making decisions on behalf of individuals who lack the mental capacity to make decisions. This includes: • the capacity to consent to/ refuse treatment • promoting the best interests/advocacy of the individual • supporting individuals appropriately in the decision making process Under the Act it is a criminal offence to ill treat any person who lacks capacity, with the punishment possible imprisonment.	English and Welsh Legislation
Mental Health (Care and Treatment Act) Scotland 2003		Similar requirements to England.	Scottish Legislation
Care Standards Act (2000) and the Protection of Vulnerable Adults (POVA) Scheme	www.dh.gov.uk	The Care Standards Act established a major regulatory framework for social care, to ensure high standards of care and improvement in the protection of vulnerable people by the use of the POVA scheme. This scheme provides an effective, workable measure to safeguard vulnerable adults from people who are unsuitable to work with them. From 26 July 2004, individuals should be referred to, and included on, the POVA list if they have abused, neglected or otherwise harmed vulnerable adults in their care or placed vulnerable adults in their care at risk of harm. By making statutory checks against the list (with the Criminal Records Bureau, CRB), providers of care must not offer such individuals employment in care positions.	UK Legislation
Regulation of Care (Scotland) Act 2001		In Scotland the Care Commission regulates and inspects all care services in Scotland. It uses National Care Standards to ensure that patients receive the same standard of care wherever they live in Scotland. The *Codes of Practice for Social Service Workers and Employers* sets out the standards that all social care workers in Scotland must meet. Social service workers and those working in social care will be registered with the Scottish Social Services council.	
Disability Discrimination Act (2005)	www.dh.gov.uk	It is unlawful for a provider of services to discriminate against a disabled person, in terms of employment or in the provision of services. Employers must make reasonable adjustments to the physical environment to accommodate those with disabilities, either employees or disabled users of the service.	Treaty of Amsterdam (1997)
Community Care and Health (Scotland) Act 2002		On 1 July 2002 free nursing and personal care for elderly people was introduced in Scotland. Older people who qualify receive payments of £145 per week depending on their needs.	

The Nursing and Midwifery Council (NMC) was established under The Nursing and Midwifery Order (2001). Its core function is to establish and improve standards of nursing and midwifery care in order to serve and protect the public. One way in which these standards are up held is by ensuring all nurses adhere to the Code of Practice for the NMC. There is currently no official registration of healthcare assistants in the UK and therefore there is no specific Code of Conduct for them. the table below utilises two Codes of Conduct that healthcare assistants could refer to.

Please note many health Trusts have Code of Conduct for health care assistants so please make sure you are fully aware of the one within your own Trust.

Code of Conduct	Website	Content
Nursing and Midwifery Council Code of Conduct (2008) (relates only to nurses, midwifes or specialist community public health nurses registered with the Nursing and Midwifery Council but is a useful point of reference for all healthcare assistants)	www.nmc-uk.org	As a registered nurse, midwife or specialist community public health nurse, you must: • respect the patient or client as an individual • protect confidential information • obtain consent before you give any treatment or care • co-operate with others in the team • maintain your professional knowledge and competence • be trustworthy • act to identify and minimise the risk to patients and clients. This applies to all nurses working in England, Scotland, Ireland and Wales.
Unison Code of Conduct (2005)	www.unison.org.uk	As a healthcare assistant you must: • maintain patient confidentiality and to seek guidance from someone senior about any confidence that they are concerned about • ensure that they communicate effectively with patients in their care and take time to listen to their concerns • treat every patient as an individual and respect their rights and beliefs, even where they differ from their own • document care - ensure that observations and changes are recorded clearly in black ink and, where appropriate, that changes in patients' conditions are reported.

Identify the individual at risk from skin breakdown; undertake risk assessment and pressure area care, move, and position individuals

Introduction

While working in the health care industry you may have cared for individuals with serious conditions such as liver failure, kidney failure or even heart failure. These conditions all involve major organs of the body and are all potentially life threatening. The skin is also a major organ, one that can cause death if it fails. When you think about the condition of skin breakdown or pressure sores, think of the condition as an organ failure, because that is exactly what it is. Skin breakdown is very serious – the prevention and treatment of it is vital for the individual's life.

Treating individuals with skin breakdown costs the NHS millions of pounds every year. As a health care assistant, you can contribute to reducing this cost, not only in monetary terms but also the cost to the individual in terms of pain, discomfort and poor health. In preventing the breakdown of skin, you prevent the potentially life-threatening condition of pressure sores and all the problems associated with them.

In this section we have combined three units: CHS 4, 5 and 6. These units look at: identifying the individual whose skin integrity is at risk and undertaking the appropriate tissue viability risk assessment; undertaking agreed pressure area care; and moving and positioning individuals.

In these units you will look at those individuals who are at risk from skin breakdown and identify the factors that create the risks. You will also develop an understanding of what pressure sores are, discover how you should prepare and carry out risk assessments and learn how to undertake pressure area care using safe moving and position techniques.

What you need to learn

- Anatomy and physiology of the human body
- Individuals at risk from skin breakdown
- External factors to skin breakdown
- What pressure sores are
- Involving the individual
- Assessment tools used to identify risk of skin breakdown
- Assessment procedures
- Undertaking pressure area care
- Recording, reporting and reviewing risk assessments

What evidence you need to generate for your portfolio

The main type of evidence you need to produce for your award is observation. Your assessor will observe you undertaking real life activities to cover the performance criteria and scope. This can be supported by witness testimonies from your colleagues who have seen you working. In addition to this you will need to demonstrate your knowledge and understanding. You can do this by providing written accounts, answering verbal or written questions and completing assignments.

Anatomy and physiology of the human body

(CHS 4 K13; CHS 5 K9, 12; CHS 6 K10)

Before you can begin to learn how to identify individuals at risk of skin breakdown, it is important that you develop an understanding of healthy skin, muscles, bones and joints. Once you develop your knowledge of these areas you should be able to identify more easily those individuals at risk from skin breakdown.

Firstly, you will look at how the body is made up of bones, joints and muscles. You will then look at what healthy skin is, the individuals at risk from skin breakdown and the external factors that can cause the skin to breakdown. You will also look at how and why you should involve the individual from the beginning in preventing skin breakdown.

Muscles bones and joints

The human body has 206 different bones and four main types of **joints.** Without bones and joints you would not be able to stand, sit, walk or run. You would just be a lump of jelly! It is your bones that give your body shape and support. Your bones and joints are connected to **muscles** and **ligaments**, which also help your body to move.

Key terms

Joints Where two bones meet.

Muscles Strong fibrous tissues, which shorten to give the body strength.

Ligaments Fibrous tissue that connects muscle to bones.

The four main joints in your body are:

- hinge joints
- pivot joints
- ball and socket joints
- glide joints.

Hinge joints You have hinge joints in your knees, elbows fingers and toes. A hinge joint lets your **limb** bend. Think of a hinge joint as a door opening or closing. A door cannot open or close more than the hinge will let it. This is just like your knee or elbow. When you bend and straighten your leg, it bends at the knee and will only straighten so far. A hinge joint is very strong. When you walk your knees straighten and take the weight of your body.

Key term

Limb An arm or leg.

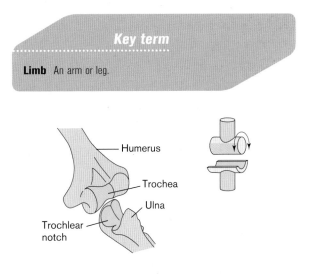

Humerus
Trochea
Ulna
Trochlear notch

Pivot joints The joint in your neck is a pivot joint. It lets you rotate or turn your head. You also have a pivot joint in your elbow. This allows you to turn your lower arm. You cannot turn your head or lower arm all the way around because there are muscles and ligaments that stop this.

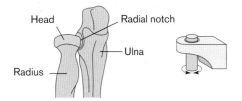

Head
Radial notch
Ulna
Radius

Ball and socket joints This type of joint gives you the most range of movement. You have a ball and socket joint in your hips and shoulders. This type of joint lets you move your limb up and down, from side to side and round in a full circle. A ball and socket joint is where the end of one bone sits in the hollow of another bone.

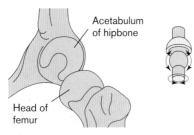

Acetabulum of hipbone
Head of femur

Glide joints These can be found in your spine or backbone. They can give you a lot of movement but not as much as the ball and socket joint. A glide joint is where bones glide or move over each other. To help the bones move over each other easily, there is a disc or pad of cartilage. Cartilage is a tough flexible tissue, which also acts as a shock absorber between the bones in your back.

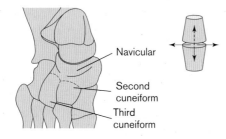

Navicular
Second cuneiform
Third cuneiform

A special fluid called **synovial fluid** protects most of the joints in your body. This fluid helps your joints to move smoothly and without pain.

The skin

Functions of the skin

The skin provides protection by:

- acting as a barrier to infection
- keeping body tissues moist, preventing them from drying out
- registering sensations such as pain, texture and temperature through nerve endings
- helping to regulate body temperature through sweat glands
- storing fat as an essential requirement to the body's functioning
- making vitamin D
- excreting waste through the skin's pores.

Structure of the skin

There are three main layers to the human skin:

- the epidermis or outer skin
- the dermis or inner skin
- subcutaneous fatty tissue.

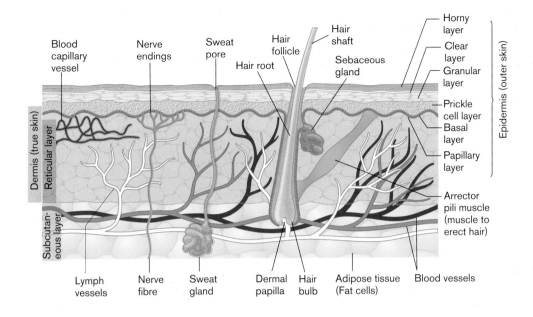

The structure of the skin.

The epidermis

The epidermis is the outermost layer of the skin. It is constantly dying and shedding itself. In the healthy individual, this outer layer of skin replaces itself on a daily basis with the growth of new skin cells. The epidermis is waterproof, which keeps the skin dry on the outside while ensuring that the body's internal tissues remain moist. The epidermis does not contain any blood vessels, which is why you do not bleed when you scratch the epidermis.

> **Did you know?**
>
> Most dust particles in the home are made up from dead skin cells.

The dermis

The second layer of skin is known as the dermis. This inner skin is a thick layer of tissue containing:

- sebaceous glands (otherwise known as oil glands)
- sudoriferous glands (also known as sweat glands)
- hair follicles
- blood vessels
- nerve endings.

The nerve endings send information to the brain letting the body know of pain, touch, pressure, temperature and irritation. If you cut yourself, you will only bleed if you cut through the epidermis and into the dermis. Within the dermis there are also elastic fibres that help the skin regain its original shape after stretching or moving.

Subcutaneous fatty tissue

The third and innermost layer of the skin is known as subcutaneous fatty tissue. This collection of fatty tissue cells is vital in cushioning the body from any excess pressure placed on it. This layer also keeps the body warm and is a source of nutrition. People who are on extreme diets or who are underweight will feel the cold more because of the reduction of this important fatty layer.

What is healthy skin?

Skin that is healthy should be smooth, with no breaks or cracks. It should be warm to touch but not hot or red; it should be neither dry nor moist, neither taut nor wrinkled.

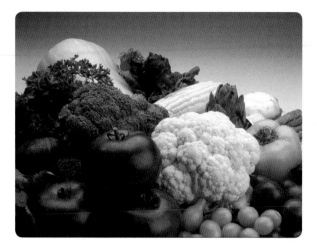

Fresh foods contain more nutrition than processed foods, so are better for you.

For skin to remain healthy, it requires nutrition, fluids and oxygen. Look at the skin of a healthy newborn baby: it is soft and smooth, warm to the touch and has a delicate sheen to it. This is because the skin had everything it required in the mother's womb. As a child grows into an adult, the skin can begin to show signs of wear. As the adult ages, the signs become more apparent – wrinkles begin to appear on the face, especially around the eyes and mouth. Many women prefer to call them 'laughter lines' as wrinkles can be generally seen as a sign of becoming old.

Maintaining healthy skin

Regardless of the age of an individual, in order to maintain healthy skin you need to ensure three essential ingredients: nutrition, fluids and oxygen.

Nutrition

A well balanced diet will give the body all the nutrition it requires to remain healthy. A well balanced diet must contain the following nutrients.

- Proteins – for example, lean meat, fish and dairy products.
- Carbohydrates – for example, bread and cereals.
- Vitamins and minerals – for example, fresh fruit and vegetables.
- Fats – for example, nuts and seeds.
- Fibre – for example, wholegrain breads, cereals and potato skins.

All of the above forms of foods need to be eaten in moderation and not in excess.

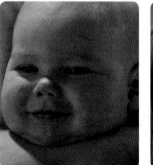
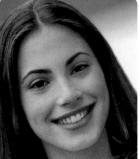
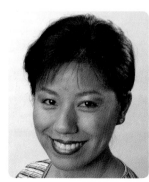
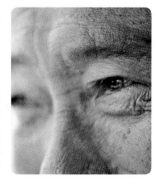

As a person ages, the skin begins to show signs of wear.

Fluids

The human body requires at least 2 litres (4 pints) of water per day to maintain healthy tissues including the skin. Beverages such as tea and coffee can cause the body to dehydrate (to lose valuable fluids) when taken in large quantities. For this reason it is important for the individual to drink water in addition to tea and coffee. Fluids help the skin maintain its elasticity so it is essential that you drink plenty of fluids to keep the skin supple and moving freely.

Oxygen

Oxygen is an essential requirement in keeping the body alive. Without oxygen, your body's organs will suffocate and die. Blood vessels are responsible for transporting oxygen around the body so you need to ensure these remain healthy.

Blood vessels that become constricted (made smaller) or blocked will not be able to carry oxygen to the body's organs, including the skin. Smoking is one of the major causes of constriction. Another cause is high cholesterol, which is a build up of fats in the bloodstream. Both of these reduce or prevent the amount of oxygen getting to the skin and other essential organs.

Exercise helps to maintain healthy oxygen levels in the body by keeping the lungs, heart and circulation system in tip-top condition. The good work gained through exercise will, however, be lessened if the individual continues to smoke and eat fatty foods.

Remember

Nutrients + oxygen + fluids = healthy skin.

Evidence in action
(CHS 4 – K12, 13; CHS 5 – K2, 9)

Design and produce a leaflet showing the anatomy and physiology of skin, what skin needs in order to be healthy, and how individuals can achieve this. Show this to your assessor: explain how you could use the leaflet to inform an individual's knowledge and why this is important.

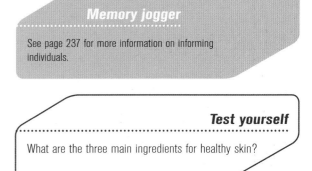

Memory jogger

See page 237 for more information on informing individuals.

Test yourself

What are the three main ingredients for healthy skin?

Individuals at risk from skin breakdown

(CHS 4 – K9, 16, 17; CHS 5 – K10, 12; CHS 6 – K11)

You have examined what makes skin healthy, including nutrition, fluids and oxygen. The breakdown of skin occurs when these factors are compromised.

When considering the risk of skin breakdown, you need to look at the individuals themselves. The individual's age, ability and general health are major factors in the risk of their skin breaking down, because they affect how much pressure that individual puts on particular parts of their body.

Before you look at the different groups of **individuals at risk**, you need to understand the areas of the body involved in pressure.

Key terms

Individuals at risk People whose health is particularly vulnerable, because they are:
- unconscious
- very elderly
- people with reduced mobility or immobility due to surgery, stroke, etc.
- suffering from malnutrition, dehydration, skin conditions, sensory impairment, acute illness, vascular disease, severe chronic or terminal illness
- people with a previous history of pressure damage or incontinence
- people with diabetes
- those with an altered mental state.

Mental state The mental condition of an individual. This can include the individual being withdrawn, depressed, agitated or confused.

Pressure areas

All individuals have areas on their body that come under pressure from external sources on a regular basis. Take sitting down, for example. You may have experienced the sensation of your buttocks becoming numb after sitting in one place for a long time without moving. This is because of the constant pressure placed on your buttocks during the process of sitting. Providing the individual is healthy, this pressure should not result in any skin breakdown.

The most common areas prone to pressure damage on the body include:

- head – back of head or ear
- shoulder – back of shoulder or side
- rib cage – front of chest
- elbow – back of elbow or side
- spine – along the bones which are prominent
- hip
- buttocks and sacrum (lower spine)
- thigh – inner and outer, front and back
- knees – front and side
- calves – back of
- heels
- toes.

The pressure comes from sitting or lying. If an individual puts prolonged pressure on one area of their body, and the individual has poor nutrition, oxygen and fluid intake, that individual is at a greater risk of skin breakdown.

Reflect

Take a few minutes to think of your body position while you are reading this book.

- What areas of your body are under pressure?
- How do you know that they are under pressure?
- Are any areas of your body under more pressure than others?

Evidence in action (CHS 4 – K 17; CHS 5 – K 10)

Using a full-size model, a volunteer or yourself, show your assessor where on the body pressure damage is most likely to occur. Explain why this is so.

Individuals most at risk

If you consider that the risk of skin breakdown is associated with remaining in one position for a long period of time, this will give you a good indicator of those at risk. Combine this with individuals who do not meet the requirements for having healthy skin and you should begin to have a clearer understanding of all the groups of individuals at risk of skin breakdown.

Activity

Using the knowledge you have gained so far, which groups of individuals do you think would be at risk of skin breakdown? List as many as you can.

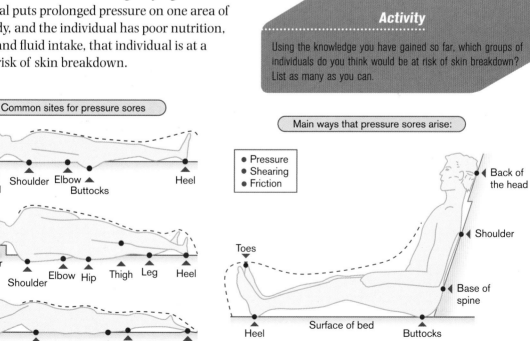

Common sites for pressure sores – lying on back, front, side and sitting (Source: Tissue Viability Society).

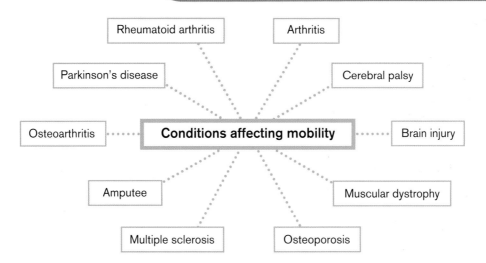

```
              Rheumatoid arthritis        Arthritis

   Parkinson's disease                          Cerebral palsy

Osteoarthritis  ·····  Conditions affecting mobility  ·····  Brain injury

        Amputee                              Muscular dystrophy

            Multiple sclerosis       Osteoporosis
```

People who have reduced mobility are also at risk of skin breakdown.

Groups of individuals who would be at risk of skin breakdown include those who:

- are immobile
- have reduced mobility
- are acutely ill
- have an altered mental state
- have a sensory impairment to the body.

Immobility

Immobility is a state of not being able to change position or move around the environment at all. This will affect individuals who are both conscious and unconscious, including people undertaking or recovering from an operation or those under sedation.

The individual who is immobile will be placing constant pressure on one particular area. This is because the person will not be able to change his or her position. This pressure and the inability to relieve it will put the individual at risk from skin breakdown.

Reduced mobility

Individuals with reduced mobility may have some movement but not sufficient to move freely around their environment or to take regular exercise. People in this group include those who have recently had surgery or have a mobility-reducing condition such as osteoarthritis, Parkinson's disease, a stroke or another brain injury. Individuals over the age of 70 years may also come under this group when their mobility and skin elasticity begin to decrease.

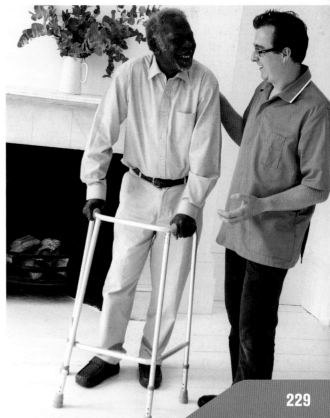

Test yourself

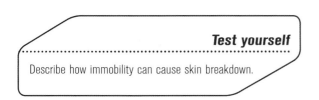

Describe how immobility can cause skin breakdown.

As long as the individual is able to maintain a well balanced diet, take in plenty of fluids and has a good level of oxygen intake, their risk of skin breakdown will be reduced, but not eliminated. If, however, these factors cannot be maintained, the risk of skin breakdown will be increased.

Acute illnesses

Individuals with an acute illness such as pneumonia can be confined to bed for long periods, and this increases the risk of skin breakdown. Poor food intake can cause the body's nutritional levels to fall. In addition, a high body temperature or vomiting associated with an illness can result in the individual losing bodily fluids, and this can lead to dehydration. Combined, these factors will put the individual at a higher risk of skin breakdown.

Reflect

Think of a time when you have had an illness that required you to spend some time in bed. Did it cause you to go off your food?

Remember

Illness + poor nutritional/food intake + fluid loss = increased risk of skin breakdown.

Other illnesses, such as vascular disease, can increase the risk of skin breakdown. Vascular disease is a condition affecting the blood vessels and it reduces the flow of oxygen and nutrients to the body's organs, including the skin. This causes the skin tissues to become starved of essential requirements, leaving it at greater risk of breakdown. Atherosclerosis is a form of vascular disease that affects the legs. The blood vessels in the legs become blocked with fatty tissue. This decreases the blood supply to the legs muscles, causing severe cramping. A complete blockage of the blood vessels can result in constant leg pain, leg ulcers and gangrene, leading to possible amputation of the limb.

Altered mental state

Individuals with depression, or who are withdrawn or confused, can be at risk of skin breakdown. The altered mental state of an individual can reduce the person's mobility if he or she sees no point in moving about or undertaking activities. The individual may feel that there is no point to life and may spend many hours in bed or sitting motionless in a chair.

Evidence with a case study

Bernadette is 58 years old and recently separated from her partner. She does not have any children and retired from work two years ago due to ill health. Bernadette's only close friend passed away recently. She used to go out with her friend every day, either into town shopping or out for a meal. Since the death of her friend one month ago, Bernadette has not left the house. She now tends to spend most of her time sitting in her armchair looking out of the window. She has often woken in the morning still sitting in the chair from the night before.

1 What are the main factors that might lead Bernadette to develop a pressure sore?

2 What do you think Bernadette's nutritional state has become?

3 How can Bernadette's nutritional state affect the chances of developing a pressure sore?

How many times have you been at home alone and thought it was not worth cooking a meal just for you? Eating is generally a sociable activity and, if a person lives alone, he or she may not want to eat alone. If a person is depressed, confused or withdrawn, the individual may not be bothered to cook for him or herself, or may lose interest in eating altogether.

Did you know?

In the later stages of dementia, the individual often loses motivation and does not move for long periods. This lack of movement can lead to pressure sores.

If the individual does not eat properly, he or she will not receive the nutrients required to keep the skin healthy. If the individual does not mobilise, he or she runs a greater risk of skin breakdown.

Sensory reduction

A sensory reduction is one where the individual has no sense of feeling on areas of his or her body. This could be caused by illness, accident or a condition from birth in which the nerves responsible for transmitting sensations to the brain are damaged.

Having a sensory reduction means that the individual will not be able to feel pain or discomfort and so will not recognise when the skin becomes sore (if this occurs on an area where no sensation is felt). This could lead to further skin breakdown if the sore area continues to be damaged without the individual realising.

Medication

As you have seen (page 227), the skin is maintained by a blood supply that feeds it oxygen and nutrients from the body (gained from the air during breathing and by the digestion of food). Some medication can cause nutritional deficiencies in the individual, by preventing essential nutrients from being absorbed into the bloodstream or by increasing the body's tendency to eliminate waste. These medications include:

- cytotoxics (used in the treatment of cancer) e.g. cyclophosphamide
- lipid lowering medicines (those which reduce cholesterol) e.g. cholestyramine
- diuretics (those that help the body to eliminate fluids) e.g. furosemide
- anti-inflammatory medicines (to reduce swelling) e.g. Ibuprofen
- antacids (these create a lining on the stomach wall) e.g. Milk of Magnesia
- laxatives (medicines to aid the elimination of body waste) e.g. Bisacodyl

Medication that prevents the absorption of nutrients or helps the body to pass fluids or waste can cause essential nutrients to be lost from food. This reduces the skin's healthiness, exposing it to the risk of skin breakdown.

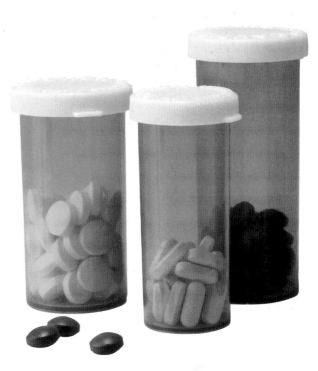

Moisture

The skin requires fluids to be healthy, but excess moisture on the skin caused by sweat or incontinence can increase the risk of skin breakdown.

An individual who wears incontinence pads may have excess moisture caused by sweat and urine around the buttocks for long periods of time. This excess moisture may irritate the skin, causing it to breakdown. If the individual has reduced mobility and remains seated, this will only compound the problem, greatly increasing the risk of skin breakdown.

Evidence in action (CHS 4 pc 3 K16)

Create a chart to show the factors that put individuals at risk of skin breakdown. Show this to your assessor as evidence, explaining how these factors can put individuals at risk of skin breakdown.

External factors contributing to skin breakdown

(CHS 4 – K15; CHS 5 – K12, 13; CHS 6 – K6, 7, 26)

External factors are those things outside of the individual's body that can cause skin breakdown. You have looked closely at individuals at risk of skin breakdown and predisposing factors, including excess moisture and medication. You now need to consider external factors, all of which are preventable, providing you work with the individual to the correct standard and use the correct practices.

External factors to skin breakdown include:

* shearing
* friction
* poor handling
* poor hygiene
* knocks to the skin.

Shearing

Poor posture when sitting up in bed or slouching in a chair can cause what is known as shearing forces. Shearing is when the skin slides over muscles and bones and become stretched in one area and wrinkled in another, decreasing the blood supply to the skin. It is the underlying tissues of the skin that become damaged, and the true damage is not always immediately apparent: it may only be recognised when it has become extensive.

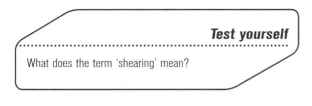

Test yourself

What does the term 'shearing' mean?

Reflect

Most people are guilty of slouching in a chair, especially in front of the television after a hard day. But did you realise the potential damage you are causing, not only to your posture but to your skin as well? Think about the times you might slouch like this, and the circumstances in which you might do it.

The shearing force is created by the natural gravity of the body pulling in a downward motion. While sitting in a bed or chair, your body is naturally pulling itself downwards. If an individual is unable to maintain their seated position, they will begin to slip downwards, causing shearing. The shearing force places additional risk of damage on the skin and can be reduced by ensuring appropriate seating positions.

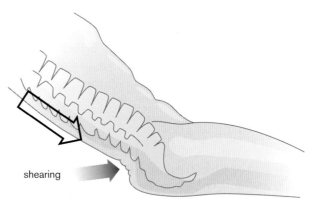

shearing

Shearing force due to poor posture, showing how natural gravity contributes to the risk of skin damage.

Remember

Where shearing forces are present, it only takes half of the amount of pressure to create the same amount of damage.

Friction

Friction is the rubbing of the skin on rough or uneven surfaces. You may have experienced damage to the skin caused by friction when wearing new shoes, for example, which can be very painful.

Friction is associated with shearing and can therefore occur when slipping down a bed or chair when sitting in an inappropriate position. The skin rubbing on man-made fibres such as nylon or polyester can also cause friction.

Poor handling

Individuals who require support in moving can be put at risk of skin breakdown by the way you or other staff handle them. Dragging the individual up a bed or chair to reposition him or her can cause shearing and friction. The individual's skin may be pulled against the bedsheets or seat covering, which can damage the delicate skin tissue.

Fingernails catching on the individual's skin can also cause it to break down. It is vitally important as a health care assistant that you keep your fingernails trim and do not wear jewellery, in order to avoid scratching individuals when providing personal care.

Poor hygiene

The human body has a number of areas that require particular attention when cleansing. Any area of the body that has a natural skin fold, or where one skin surface lies against another, can be susceptible to breakdown if not cleansed and dried thoroughly.

Bacteria grow where there is moisture, warmth and food. Between the natural folds of the skin, warmth and moisture occur naturally; the food supply is the dead skin cells, which have been shed by the body. The bacteria will grow and multiply quickly, providing they continue to have the moisture, warmth and food they require. It is this build-up of bacteria that causes body odour. If left, the area can become infected, causing the skin to break down. Skin that is also constantly moist from sweat, urine or faeces can become irritated, resulting in damage.

Knocks to the skin

A simple bump to the skin for most people would often go unnoticed and does not generally create any major problems. However, for some groups of individuals, any bump or scrape to the skin can lead to serious conditions of breakdown.

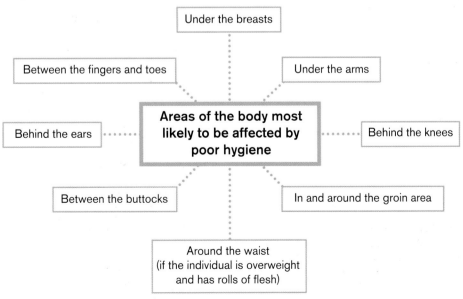

Areas of the body most likely to be affected by poor hygiene:
- Under the breasts
- Between the fingers and toes
- Under the arms
- Behind the ears
- Behind the knees
- Between the buttocks
- In and around the groin area
- Around the waist (if the individual is overweight and has rolls of flesh)

This is particularly the case for people with diabetes or leukaemia, because their skin takes longer to heal. In diabetes, this is because high blood sugar levels prevent the white blood cells from doing their job of fighting against infections, diseases and bacteria. In leukaemia, the body makes too many abnormal white cells, which leaves the body's defence against infection low. Because cuts and abrasions on the skin do not heal as quickly, they can become infected. Infected wounds to the skin take even longer to heal, and so the problem continues.

It is vitally important for individuals who heal slowly to be extra careful in preventing injuries to the skin, to avoid any serious skin breakdown. As a health care assistant, you can contribute to this prevention by: encouraging good posture when the individual is sitting; promoting good standards of hygiene; and ensuring you handle the individual correctly without dragging their skin.

Test yourself

Describe how the condition of diabetes can increase the risk of skin breakdown.

Best practice

✔ In your daily practice, remember that nutrients, oxygen and fluids are the three main ingredients for healthy skin.

✔ Help patients to keep mobile wherever possible – immobility is the leading cause of skin breakdown.

✔ Be aware of the medication your patients are taking, as certain medicines can increase the risk of skin breakdown.

✔ Take all appropriate measures to prevent poor hygiene, poor handling, friction and shearing, as these external factors can all increase the risk of skin breakdown.

Evidence in action (CHS 4 pc 2 K16)

From the individuals you work with, identify who is at risk from skin breakdown. Explain in detail to your assessor why you feel these individuals are at risk from skin breakdown.

Pressure sores

CHS 4 – K9, 14; CHS 5 – K11

Pressure sores – otherwise known as pressure ulcers, bedsores or (more technically) decubitus ulcers – are injuries to the skin or underlying tissues caused by insufficient blood flow to the area for a prolonged period.

You have looked at individuals at risk from skin breakdown and established that individuals with little or no mobility are more likely to develop this condition. This is because, for skin to be healthy, it requires oxygen from the blood; individuals who do not relieve the pressure from areas of the skin through moving or turning on a regular basis will cause a disruption of the blood vessels, cutting off the supply of oxygen to the skin.

Did you know?

95 per cent of pressure sores are preventable.

Activity: Reducing blood supply

To develop a good understanding of the disruption of blood to areas of skin caused by pressure, try this simple activity.

- Gently place together your thumb and index finger as though you are picking up a tiny object. You will see the change in your skin colour with just a small amount of pressure.

- Now squeeze your thumb and finger together tightly for no longer than 10 seconds and you will see a greater colour change. This is because your blood supply is being prevented from reaching the tip of your finger.

- Now imagine the pressure you exert on your buttocks when sitting for hours on end without moving and the damage this is causing due to lack of oxygen.

You could use this as an activity to inform your patients' knowledge and understanding as to what contributes to skin breakdown – see page 237 for more information on informing individuals.

The development of a pressure sore

There are four stages in the development of a pressure sore.

Stage one pressure sore

- The area of skin affected becomes red or discoloured. Darkly pigmented skin becomes purplish/bluish.
- The area of skin is not broken but may feel warmer than the skin around it.
- The redness or change in colour does not fade within 30 minutes of removing the pressure.

At this stage, the pressure sore can be prevented from developing further by removing the pressure from the affected area and involving the individual. Involving the individual is covered in more depth on the next page.

Stage two pressure sore

- Both the epidermis and dermis (outer and inner layers of the skin) are affected.
- The epidermis may blister or break, creating a shallow pit into the dermis.
- The sore may be weeping or leaking fluid.

At this stage, the damage to the skin and underlying tissues is greater than you can see.

Stage three pressure sore

- The break in the skin extends through the dermis into subcutaneous fatty tissue.
- The sore is deeper than stage two.
- Weeping will be evident.
- The sore is likely to be infected.

Stage four pressure sore

- The breakdown extends into the muscle, and can extend down to the bone.
- The area of skin blackens from dead and rotting tissue.
- Weeping will be evident.
- Surgery is usually required.

At this stage, the sore can create a life-threatening condition such as septicaemia (blood poisoning) or osteomyelitis (infection of the bone).

Did you know?

62 per cent of stage four pressure sores never heal; 38 per cent take more than one year to heal.

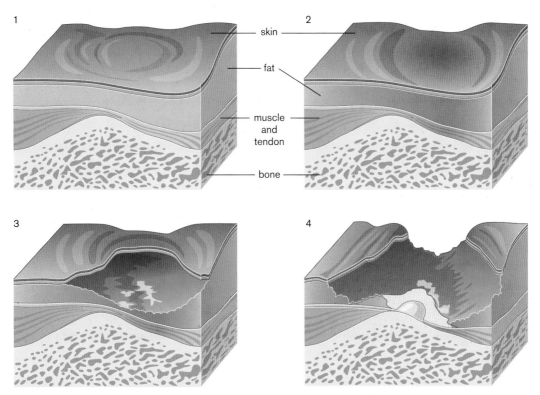

The four stages in the development of a pressure sore (Source: Spinal-Injury Network).

Evidence in action
(CHS 4 – K9, 14; CHS 5 – K11)

Describe to your assessor what you need to look for at each stage of pressure sore development, and the changes that would be present in the skin's appearance at each stage. To demonstrate your knowledge fully, you will also need to state why the appearance of the skin changes at each stage.

Involving the individual

(CHS 4 – K 1, 2, 5, 6, 8; CHS 5 – K1, 2, 19)

Supporting knowledge

When working with individuals, you have a responsibility to support their knowledge and understanding of how they can maintain and improve their own health, including pressure sores. It is essential from the outset to inform and support the individual's knowledge of the risk factors involved in the breakdown of skin; in fact, this can help to reduce the incidence of skin breakdown.

Reflect

How do you meet your responsibilities to inform and support an individual's knowledge on their health and skin care?

In 2001, the Department of Health (DoH) published the document *Essence of Care* in response to concerns about the quality of care individuals were receiving in the National Health Service (NHS). One of the areas of concern was the prevention of pressure sores. The NHS set 'benchmarks' or standards for all NHS Trusts to use, to compare with their current practice and then help them develop plans for improvement. For pressure sores the benchmark was:

> 'Patients and/or carers have ongoing access to information and have the opportunity to discuss this and its relevance to their individual needs, with a registered practitioner' (Essence of Care, NHS 2001).

In March 2006, the DoH published a new benchmark, which moved the focus of care to promoting healthier life choices. The document *Essence of Care: benchmarks for promoting health* suggests that health care workers measure 'benchmark Factor 1' ('empowerment and informed choice') by considering whether 'individuals have the knowledge, skills and opportunities to maintain and improve their own health.'

A study published in the *Nursing Standard 14, 26, 49-52 February 7 2000* demonstrated the need for individuals to have further education in this area. The study, funded by South Thames NHSE, consisted of responses to a simple questionnaire on pressure sores. It was posted to a local Patients and Carers Association and some of the results were as follows:

53% stated that they had seen a pressure sore

27% thought that pressure sores could be avoided

95% thought pressure sores were caused by a lack of regular turning

13% related pressure sores to poor nutrition

36% related pressure sores to incontinence

24% believed that not using talcum powder or creams after bathing contributed to pressure sores

45% recognised the relationship between sitting for long periods and the development of pressure sores

10% recognised the relationship between lying on a hospital trolley and the development of pressure sores

4% recognised the relationship between lying on an operating table and the development of pressure sores

As the results of this study show, individuals needed to develop a greater understanding of the risks to skin breakdown.

As a health care assistant, you need to support the knowledge of individuals if they are to play a role in helping to reduce the risk of skin breakdown. The following text will show you how this can be done.

Informing the individual

Individuals should be encouraged to identify their own risk to skin breakdown wherever possible. To do this, they need to know what is needed for healthy skin. Informing the individual on the maintenance of healthy skin including nutrition, oxygen and fluids will not only reduce his or her risk of skin breakdown, but will support the health of the individual in general.

Educating the individual in all areas of risk to skin breakdown can be achieved in a variety of ways, depending on the person's understanding and communicative abilities. Methods include:

- menus (pictorial or written) to show choices of healthy foods
- books or videos to show different forms of exercise
- individual or group discussions to identify good and bad practices in maintaining a healthy lifestyle

- educational games relating to maintaining a healthy lifestyle
- supported shopping trips to purchase healthy foods.

The information shared with individuals needs to be relevant to them and provided in a format that they will be able to understand and accept. All individuals need to be aware of the requirements of a healthy diet, exercise and fluid intake, but, for example, someone who does not have continence difficulties may not need to be made aware of the problems created by incontinence. Not all individuals have the ability to read; for those who cannot, providing the information in written format would be of no use and you may need to use alternatives such as picture symbols or audiotape.

In addition to a healthy lifestyle, the individual should be educated and supported in understanding the predisposing and external factors that increase the risk of skin breakdown, including:

- how medication can affect nutritional intake and thus the skin
- the effects of excess moisture (including sweat, urine and faeces) on the skin
- mobility – the risks of sitting or lying in one position for long periods

Educating the individual about skin breakdown can be achieved simply by talking.

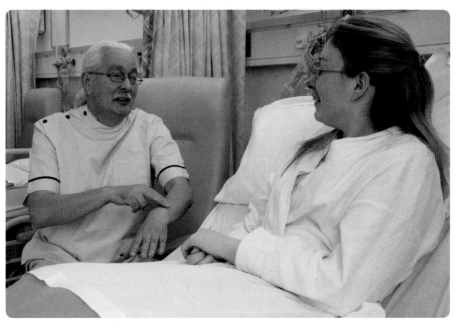

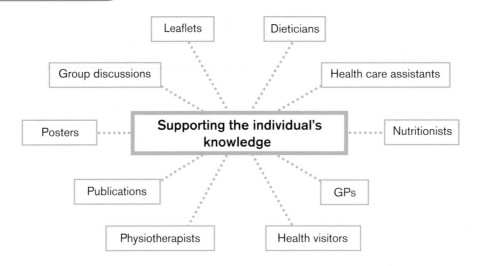

There are different ways to support an individual's knowledge and understanding of their health.

- friction and shearing forces and the requirement for the maintenance of a good seating position; wearing new shoes, callipers or splints
- the importance of good hygiene practices, particularly when cleansing and drying the skin
- the effects of knocks to the skin for some groups (diabetics and those with leukaemia)
- the need to check the skin regularly for any injuries or skin breakdown.

The National Institute for Health and Clinical Excellence (NICE) have produced a document called *Working together to prevent pressure sores – A guide to patients and their carers*. It is an easy-to-read document and avoids the use of technical words. Unfortunately, it is not available in any format other than the written word, but it can be easily adapted for use with the individuals you work with if required.

Evidence with case studies

Michelle is a 39-year-old woman with Down's Syndrome and diabetes who lives at home with her elderly parents in the community. Michelle does not attend any daytime activities and spends most of her time watching television while eating. She has put on a large amount of weight during the past twelve months, which is affecting her mobility and breathing. You meet with Michelle for the first time when she attends the diabetic clinic where you work.

1 What risk factors does Michelle have in contributing to skin breakdown?

2 How can you help Michelle to reduce these risks?

3 Who else should you involve to help reduce these risks?

4 What format would you use to inform Michelle of the health information she requires?

Activity

Get some copies of *Working together to prevent pressure sores – A guide to patients and their carers* and give them to the individuals who took part in the survey you carried out for the earlier activity. Ask them to read the document and encourage them to answer your survey again a few weeks later. Collate the results and identify whether the document has helped to improve the individuals' knowledge.

Evidence in action (CHS 4 pc 8)

Give an individual you provide care for the knowledge and understanding of the risks about pressure sores and ask them to assess their own risk. You can do this whilst being observed by your assessor, or you could ask a colleague to observe and then provide you with a witness testimonial.

Assessment tools used to assess risk of skin breakdown

(CHS 4 – K1, 2, 5, 7, 10, 18; CHS 5 – K1, 2, 5, 6)

Now that you know what to look for in an individual at risk of skin breakdown, you can begin to develop your knowledge of the assessment tools used to identify that risk.

Under the NHS document *Essence of Care* (2001), the benchmark of best practice is 'for all patients identified as "at risk" to progress to further assessment.' This means that, once you have identified an individual at risk through informal assessment, a formal assessment must be carried out. In September 2005 NICE in its publication *Pressures ulcers – prevention and treatment* recommended: 'Patients should receive an initial and ongoing pressure ulcer assessment. This should be supported by photography and/or tracings (ruler for calibration).' Further reading on this can be found at www.nice.org.uk/CG029.

Assessment for pressure sores requires a holistic approach – one that looks at the individual as a whole rather than at a specific area. In the UK, the most widely used risk assessment tool for pressure sores is the Waterlow Scale. There are also other forms of assessment tools, including the Gosnell Scale, Norton Scale and the Braden Scale. You will be examining all of these assessment tools in this element.

The Gosnell Scale

Devised by DJ Gosnell, the Gosnell Scale looks at the risk to the individual of pressure sores developing using five particular areas:

- mental status – an assessment of the level of response to the environment
- continence – the amount of bodily control of urination and defecation
- mobility – the amount and control of movement of the body
- activity – the ability to ambulate (walk)
- nutrition – the process of food intake.

In addition, evaluation includes recording of:

- the vital signs of temperature, pulse, respirations and blood pressure
- skin appearance
- diet
- medication
- 24-hour fluid intake and output.

Each of the areas is scored with points from 1 up to 5. The minimum score an individual can attain is 5 and the maximum score is 20. These are worked out as shown in the table.

Each of the expected findings per area comes with a clear description of the definition of what the health care assistant should be looking for. This can aid the worker in his or her understanding and ensures that everyone assesses individuals following the same criteria. Individuals scoring 5 are said to be at a very low risk of developing pressure sores; those scoring 20 are said to be at a very high risk of developing pressure sores.

Key term

Assessment tool In relation to skin breakdown, a process of assessment using a variety of risk factors, including continence, weight and nutritional status, against which a score is identified, clarifying the degree of risk that an individual's skin will break down. Assessment tools have various names according to their authors or developers.

Area	Finding	Description	Points
Mental status	Alert	Responsive to all stimuli; understands explanations	1
	Apathetic	Forgetful, drowsy; able to obey simple commands	2
	Confused	Disorientation to time, person and place	3
	Stuporous	Does not respond to name or simple commands	4
	Unconscious	No response to painful stimuli	5
Continence	Fully controlled	Total control of urine and faeces	1
	Usually controlled	Incontinence of urine or faeces no more than once every two days	2
	Minimally controlled	Incontinence of urine or faeces at least once every 24 hours	3
	Absence of control	Consistently incontinent of both urine and faeces	4
Mobility	Full	Able to move at will	1
	Slightly limited	Movement is restricted slightly and requires assistance, but will initiate movement	2
	Very limited	Unable to initiate movement but can assist a person who helps them to move	3
	Immobile	Unable to move without assistance	4
Activity	Ambulatory	Can walk unassisted	1
	Walks with help	Walks with help from another person, braces or crutches	2
	Chairfast	Walks only to chair (or is confined to wheelchair)	3
	Bedfast	Confined to a bed 24-hours a day	4
Nutrition	Regular intake of food	Eats some food from each basic food category each day	1
	Occasionally misses food	Occasionally refuses a meal or frequently leaves more than half of meal	2
	Seldom intakes food	Seldom eats a complete meal and only a few bites of food	3

The Gosnell Scale.

The Norton Scale

Devised by Doreen Norton, the Norton Scale looks at the risk of the individual to pressure sores using five particular areas:

- physical condition
- mental condition
- activity
- mobility
- incontinence.

Each area is scored on a points system from 1 to 4. Unlike the Gosnell scale, the higher point is awarded for the positive findings, as shown in the table below. Individuals are seen to be at risk of developing pressure sores if their overall score is below 14. The lower the individual's score, the greater he or she is at risk.

Area	Finding	Points
Physical condition	Good	4
	Fair	3
	Poor	2
	Very bad	1
Mental condition	Alert	4
	Apathetic	3
	Confused	2
	Stupor	1
Activity	Ambulant	4
	Walks with help	3
	Chairbound	2
	Bedbound	1
Mobility	Mobility	4
	Slightly limited	3
	Very limited	2
	Immobile	1
Incontinence	None	4
	Occasional	3
	Usually urine	2
	Urine and faeces	1

The Norton Scale.

The Braden Scale

Devised by Barbara Braden and used widely in the United States, the Braden Scale looks at the risk to the individual of pressure sores using six particular areas (one more than the Norton Scale and the Gosnell Scale):

- sensory perception – the ability to respond meaningfully to pressure-related discomfort
- moisture – the degree to which skin is exposed to moisture
- activity – the degree of physical activity
- mobility – the ability to change and control body position
- nutrition – the usual food intake pattern
- shear and friction (see page 232).

As with the previous scales, each area is broken down into findings, with points awarded. Like the Norton Scale, the higher point is given to the most positive finding. Individuals with a total score of 16 or less are considered being at risk of developing pressure sores:

- a score of 15 or 16 is considered mild risk
- a score of 13 or 14 is considered moderate risk
- a score of 12 or less is considered high risk.

Braden Scale research studies

Several studies have been made on the Braden Scale, including Bergstorm et al (1998) and Nixon & McGough (2001). Both of these studies looked at the validity of the Braden Scale in predicting individuals at risk from pressure sores.

Bergstorm et al (1998) randomly sampled 843 inpatients from three different care settings; some of the inpatients were free from pressure sores on admission, although it has been acknowledged that pressure damage to tissues can take three days to become visible. Research nurses were used to collect the information from the three care settings and were regularly monitored to ensure they were using the assessment tool correctly. From the studies made, Bergstorm et al (1998) identified that the mean (average) age of those who developed pressure sores was higher than those who did not. From this it could be concluded that age is a risk factor, which needs to be considered within the assessment tool. It was also suggested that scoring 18 on the Braden Scale should indicate the risk of pressure sores (the original 'mild risk' score is 16). It was explained that, by raising the score

Area	Finding	Points
Sensory perception	No impairment	4
	Slightly impaired	3
	Very limited	2
	Completely limited	1
Moisture	Rarely moist	4
	Occasionally moist	3
	Very moist	2
	Constantly moist	1
Activity	Walks frequently	4
	Walks occasionally	3
	Chairfast	2
	Bedfast	1
Mobility	No limitations	4
	Slightly limited	3
	Very limited	2
	Completely immobile	1
Nutrition	Excellent	4
	Adequate	3
	Probably inadequate	2
	Very poor	1
Friction and shear	No apparent problem	3
	Potential problem	2
	Problem	1

The Braden Scale.

to 18 to identify those at risk, more individuals would be identified, but equally, more individuals would be falsely identified. This would be beneficial to the individual, but could create an increase in expenditure to the care organisation.

The Waterlow Scale

The Waterlow Scale, devised by Judy Waterlow in 1985 and revised in 2005 to incorporate research undertaken by Queensland Health, is a comprehensive assessment tool widely used within the UK. You may already be familiar with this scale if it is used within your organisation. However, many organisations have adapted the format to suit the area in which it is used, while retaining many of the original scoring areas.

The Waterlow Scale looks at a total of ten areas potentially contributing to risk of pressure sores, more so than the Braden, Gosnell and Norton scales. These areas include:

- build/weight for height ratio
- continence
- skin type, visual risk areas
- mobility
- sex and age
- malnutrition screening tool
- tissue malnutrition
- neurological deficit
- major surgery or trauma
- medication.

A version of the table is shown below.

The Waterlow Scale, designed to be used with its accompanying prevention and treatment policy,

also has a manual to inform the user on how to interpret and use the assessment tool correctly. This manual was updated in 2005 to incorporate clarification on the areas assessed.

To ensure your understanding of the Waterlow Scale, here are some definitions of the terms used.

- BMI – Body Mass Index (the amount of fat within the body), calculated using a formula Body Mass Index = weight (kg) ÷ height (m)^2
- Oedematous – collection of watery fluid in the body's tissues
- Pyrexia – raised body temperature above 37°C
- Apathetic – lacking in interest
- Terminal cachexia – life-threatening muscle wastage
- Peripheral vascular disease – build up of plaque (atherosclerosis) in the arteries outside the heart, reducing blood flow
- MS – multiple sclerosis
- CVA – cerebral vascular accident

Build/weight for height	♦	Skin type visual risk areas	♦	Sex Age	♦	Malnutrition screening tool (MST) (Nutrition vol. 15, No. 6 1999 – Australia)	
Average BMI = 20–24.9	0	Healthy	0	MALE	1	A – Has patient lost weight recently?	B – Weight loss score
		Tissue paper	1	FEMALE	2	YES – Go to B	0.5–5 kg = 1
Above average BMI = 25–29.9	1	Dry	1	14–49	1	NO – Go to C	5–10 kg = 2
		Odematous	1			UNSURE – Go to C	10–15 kg = 3
Obese BMI >	2	Clammy, pyrexia	1	50–64	2	and score 2	> 15kg = 4
							Unsure = 2
		Discoloured grade 1	2	65–74	3	C – Patient eating poorly or lack of appetite	NUTRITIONAL SCORE
Below average BMI < 20	3			75–80	4	NO = 0	If > 2 refer for nutrition assessment/intervention
		Broken/spots grade 2–4	3	81+	5	YES = 1	
BMI = Wt(kg)/Ht(m^2)							

Continence	♦	Mobility	♦	Special risks			
Complete/ catheterised	0	Fully	0	**Tissue malfunction**	♦	**Neurological defecit**	♦
		Restless/fidgety	1	Terminal cachexia	8	Diabetes, MS, CVA	4–6
Urine incontinent	1	Apathetic	2	Multiple organ failure	8	Motor/sensory	4–6
Faecal incontinent	2	Restricted	3	Single organ failure (respiratory, renal, cardiac)	5	Paraplegia (max of 6)	4–6
Urinal and faecal incontinence	3	Bedbound, e.g. traction	4			**Major surgery or trauma**	
				Peripheral vascular disease	5	Orthopaedic/spinal	5
		Chairbound, e.g. wheelchair	5			On table > 2 hr#	5
				Anaemia (Hb < 8)	2	On table > 6 hr#	8
				Smoking	1		

MEDICATION – cytotoxics; long-term/high dose steroids; anti-inflammatory
Max of 4

#Scores can be discounted after 48 hours provided patient is recovering normallly.

The Waterlow Scale.

Memory jogger

Can you remember how BMI is calculated? Look back at page 242 to check your answer.

Activity

Using the formula, calculate your own BMI.

- Cytotoxics – medication used in the treatment of cancer
- $\geq$ – more than
- $\leq$ – less than.

Waterlow research studies

Studies conducted by Dealy (1989), Edwards (1995), Watkinson (1996) and Cook et al (1999) all assessed real patients using the Waterlow Scale. The outcomes of these studies have shown that the tool lacks inter-rater reliability. Inter-rater reliability is when two assessors, assessing independently, rate the same score for the areas assessed. It is difficult to determine if the outcomes of the studies made were as a result of the different perceptions of the patients by the assessor or because of the different interpretations of the Waterlow Scale itself.

To try to identify Waterlow's inter-rater reliability more accurately, another study was conducted of 110 qualified nurses all experienced in using the Waterlow Scale. Each nurse was given the same case study to assess using the scale. The case study was fairly detailed, sufficiently to determine if there was a risk of pressure sores and the level of that risk. Having read the case study and completed the Waterlow Scale:

- 65 per cent of the nurses overrated the risk
- 23 per cent underrated the risk
- only 12 per cent correctly rated the level of risk.

One difficulty the nurses faced was accurately working out the case study's BMI. Without a calculator, this can be fairly difficult to do – without knowing the formula it would be impossible. Waterlow addressed this difficulty in her revision of the scale in 2005 by giving the formula for calculating BMI and the ranges for each score. The use of a BMI conversion table, like the one below, should also help.

Waterlow has also addressed other difficulties encountered by the nurses in her revision of the scale, including clarification on skin types, malnutrition screening tool and major surgery or trauma scoring.

The conclusion of this study showed that, as an assessment tool, it was successful at identifying the individual at risk, if not entirely accurately in terms of the *level* of risk. Not using the tool in

Body Mass Index (BMI) Table																	
BMI	19	20	21	22	23	24	25	26	27	28	29	30	31	32	33	34	35
Height	Weight (in pounds)																
4'10" (58")	91	96	100	105	110	115	119	124	129	134	138	143	148	153	158	162	167
4'11" (59")	94	99	104	109	114	119	124	128	133	138	143	148	153	158	163	168	173
5' (60")	97	102	107	112	118	123	128	133	138	143	148	153	158	163	168	174	179
5'1" (61")	100	106	111	116	122	127	132	137	143	148	153	158	164	169	174	180	185
5'2" (62")	104	109	115	120	126	131	136	142	147	153	158	164	169	175	180	186	191
5'3" (63")	107	113	118	124	130	135	141	146	152	158	163	169	175	180	186	191	197
5'4" (64")	110	116	122	128	134	140	145	151	157	163	169	175	180	186	192	197	204
5'5" (65")	114	120	126	132	138	144	150	156	162	168	174	180	186	192	198	204	210
5'6" (66")	118	124	130	136	142	148	155	161	167	173	179	186	192	198	204	210	216
5'7" (67")	121	127	134	140	146	153	159	166	172	178	185	191	198	204	211	217	223
5'8" (68")	125	131	138	144	151	158	164	171	177	184	190	197	203	210	216	223	230
5'9" (69")	128	135	142	149	153	160	167	174	181	188	195	202	209	216	223	230	236
5'10" (70")	132	139	146	153	160	167	174	181	188	195	202	209	216	222	229	236	243
5'11" (71")	136	143	150	157	165	172	179	186	193	200	208	215	222	229	236	243	250
6' (72")	140	147	154	162	169	177	184	191	199	206	208	215	222	229	236	243	250
6'1" (73")	144	151	159	166	174	182	189	197	204	212	219	227	235	242	250	257	265
6'2" (74")	148	155	163	171	179	186	194	202	210	218	225	233	241	249	256	264	272
6'3" (75")	152	160	168	176	184	192	200	208	216	224	232	240	248	256	264	272	279

the way it was intended, however, created part of this problem. With sufficient training, this could be excluded, but additional studies will need to be put in place to show any improvement on the Waterlow's inter-rater reliability.

Activity

Ernest was born on 12 June 1928. He is 5 feet 8 inches tall and currently weighs 12 stone 4 pounds; he did weigh 14 stone 3 pounds five weeks ago. Ernest is in the later stages of dementia and is very confused and withdrawn, often spending one or two days in bed not wanting to get out. He is incontinent of urine and faeces and has dry skin. Blood tests show his haemoglobin levels are 7.2 and he has traces of protein in his urine. Using the Waterlow Scale:

1 What score would you give Ernest under the heading sex/age?

2 What is Ernest's BMI?

3 What total score would you give Ernest under mobility, malnutrition and special risk?

4 How would you score Ernest overall in terms of risk?

Evidence generator (CHS 4 pc 7)

Identify and obtain the assessment tool used within your organisation and show this to your assessor.

Best practice

✔ Develop a good knowledge of the factors contributing to healthy skin.

✔ Know what healthy skin should look like for individuals of different skin pigmentation.

✔ Know what signs to look for indicating skin breakdown.

✔ Know what the four stages of pressure sores look like.

✔ Have an in-depth knowledge of your organisation's pressure area risk assessment tool and practise how to use it correctly.

Assessment procedures

(CHS 4 – K1, 2, 3, 4, 6, 8, 10, 19; CHS 5 – K1, 2, 3, 4, 7, 8, 13, 19; CHS 6 – K1, 2, 3, 9, 13, 14, 19, 20, 21)

As with any assessment you undertake as a health care assistant, there are certain criteria you must follow to ensure an accurate outcome. For risk assessments on skin breakdown these include:

- using assessment tools
- taking standard precautions
- following timescales
- using safe handling techniques
- working within your own sphere
- including the individual.

Pressure area risk assessment tools are not designed to replace the clinical judgement of the professional. They are there to support the care given to the individual in conjunction with the expertise of the multidisciplinary team.

Using assessment tools

Using the appropriate assessment scale is essential. The tool you use should also be one that has been approved by your organisation for this use. The assessment scale should be:

- valid – it accurately assesses what it claims to assess
- reliable – when used by different people, it gives the same outcome
- culturally sensitive – it does not unfairly discriminate against any individual because of their ethnicity or preferred language.

The DoH, in its *Guidance on the single assessment process* (2004), suggest the Waterlow Scale as being an assessment tool to use in assessing risk of skin breakdown. However, it is important to add that they do not endorse this or any of the suggested assessment scales used within the National Health Service.

Taking standard precautions

To prevent infection and cross-infection, you must ensure you take **standard precautions** with hand washing before undertaking the assessment, during it and after it. You should also wear the appropriate protective clothing, such as disposable gloves and aprons, ensuring that they are removed after interaction with one individual and replaced with clean protection before interaction with another individual. Failure to follow these actions could result in individuals being exposed to infection transmitted from one individual to another. Some of these infections could increase the risk to the individual of skin breakdown, especially if the infection affects the person's health: for example, if it involves vomiting and diarrhoea.

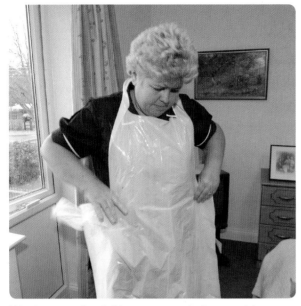

Wearing protective clothing can protect both you and the individual from infection.

Key terms

Standard precautions and health and safety measures A series of interventions that minimise or prevent infection and cross-infection, including: hand washing/cleansing before during and after the activity, and the use of personal protective clothing and additional protective equipment when appropriate.

- **personal protective clothing** Items such as plastic aprons, gloves (both clean and sterile), footwear, dresses, trousers and shirts, and all-in-one trouser suits. These may be single use disposable clothing or reusable clothing.
- **additional protective equipment** Types of personal protective equipment such as visors, protective eyewear and radiation protective equipment.

For individuals who already have open sores, the risk of infection is even greater. The health care assistant who has not followed health and safety guidelines appropriately can transfer infection from one individual to another. This infection can enter the individual's bloodstream through the open sore and cause serious illness, or even death.

Remember

Protect yourself to protect the individual.

Timescales

As the old saying goes, 'a stitch in time saves nine'. As with many things, the sooner something is carried out the better. Individuals can be prevented from long-term suffering of pressure sores if they are assessed and appropriate treatment is put in place sooner rather than too late.

Following NICE guidelines (2005), all individuals should be assessed for the risk of pressure sores on admittance to the care environment. This could be undertaken immediately on an informal basis and, if the individual is felt to be at risk, a more formal assessment should be carried out within six hours of admittance. For individuals living in the community, the risk assessment should be carried out during the first home visit.

Remember

Failure to assess an individual in time potentially puts the person's life at risk.

Using safe handling techniques

To avoid creating additional factors conducive to getting pressure sores within the individual, such as friction and shearing, you must ensure during your risk assessment and at any other time that you handle the individual using safe techniques. Under the Health and Safety at Work Act 1974, as stated by the Manual Handling Regulations 1992, all employees carrying out manual handling tasks must be suitably trained in this area and then given regular updates to training as required.

Friction and shearing are contributory factors to skin breakdown. As the health care assistant, you can cause both of these if you use inappropriate methods of moving and handling. When supporting or moving an individual, you must always ensure that his or her body is lifted clear of the bed or chair. This is to prevent the skin being dragged against the mattress or seat creating friction and shearing. You must follow the manual handling guidelines in the individual's care plan and use any equipment provided, such as a hoist, to assist in the move appropriately and as trained.

Memory jogger

What is the difference between shearing and friction? Look back at page 232.

There are three main types of moving and handling equipment:

- those that take all of the person's weight
- those that take some of the person's weight
- those that help the individual to move on their own.

The type of equipment that is used depends on the individual's ability.

Ability of individual	Type of equipment	Examples of equipment
Unable to help themselves	Takes all of the person's weight	Hoists Slings Slide sheets
Can help themselves a little	Takes some of the person's weight	Slide boards Slide sheets
Can help themselves just need support	Helps the individual to move on their own	Grab handles Lifting handles Handling belt

It is important to always prepare moving and handling equipment before you use it. Always follow a simple checklist when preparing moving and handling equipment:

Checklist: moving and handling equipment

✔ Is it clean?
✔ Does it have a safety check label in date (mechanical equipment)?
✔ Are there any rips or tears (slings or slide sheets)?
✔ Has any of the stitching come undone (slings, slide sheet, handling belt)?
✔ Are there are sharp edges (slide board, hoist)?
✔ Are there any loose or exposed wires (electrical equipment)?
✔ Has the battery been charged (electric hoist)?

After you have prepared the equipment, you then need to prepare the environment. This may include moving any furniture that could create an obstacle in your safe movement of the patient.

It is vitally important that you also prepare the patient prior to moving and handling. The Human Rights Act (1998) says that everyone has a right to choice. This is covered in more detail on page 106. The right to choice includes moving and handling. The individual has a right to choose, as much as possible, how they prefer to be moved and handled. An individual's choice may come from:

- personal beliefs – what the individual believes in, e.g. a Muslim woman not allowing a male to support her
- preferences – what the individual prefers, e.g. he or she may prefer to be lifted by a care worker rather than use equipment
- fear – what the individual is frightened of, e.g., heights, loss of control.

There may be times when you face **conflicts** or difficulties when preparing the individual for moving and handling. A conflict can happen when the individual's choice goes against safe practice, risk assessment or the care plan.

Key term

Conflict Clash or difference of viewpoints.

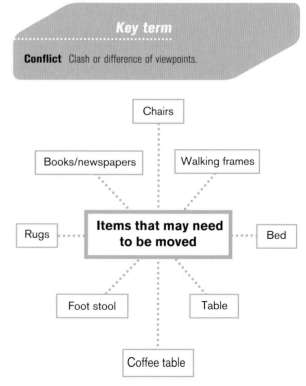

You may need to prepare the environment before moving a patient.

Working within your own sphere

To ensure the individual receives the best care or treatment, this should be given by those who have the ability through appropriate training and experience. It is highly unlikely that you would ask or even trust your local vet to remove your painful tooth, even though your vet may be very experienced in removing animal's teeth.

As a health care assistant, you have a responsibility to work at the level of your own competency, without exceeding that level: to do so could place yourself and the individual at harm through misjudgement.

The NICE guidelines state that all staff undertaking risk assessment in pressure area care should be suitability trained in the use of the assessment tool and have a good knowledge of appropriate preventative measures. If you have any difficulties assessing individuals at risk it is important that you seek support from someone more senior to you.

Asking for help or support is not a sign of weakness; in fact it is the opposite. It is a positive strength to admit you need help. Seeking the help and support you need will develop you as a person and in turn help the individual you are caring for. Failure to seek support could put the health of the individual at severe risk. There are a number of other health care staff you could turn to.

- Tissue Viability Nurse – a qualified nurse who has been specially trained in the role of assessing skin and the risks of breakdown. The Tissue Viability Nurse is usually employed by the health service to work in hospitals, clinics and in the community alongside community nurses and health visitors.
- Manager – the person responsible for staff within his or her team. This person leads through advice and example. If you need support, your manager should be the first person to turn to. If he or she cannot offer the expertise a situation requires, then he or she will be able to refer any difficulties to other professionals.
- GP (General Practitioner) – the GP will have the individual's medical history, including any current medications, health conditions or disabilities that could contribute to the individual's risk of skin breakdown.

Involving the individual

The NICE (2001) guidelines state that 'individuals who are willing and able should be encouraged, following education, to inspect their own skin. Individuals who are wheelchair users should use a mirror to inspect areas that they cannot see easily or ask others to inspect them.'

These guidelines go back to the importance of supporting and educating individuals in recognising what is healthy skin. The individual and his or her carer worker should also be informed of what to look out for as indicators to skin breakdown. This can be done through the use of pictures or a checklist of initial indicating factors, such as reddening skin, skin that is warm to the touch, swelling or skin loss.

What to look for	What to do
1 An area of the skin becomes pale or lighter in colour.	Keep moving your body position so that you do not stay in one position for too long.
2 Skin becoming red, warm or swollen.	Stay off areas of redness until skin returns to normal colour. Do not rub the area or put anything on it.
3 A blister appears over the red area of skin.	Stay off the area. Call your doctor or nurse.
4 The centre of the blister turns brown or black and is leaking fluid.	Stay off the area. Cover area with a sterile dressing. Call your doctor.

Pressure area care checklist for individuals and their carers.

If you are assessing an individual, it is important that you inform the person what actions you need to take and obtain his or her permission before undertaking those actions. Pouncing on an individual and starting to prod and poke him or her will not help you to obtain the information you need. Apart from startling the unsuspecting individual and appearing very rude, you will also be breaching the person's rights and many of your organisation's policies, procedures and codes of conduct.

Individuals must be given appropriate information in the most suitable format to their needs to enable them to make informed decisions. Approaching the individual and explaining to him or her what you need to do and why will help the person to be involved in his or her care. Obtaining consent from the individual to assess the risk of skin breakdown will supply you with the accurate information you need. The consenting individual will be more willing to answer your questions and will have a better understanding of what information you are requesting if he or she knows why you need the information.

Best practice

When undertaking a risk assessment ensure that you:

✔ use the appropriate assessment tools

✔ take standard precautions

✔ carry it out in required timescales

✔ use safe handling techniques

✔ work within your own sphere

✔ always include and involve the individual.

Evidence in action
(CHS 4 pc 1, 5, 6, 8, 9, 10, 11, 12)

Describe in detail how you have followed your organisation's pressure area risk assessment procedure. Include:

• assessment tools

• standard precautions

• timescales

• safe handling techniques

• working within your own sphere

• including the individual.

Undertake pressure area care

(CHS 5 – K14, 15, 16, 17, 18; CHS 6 – K5, 8, 12, 16, 17, 18, 22, 23, 24, 25, 26, 27, 28, 29)

When undertaking pressure area care, it is important that a number of procedures are followed. Some of these have already been covered in other sections of this book so you should make sure that you look at these pages again. The procedures you need to follow when undertaking pressure area care include:

• following the care plan

• team working

• using appropriate pressure relieving aids

• using appropriate moving and handling techniques.

Following the care plan

As a health care assistant, it is part of your role and responsibility to read an individual's care plan before you provide any care or support, and to follow the plan when you do. In relation to pressure area care, you must do this to ensure that you give the correct treatment. If you do not read the care plan, you do not know what care should be given or indeed how the care should be given. More information on care plans can be found on page 255.

Team working

Team work is what happens when a group of people work together towards one aim. Within health care, it is about different professions and disciplines working together to promote the health of the individual. As with many teams, each health team has a leader – one who guides and supports the team. This may be your manager.

Together, as a team, you need to ask questions, discuss the patient's care, listen to each other and respect and support each other's ideas. You need to communicate with each other effectively. As a health care assistant, you need to observe and talk with the patient, and assess his or her condition. You then need to communicate this effectively to other members of the team to enable them to play their role in providing the appropriate care to the individual.

Looking at what is involved in team work, you should be able to identify that communication plays a major role: effective communication is key to effective teamwork. More information on communication can be found in HSC 31on page 2.

Using appropriate pressure-relieving aids

There are many different ways pressure can be relieved from areas of the body, the main ones being mattresses and cushions. As with any form of care, the individual must first be assessed for the best possible treatment or aid to be identified.

Judy Waterlow has suggested specialist equipment depending on the outcome of the Waterlow score.

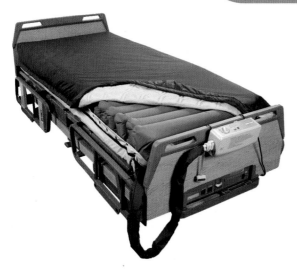

A low air loss mattress can be used by individuals at high risk of pressure sores.

Waterlow Score	Special mattress/bed	Cushions
10+	Overlays or specialist foam mattresses	100 mm foam cushion
15+	Alternating pressure overlays, mattresses and bed systems	Specialist gel and/or foam cushion
20+	Bed systems: Fluidised bed, low air loss and alternating pressure mattresses	Specialised cushion, adjustable to individual

Evidence in action (CHS 5 pc 8)

Identify the types of pressure relieving equipment used by your organistaion and research how they benefit the individual.

NICE (2005) suggests that the decision about which pressure-relieving device to use should be based on the cost of equipment and an overall assessment of the individual. They suggest the assessment should be holistic and include all of the following factors:

- identified levels of risk
- skin assessment
- comfort
- general health state
- lifestyle and abilities

- critical care needs
- acceptability of the proposed pressure-relieving equipment to the patient and/or carer.

NICE (2005) has stated the following **should not** be used as pressure-relieving aids:

- water-filled gloves
- synthetic sheepskins
- doughnut-type devices.

Using appropriate moving and handling techniques

Some individuals can have difficulties moving themselves because of their physical health. The difficulties may be temporary or short-term, or they may be permanent or long-term. Short-term problems could be people getting over an operation or illness; long-term difficulties could be due to an illness or disability such as multiple sclerosis.

Some individuals need to have their position changed regularly because of their physical health. If they do not move positions, these individuals may develop pressure sores. To help prevent individuals getting pressure sores, you need to encourage and support them to change position regularly. The type of help or support you give to an individual will depend on the type of disability they have.

Whatever support you give a patient with moving and handling, you need to ensure you have received the correct training. The Manual Handling Operations Regulations (2007) state that all individuals undertaking manual handling tasks must be suitably trained. This is to prevent you from hurting yourself and the individual. You must also ensure that you adhere to risk assessments and read and follow the individual's care plan.

Before beginning moving and handling, you may need to move any pieces of equipment or furniture that are not being used to make the area safe and clear from obstacles. This is to prevent you from tripping over items or bumping into furniture and hurting yourself.

Some moving and handling techniques, such as rolling the individual over, may require more than one person to be involved in moving the patient.

Where this is required, it is important that you work as a team: you need to work together and move the individual at the same time as each other. This is known as 'coordinating the move'. You should do this by following four steps.

1. Decide who will 'lead' the move

2. The leader checks everyone is ready, including the individual.

3. The leader says 'Ready, steady, move.'

4. On the word 'move', everyone moves the individual.

If the move is not coordinated, you could seriously hurt yourself, other members of the team and/or the individual.

When you move or handle individuals, you need to be very careful not to damage their skin. This could happen in the following types of move:

- moving up or down the bed/up a chair – the individual's bottom, heels or elbows could be dragged on the mattress or bedclothes. Lifting the individual clear of the bed can prevent this. Individuals whose skin is damaged in this way could develop a pressure sore.

- Supporting an individual to walk or stand – holding onto the individual's arm can cause them to have bruises, especially if they bruise easily. To avoid causing pain and bruising, you should use a handling belt.

Activity: Moving and handling

Identify all the moving and handling techniques used within your organisation. State which of them should be undertaken by more than one member of staff and why.

Wherever possible it is important to encourage the individual to contribute to the move. This will help them to develop more independence and make the task easier for you. You could encourage individuals to help themselves as much as possible if they are physically able. You could do this by helping them to help themselves out of bed using the following illustrations.

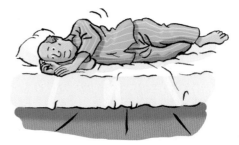

1 *Encourage the individual to roll to the edge of the bed, but not too close to the edge, as you do not want them to fall out. Their hand should be up by their shoulder, and facing down on the mattress.*

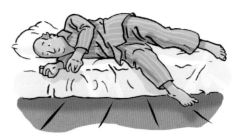

2 *Encourage the individual to swing their legs over the side of the bed.*

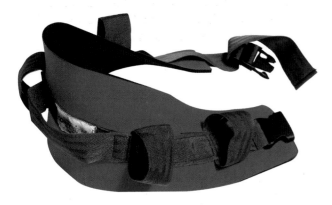

Handling belts prevent you harming the individual when supporting mobility.

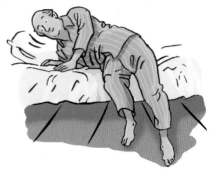

3 *Finally, the individual should sit up, with their hands pushing down on the mattress, before moving their feet towards the floor.*

Throughout any moving and handling procedure you need to provide the individual with verbal support both as encouragement and as a form of reassurance. It is also important that you return the environment back to its original state. You should put back furniture from where you moved it so that the individual knows exactly where it is and gives reassurance through familiarity. This is especially important when working with individuals who have visual disabilities or mental health issues.

Recording, reporting and reviewing risk assessments

(CHS 4 – K1, 11, 20, 21, 22, 23, 24; CHS 5 – K2, 20, 21, 22)

A risk assessment, however well carried out, will only be as good as the information recorded and reported from it. You could assess an individual following all the required criteria of the assessment but fail to record it appropriately. The recording and reporting of risk assessments and how this is done is vitally important, as is the regular reviewing of the condition of skin.

Frequency of reviewing risk assessments

Risk assessments should not be carried out once and then forgotten about. To ensure the individual receives the appropriate ongoing care, risk assessments should be reviewed or repeated at intervals agreed by the team and your organisation.

If an individual is identified as being at risk to pressure sores, a formal reassessment should be carried out as follows:

Waterlow Score	Frequency of reassessment
< 10	Weekly
10–15	Every 72 hours
16–20	Every 72 hours
> 20	Every 48 hours

The individual should also be reassessed:

- following any surgical or medical procedure
- after receiving an epidural (injection into the spinal cord to produce a loss of sensation below the waist)
- following signs of deterioration or improvement in his or her condition
- upon transfer to a new ward or care environment.

Activity: Policy at your workplace

Identify your organisation's policy on pressure area risk assessment. What timescales does it state for reviewing and reassessing individuals at risk?

Did you know?

Approximately 65 per cent of individuals hospitalised with hip fractures develop pressure sores.

As a health care assistant you should assess the individual's skin condition informally on a regular basis during general care procedure interactions, such as changing dressings or incontinence aids. You should also examine the individual's skin each time you change his or her position. This information should be recorded on a chart such as the example given on the next page.

Some individuals may be identified as not being at risk of skin breakdown. However, this could change if the individual's condition changes and so should be reassessed accordingly.

PATIENT TURNING CHART

Frequency of patient turning should be agreed by the team and recorded in the patent care plan.

Name: Phillip Young

Hospital number: JL56002316

Date: 21.08.06

Time	Position	Skin Grading	Signature	Status
01.00				
02.00				
03.00				
04.00				
05.00				
06.00				
07.00				
08.00				
09.00	B	2 – on admission	L Harding	SW
10.00				
11.00	R	2	L Harding	SW
12.00				
13.00	P	2	L Harding	SW
14.00				
15.00	L	2	N Green	Staff Nurse
16.00				
17.00	B	2	N Green	Staff Nurse
18.00				
19.00	R	2	N Green	Staff Nurse
20.00				
21.00	P	2	Andrew Pitts	B Grade
22.00				
23.00	P	2	Andrew Pitts	B Grade
24.00				

Patient position key:
SM – Self mobilising
L – Left side
R – Right side
P – Prone

B – Back
AC – Arm Chair
T – Therapy
I – Investigation

Plan of positions:
1. Change position every 2 (two) hour/s.
2. Patient can sit in arm chair for 1 (one) hour/s only.

Patient turning chart.

Information to be reported and recorded

All formal and informal risk assessments relating to skin breakdown should be reported, recorded and made available to all members of the care team. This is to ensure that all staff involved in the individual's care are kept up to date with any changes in the individual's condition.

Individuals with stage 1 pressure sores and above should have in depth recordings made of the following information:

- Grade of pressure sore (e.g. Waterlow Grade 2): when monitoring and recording on pressure sores which are healing it is important to record the grade of the sore as it originally was and to state on the record that it is healing. Pressure sores can deteriorate from a grade 3 to a grade 4 but should not be graded back up when healing.
- Cause of the pressure sore (e.g. rubbing on splint).
- Area affected (e.g. upper left calf, elbow).
- Size of the pressure sore (e.g. 2cm x 1cm).
- Any signs of infection (e.g. skin red 1cm out from edge of sore).
- Odour emitting from sore (e.g. no odour detected).
- Pain (e.g. individual complaining of moderate pain).

A photograph of the pressure sore should be taken to help identify healing or further breakdown.

An example review is shown on the next page.

Did you know?

NICE (2005) recommend all pressure ulcers graded 2 and above should be documented as a local clinical incident.

Any change within an individual's condition should be reported and recorded immediately. The change in an individual's condition may require that the person's care plan is reviewed and altered accordingly. Changes that need to be reported and recorded include:

- changes to the skin – e.g. colour, spots, dryness
- rise in temperature – the individual can become sweaty, increasing the risk
- change of continence ability – e.g. the insertion or removal of a catheter
- development of health condition – e.g. cancer, anaemia, diabetes, MS
- changes to mobility – becoming ambulant or losing mobility
- changes to appetite – an increase or decrease in appetite
- weight loss or weight gain
- prescription of risk-increasing medicines – e.g. steroids, cytotoxics.

PATIENT PRESSURE AREA REVIEW RECORD

Name: MarionSpierrs

Ward: Ward 17 Rehabilitation

Hospital number: JJ4235633

TO BE COMPLETED FOLLOWING REASSESSMENT USING THE FOLLOWING TIMESCALES

Waterlow score:	Frequency of review:
< 10	Weekly
10 – 15	Every 72 hours
16 – 20	Every 72 hours
> 20	Every 48 hours

AFFIX PHOTOGRAPH HERE

Grade of pressure sore	1	2	3	4
Area affected	$\geq$ Left heel			
Cause of the pressure sore	Rubbing on splint			
Size of the pressure sore	2cm by 2cm			
Any signs of infection	No signs indicated at present			
Odour emitting from sore	No odour detected			
Pain	Marion states she only has pain when pressure is put onto the heel			

Completed by: Lucy Harding   **Status:** Support Worker

Date of last review: Not applicable

Date of this review: 19.8.06

Patient pressure area review record.

Activity

Find out what your organisation's policy is for reporting and recording on pressure area risk assessments for the individual and collectively.

Some organisations, especially larger ones such as the NHS, may have a collective report form that needs to be completed. This form enables the organisation to collect information relating to the incidence or number of individuals developing pressure sores whilst in the care of the organisation. This information would be collated by the Tissue Viability Service on a weekly basis and aids them to identify any increase or decrease in individuals developing pressure sores.

An increase in the incidence of pressure sores does not necessarily indicate that staff are not doing their job – this may be due to the susceptibility of the individuals receiving treatment at that time. However, regular increases may need to be looked into to ensure that staff are suitably trained and are following the guidelines correctly.

NHS Trust
Weekly Pressure Report Form

Unit/Ward: Ward 17 Rehabilitation

Week Ending: 20 August 2006

Total number of patients on ward: 18

Total number of patients with pressure sores: 3

Patient's Name	Hospital Number	Date of Admission	Waterlow Score	Grade of Pressure Sore
OR Hospital Sticker				
Joseph Wilson	HR2758921	02.08.06	21	2
Marion Spierrs	JJ4235633	19.08.06	14	1
Joy Masters	MJ4530076	19.08.06	18	1

Name: Lucy Harding

Status: Support Worker

Signature: Lucy Harding

Signature: 20.08.06

A weekly report form.

> **Did you know?**
>
> Up to 80 per cent of individuals with a spinal cord injury will develop a pressure sore and 30 per cent will develop more than one.

> **Remember**
>
> A risk assessment will only be as good as the information recorded and reported from it.

The importance of recording and reporting risk assessments

The passing on of information within a healthcare environment is important to enable the continuity of care for that individual. If information relating to an individual was not reported or passed on appropriately, staff, professionals and the individual themselves would not know what care had been given or indeed needed to be given. The environment would be chaotic – nobody would know what to do and the individual would not receive the care that he or she required.

Records relating to an individual's care are just as important as the care that is given. Records can be used:

- to collate information for the individual's treatment
- to monitor areas of change within the individual
- to inform other staff or professionals on the individual's progress
- for legal purposes – for example, a coroner's inquest.

Following the Data Protection Act 1998 all records completed by you must be accurate, legible and complete. Risk assessments on pressure areas must be recorded accurately and legibly to ensure the correct level of care is given to the individual following the assessment. If you record the assessment inaccurately or incorrectly this wrong information will be passed onto others and the individual would receive the wrong type of care.

To ensure your recording is legible you must write clearly to prevent any misinterpretation of the record. If you make any mistake whilst writing the report you should simply cross out your mistake with a single line and rewrite the word. Trying to correct your mistake by going over the word or changing the letters within the word could lead to difficulties reading it correctly. To ensure your report is complete you should include the date and your initials or signature to confirm when the report was completed and by whom. Initialling your report will allow other staff to identify you as the person completing it should they need to clarify any areas of the report.

It is just as important to report pressure area assessment outcomes to the appropriate staff, including the registered practitioner and the individual concerned, to ensure immediate care can be given as appropriate. Informing the individual of the risk assessment outcome is the person's right, it is also important to obtain the individual's understanding and cooperation with his or her treatment.

Remember

Records within a care environment are a legal requirement.

Following risk assessment, the information you identify and record will need to be incorporated into the individual's care plan. This plan would detail what care the individual requires and how it should be given. If you fail to record the outcome of the risk assessment accurately this will lead to the care plan being developed using inaccurate information and therefore the individual will be provided with the wrong treatment.

Evidence in action (CHS 4 pc 13)

Undertake a risk assessment on an individual in your care using your organisation's assessment tool. Report and record your findings and incorporate the outcome into the individual's care plan.

You should now see how important it is to record information accurately, legibly and completely. As a health care assistant you play a very important role in the care of individuals alongside other staff. If you do not follow your role completely, this will have an adverse effect on others – especially the individual.

Best practice

✔ The outcome of the risk assessment must be incorporated into the individual's care plan.

✔ You must ensure you record accurately, legibly and completely.

✔ Changes in the individual, whether positive or negative, must be reported and recorded.

✔ Assessment must be reviewed on a regular basis.

References

DoH 2001 *Essence of Care*

DoH 2006 *Essence of Care: benchmarks for promoting health*

NICE 2001 *Working together to prevent pressure sores – A guide to patients and their carers*

Further reading

NICE 2005 *Pressures ulcers – prevention and treatment*

Waterlow, J 2005 *Pressure Ulcer Prevention Manual*

Ousey, K 2005 *Pressure Area Care* Blackwell Publishers, Oxford

www.tissueviability.org

www.carestandards.gov.uk

www.doh.gov.uk

www.nursingtimes.net

www.nmc-uk.org

www.rcn.org.uk

Undertake treatments and dressings related to the care of lesions and wounds

Introduction

Caring for a patient with a wound or lesion involves much more than just understanding how wounds heal.

It is vital that you adopt a holistic approach. This means taking into consideration the patient's physical, spiritual, emotional, social and psychosocial needs, as well as the specific assessment of the wound itself. You will need to recognise and understand the specific care needs of the individual and agree with the patient the goals to be achieved. Clear, accurate and standardised documentation is vital as is the prompt referral to relevant members of the multidisciplinary team.

The information in this unit is not solely for staff working in acute care but can also be applied to other care settings including care homes, the individuals' home or other community settings such as the GP surgery.

In this unit the term 'wound' is used to cover both wound and lesion. You should read this unit in conjunction with Topic 1 *Infection Control*, Topic 2 *Aseptic Technique* and Topic 3 *Anatomy and physiology*.

What you need to learn

- What wounds are
- How wounds heal
- Undertaking procedures
- Patient observation during a procedure
- Assessing wounds
- Wound cleansing
- Wound complications
- Wound treatments and dressings

What wounds are (K11)

A **wound** is a flaw or break in the continuity of the skin. This can include bruises, cuts, abrasions and puncture wounds. A **lesion** is a pathological change in a bodily tissue. In this unit, the term 'wound' will be used to cover both wounds and lesions.

The skin consists of three main layers: the epidermis, dermis and the subcutaneous fatty tissue layers. It performs a number of functions:

- protection
- perception of stimuli
- thermoregulation
- excretion of waste
- metabolism.

When the skin becomes damaged or is broken, a wound can occur.

Memory jogger

Can you remember the anatomy and physiology of skin and how wounds heal? Look back at Topic 3 *Anatomy and physiology* on page 166 before you read on.

Types of wound

Wounds can be divided into two main groups – acute and chronic – and then further sub-divided into different types.

Acute wounds are wounds that are expected to heal within a defined period of time. These include:

- surgical incisions
- penetrating wounds, such as a stab wound

- avulsion and crushing injuries
- shearing injuries
- traumatic injuries.

Chronic wounds are wounds that are slow to heal. These include:

- leg ulcers
- pressure sores
- fungating lesions
- sinuses and fistulae.

Reflect

What wounds are you familiar with from your own experience and practice?

Which wound types are you permitted to dress and treat?

For each question, make a list of your answers.

Key terms

Sinus A blind-ended channel that permits the drainage of wound exudate. It extends from the surface of the wound to a cavity.

Description	Definition	Example of wound
Partial thickness	Involve the epidermal and/or the dermal layer of the skin and, because of this, would be expected to heal quickly. They are very painful and need the protection of a dressing.	Donor site of skin graft Some burn wounds
Full thickness	Involve the epidermis, dermis and subcutaneous layers; some can also involve tendons, muscle or bone. These wounds heal by granulation and contraction and take more resources, including time, than the partial thickness wound.	Pressure sores Third and fourth degree burns Deep lacerations Leg ulcers
Cavity wounds	Full thickness wounds in which the base of the wound is not always easy to visually determine. Could have the presence of a **sinus**.	Pressure sores Pilonidal sinuses Dehisced wound

Wound depth

When looking at different types of wounds, wound depth is a key factor. This table explains the terms used for different depths of wound.

Surgical wounds

These can be healed by two different methods.

- *Primary closure* Here the incision is closed at the end of the surgical procedure, leaving minimal distance between skin edges and with no tissue loss.
- *Secondary closure* Here the incision is purposely left open and possibly packed at the end of the surgical procedure. This type of closure is often seen when infection is present at the time of operation, or following surgery to trauma patients.

Surgical wound closures

When wounds are closed at the time of the operation or trauma, the doctor or practitioner closing the wound has a choice of different wound closures. The choice will depend on the position of the wound, the condition of the wound edges and a full holistic assessment of the patient.

Sutures

Sutures have been used for many years as a reliable method of wound closure. Here again, there is a choice of different types of suture: they may be absorbable (dissolvable) or non-absorbable, and made of a natural or a synthetic material.

Suture materials

Natural suture materials	Synthetic suture materials
Absorbable	*Absorbable*
• catgut – plain or chromic	• polyglycolic acid (Dexon)
	• polyglactin (Vicryl)
	• polydioxone (PDS)
	• polyglyconate (Maxon)
Non-absorbable	*Non-absorbable*
• silk	• polyamide (Nylon, Ethilon)
• linen	• polyester (Dacron, Ethibond)
• stainless steel wire	• polypropylene (Prolene)

Absorbable sutures are dissolved by enzymes in the body, so do not need to be removed by a member of the health care profession. Different

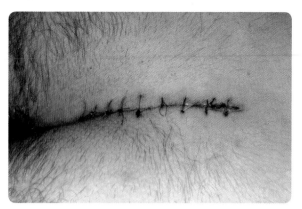
Sutures used to close a pilonidal sinus.

absorbable sutures are designed to dissolve at different rates. The choice of suture will depend on the nature and position of the wound. If the correct suture is chosen, the wound should have healed completely by the time the suture has dissolved.

A variety of non-absorbable sutures are available. The practitioner will need to choose the most appropriate one, depending on the procedure being undertaken and on an assessment of the patient's general health. These sutures do not get dissolved by the body's enzymes, so those that are externally visible will need to be manually removed later by a health care practitioner, using either a stitch cutter or surgical scissors. The time that non-absorbable sutures are left in place will depend on the material used and the position of the wound.

Some patients may return to your department from theatre with sutures in position called retention sutures. These are in place to reduce the tension (stretching) on the primary suture line. They are mainly used following abdominal surgery in obese patients, and are placed in the deep muscles and fascia of the abdominal wall, to help support the deeper tissues while the external tissues heal.

While undertaking a patient's wound care, you may be asked by the patient how long their sutures have to stay in position. Depending on your experience and the time you have spent working in your department, you may feel confident to answer the patient's query. However, you will need to check that the practitioner in charge is happy for you to give this information.

Staples

Staples come in disposable sterile packages. They are used to close wounds by bringing together the opposing edges of a clean wound. A special tool called a staple remover is required to remove the staples.

Adhesive skin closure strips

These are available in various lengths and widths, They are applied to the clean and dry edges of superficial wounds and those under little tension. Adhesive skin closure strips can also be used in conjunction with deep sutures. They are extremely effective in treating pretibial lacerations.

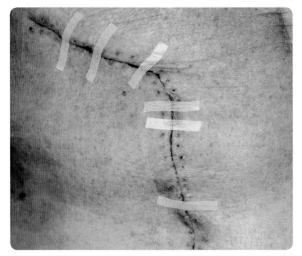

Steri-Strips® in position following removal of sutures from the wound.

Tissue adhesives

These are used mainly in Accident & Emergency departments for the treatment of simple traumatic lacerations. The glue is available in single-use vials and applied to the clean and dry tissue edges of the wound.

How wounds heal

(K12 a, b, 21, 22, 23, 24)

All wounds heal by going through four distinct stages:

- inflammation
- migratory
- proliferation (granulation)
- maturation.

In ideal circumstances, the human body is well equipped to heal a wound satisfactorily by itself, without external intervention. However, ideal circumstances very rarely occur, so wounds are prevented from healing by other factors, both **intrinsic** and **extrinsic**.

To provide an optimum wound healing environment, you must identify these factors and minimise their effects on the wound healing process. This is why it is so important to take a detailed history of the patient's social, psychological and physical wellbeing (a holistic assessment), so that interventions can commence as soon as possible.

Key terms

Intrinsic Within, on the inside.
Extrinsic Originating from the outside.

Here are just a few examples of the intrinsic and extrinsic factors affecting wound healing.

Intrinsic	
Age	As a person ages, his or her skin becomes less elastic due to the loss of collagen. An older person's skin also becomes thinner due to the loss of subcutaneous fat, and drier as secretion of sebum reduces. As people get older, the rate of cell repair also diminishes, so it generally takes longer for any wounds to heal.
Chronic health conditions, e.g. • diabetes • anaemia • peripheral vascular disease • pneumonia • COPD • Crohn's disease • ulcerative colitis	A number of diseases will affect wound healing due to their impact on; cellular metabolism, on the cells' oxygen-carrying ability and how effectively the oxygen can be transported around the body.
Nutritional status	Malnutrition, particularly in the older person, has been linked to delayed wound healing and increased risk of pressure sore development. The body requires the following for optimum wound healing: protein – for collagen production zinc –for cell division and growth. Lack of zinc reduces fibroblasts and collagen. iron – for collagen production and anaemia can lead to reduced amounts of oxygen vitamins A and C – increase the tensile strength of wounds, help with the production of collagen and the increase of fibroblasts.
Psychological	Stress and anxiety reduce the amount of chemicals called cytokines. These chemicals are partially responsible for the inflammatory process, which is necessary in the early stages of wound healing. Body image and the patient's attitude to caring for their wound will also influence wound healing.
Dehydration	The body requires 2000-2500 litres of fluid a day for efficient cellular activity. If the body is dehydrated, electrolyte imbalance occurs. Effective wound healing can only take place when the wound environment is kept moist. Many wound dressings are now designed to facilitate this.
Poor oxygenation	This is caused by disease processes or smoking. Poor oxygen levels at the wound site lead to reduced collagen formation, and hence delays in wound healing. Oxygen under pressure – Hyperbaric Oxygen Therapy – is used in some areas to treat hard-to-heal wounds.
Immunosuppression	Here the body cannot satisfactorily implement the wound healing process, as the disease and/or the patient's medication negatively impacts on the inflammatory response, leading to a lengthened healing time.
Extrinsic	
Smoking	This reduces the amount of oxygen carried in the blood, as carbon monoxide binds to haemoglobin in its place. The reduced oxygen concentration in the blood can impede wound healing. Nicotine and carbon monoxide also increase the risk of blood clotting.
Foreign material and debris	A foreign body in the wound leads to a prolonged inflammatory response, which slows down the subsequent stages of wound healing. Wounds containing necrotic tissue will not heal, so this needs to be removed.
Wound infection	Here the wound remains in the inflammatory stage for a longer period of time as the body tries to cope with the wound infection and the healing process. See the section on wound infection later in this unit, on page 276.

Medication	Some drug therapies can affect wound healing: • cytotoxics interfere with cell production • anticoagulants increase chance of bleeding and haematoma formation • corticosteriods decrease collagen growth, reduce inflammation and narrow blood vessels, reducing blood flow to the wound environment • non-steroidal anti-inflammatory drugs reduce the production of collagen.
Poor wound care and hand washing	The choice of wound dressing will impact on the rate of wound healing. Dry dressings will dry out the wound, could potentially leave particles on the wound surface and can damage the granulating tissue when removed. Bandages applied too tightly can impede the flow of blood and therefore nutrients/oxygen to the wound site. Poor hand hygiene and/or sterile technique can lead to contamination of the wound site, which could in turn lead to a wound infection.
Wound location	The location of the wound can make applying an appropriate dressing difficult. Keeping the dressing in place to provide a moist environment is difficult if it is in a location where it is constantly being rubbed or moved, e.g. sacrum. Care must also be taken with wounds that are in positions where they can easily become infected, such as the perineum, groin or anal area. Wounds in positions where it is difficult to remove pressure are also at risk of delayed healing. Pressure-relieving aids may need to be used to relieve pressure from the wound site Dressings to the scalp are also very difficult to keep in place.
Poor surgical technique	Rough handling of the wound during surgery can cause tissue damage and haematoma formation, with the possibility of secondary infection. Poor choice of suture material and suturing technique could cause tissue death at the wound edges, and potentially lead to wound infection.

Undertaking procedures

(KS 2, 3, 4, 5, 6, 7, 13, 14, 15, 18, 21, 25, 26b, 27)

Delegation and responsibility

Any procedure you undertake should have been appropriately delegated to you by the registered practitioner in charge of the patient's care. This means that the practitioner has reviewed your competence to carry out the task and has asked you whether you feel confident to proceed. If you have not been assessed as competent to undertake an activity and you do not feel confident, either before or at the time of the procedure, then you should not proceed as requested.

The activity must also be identified within your job description. If it is not one of your identified job roles, you must not proceed with the task, even if requested to do so by any member of the health care team. Politely explain that this particular activity is not within your job description and therefore you are unable to help with their request. You could, of course, offer to help in any other way that you can.

Activity

Read your job description and person specification. What are your responsibilities in the care environment? What are the limits of your role?

Checking the patient's documentation

Using the patient's written plan of care, identify exactly what dressings and treatments are required. If this is not clear or you are not completely sure, you must discuss this with the practitioner in charge of the patient's care. If the patient's dressing or treatment is one you have not used before, again you must seek guidance from the practitioner in charge.

You must check the patient's records for any documented evidence of allergies, so that you do not use any solution, treatment or dressing that may cause the patient harm or distress. Discuss allergies with the patient before undertaking the procedure, as someone may have forgotten to document this on admission.

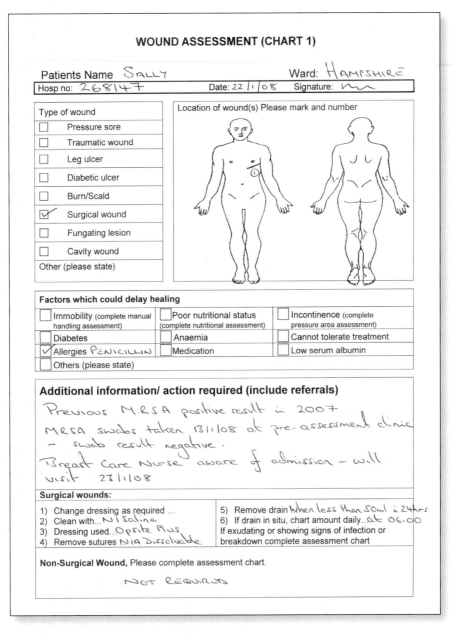

WOUND ASSESSMENT (CHART 1)

Patients Name SALLY   Ward: HAMPSHIRE

Hosp no: 268147   Date: 22/1/08   Signature: ~~

Type of wound	
☐	Pressure sore
☐	Traumatic wound
☐	Leg ulcer
☐	Diabetic ulcer
☐	Burn/Scald
☑	Surgical wound
☐	Fungating lesion
☐	Cavity wound

Other (please state)

Location of wound(s) Please mark and number

Factors which could delay healing

☐ Immobility (complete manual handling assessment)	☐ Poor nutritional status (complete nutritional assessment)	☐ Incontinence (complete pressure area assessment)
☐ Diabetes	☐ Anaemia	☐ Cannot tolerate treatment
☑ Allergies PENICILLIN	☐ Medication	☐ Low serum albumin
☐ Others (please state)		

Additional information/ action required (include referrals)

Previous M.R.S.A positive result in 2007
MRSA swabs taken 13/1/08 at pre-assessment clinic
– swab result negative.
Breast Care Nurse aware of admission – will
visit 23/1/08

Surgical wounds:

1) Change dressing as required ...
2) Clean with... N I Saline
3) Dressing used... Opsite Plus
4) Remove sutures N IA Dissoluable

5) Remove drain When less than 50ml in 24hrs
6) If drain in situ, chart amount daily.. at 06.00
If exudating or showing signs of infection or
breakdown complete assessment chart

Non-Surgical Wound, Please complete assessment chart.

NOT REQUIRED

Example of an initial wound assessment tool completed following surgery.

Check to see if the patient requires some form of analgesia or other medication before starting the procedure. If this is the case, you will need to liaise with the practitioner in charge of the patient's care, so that it can be administered at the correct time.

Memory jogger

Are you always thinking about how you are communicating with a patient? Look back at HSC Unit 31 page 2 for more detailed information on communication.

Communication

Effective communication with the patient regarding their care is seen as best practice. It ensures that the patient is fully involved in planning their own care, gives them the opportunity to offer any information that may assist in the procedure, and allows them to ask questions to clarify aspects of their care. You should refer any questions beyond your role or knowledge to a more knowledgeable member of the clinical team, so that patients are given the correct information on which to base any decisions.

Each patient is an individual with their own life history, which in turn affects the way they react to certain aspects of care. Someone who has had a bad experience while undergoing a particular treatment will be much more apprehensive this time around than someone whose experience was good. You will need to spend more time with the apprehensive patient, ensuring that all their fears are alleviated before the treatment can start.

Not everyone will react to a request or procedure in the same way. For example, people have their own pain thresholds and for some they are much lower than for others. Individuals will also react differently when asked to expose a part of their body for dressing purposes. Individuals will be influenced by their cultural background, their religion and their upbringing, as well as past events and this must always be respected.

Reflect

Think about the patients you have nursed over the past few days. Consider how each patient has reacted to you undertaking their dressing.

Have they all reacted the same in relation to pain and privacy and dignity?

If there has been a difference, do you know why this is?

Consent

Before undertaking a procedure, you must always seek consent from the patient. This includes explaining to the patient what the procedure involves and why the procedure needs to be undertaken. The information should be provided in such a way that the patient is easily able to understand all that is being said to them: in this way, the patient can make an informed decision as to whether to proceed with the treatment. The person who provides this information and seeks consent must be suitably trained and qualified to undertake the procedure:

> 'It is a general legal and ethical principle that valid consent must be obtained before starting treatment or physical investigation, or providing personal care, for a patient.

> This principle reflects the right of patients to determine what happens to their own bodies, and is a fundamental part of good practice.'

(Department of Health 2001)

See HSC Unit 31 page 34 for further detailed information regarding patient consent.

Evidence with a case study

Maud is an 87-year-old lady who had surgery yesterday. The practitioner in charge of her care has asked you to redress the wound.

1 What information would you need to access before undertaking this dressing?

2 List where you would find this information.

3 What do you need to discuss with Maud before starting the dressing?

Evidence may be gained for: CHS 12 K1, 4, 7, 9

Timing

Another important aspect to consider is the time that the procedure should be undertaken. Undertaking procedures at the wrong time or in the incorrect order could lead to an increased hospital stay, delayed rehabilitation or the potential of wound infection through cross contamination of infected to clean wounds.

Here are some examples of things you need to think about.

- *Is the wound infected? Does it need to be completed after all other cleaner dressings?*
  If you undertake the infected wound dressing first and do not follow strict standard precautions, including aseptic technique, your hands may get contaminated with pathogens that are later transmitted to the clean wound of another patient.

- *Does the patient need to go for some other form of therapy and need their wound redressed before this, e.g. physiotherapy?*
  It would be difficult for a therapist to provide treatment to a patient with a heavily exudating wound. Missing out on their therapy could lead to an increased length of hospital stay.

- *Does the wound need redressing before the application of a Plaster of Paris (POP) cast or before the fitting of a splint?*

Some patients require a splint or POP before discharge from hospital. Wounds around where the splint is being fitted may need to be redressed before the appointment time, or time may be wasted returning the patient back to the department. Always check with the practitioner in charge of the patient's care.

- *Are the doctors expected to undertake a ward round and will they want to see the wound?*

  There is no point in redressing a wound (unless there is a more important reason for doing so, such as pain or the break through of exudate) before a doctors' round if you know that they will want to review the wound. It would be a waste of your time and will, more importantly, expose the surface of the wound to potential micro-organisms unnecessarily.

- *Does the dressing need changing early in the shift as it is no longer fulfilling its purpose, e.g. exudate is leaking through, it has fallen off or the patient is in a great deal of pain due to the dressing?*

The practitioner in charge will help you to plan when the dressings should be completed. If you are unsure, you must ask their advice as it may be detrimental to the patient's care to do what you think may be correct.

Evidence with a case study

You have been allocated the following patients to care for on an early shift. The practitioner in charge has asked that you try to complete their dressings before lunchtime.

Patient 1 Steve a 20-year-old young man with a knee wound that needs redressing before his physiotherapy appointment at 9.30 am.

Patient 2 Joyce who had an open cholecystectomy yesterday. She is complaining of pain around the wound site.

Patient 3 Jane had a left breast mastectomy three days ago. At handover you were informed that a wound swab had been sent to microbiology as it was suspected that her wound was infected.

Patient 4 Paul is now two days following a repair of an incisional hernia. His consultant is expected to visit the ward at 8.30 am to review Paul's wound before he is discharged.

Describe your actions in relation to these patients, covering:

- where you could access information concerning their wound care requirements
- the order in which you would undertake these dressings and the reasons for your choice
- the potential implications of undertaking these in the incorrect order
- any other nursing care you feel is required before or following the dressing.

Evidence may be gained for: CHS 12, K 1, 5, 8, 13, 14, 15

Manual handling

Immediately before the procedure, you may need to position the patient in a certain way so that a particular part of the patient's body is made accessible. You will need to carry out a risk assessment to see whether, in order to position the patient safely and comfortably, you need the help of colleagues or should use a piece of manual handling equipment.

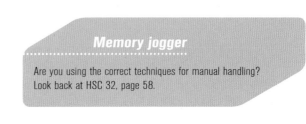

Memory jogger

Are you using the correct techniques for manual handling? Look back at HSC 32, page 58.

Before beginning the procedure, go through this checklist.

Checklist

- Can the patient help to position themselves with gentle and precise instructions from you?
- Is the patient comfortable?
- Can you help to support them using pillows or foam?
- Are your work colleagues comfortable and not at risk of a manual handling incident?
- Is the bed at the correct height?
- Can the patient help by holding on to the side rails?

Standard precautions

Refer to the section on standard precautions within Topic 1 Infection control on page 141 and Topic 2 Aseptic technique on page 159 for further information on this topic.

It is extremely important to apply the principles of standard precautions when undertaking any form of wound care. You must protect yourself from the patient's body fluids and prevent the cross-infection of pathogens from your body to the patient and/or their wound. **The primary defence against cross infection is adequate hand washing**.

Checklist: standard precautions

- Wash hands with soap and water before and after the procedure. Either use alcohol hand gel during the procedure or wash hands again with soap and water if necessary, e.g. visibly contaminated.

- Use the relevant personal protective equipment – gloves, apron and gown, along with mask and eye protection, depending on the procedure. These items may be single use disposable or reusable.

- Collect all necessary equipment before going to the patient and check all packaging for expiry dates and signs of contamination. If it is out of date or any of the packaging is damaged, dispose of it according to your organisation's policy and collect new items.

- Ensure that all the items are absolutely necessary for the procedure – once opened they immediately become contaminated and cannot be reused.

- Ensure that you have a bin or yellow bag available for the disposal of clinical waste, e.g. the old wound dressing.

- Pack up all used instruments and soiled dressings before leaving the treatment area – otherwise pathogens can be accidentally transmitted to other areas of the clinical department during disposal.

- Have a sharps bin available for the safe disposal of sharps if required.

Did you know?

Antisepsis is a process or a treatment that kills or inhibits micro-organisms. When related to hand washing, it is the process that removes transient micro-organisms from the skin and reduces the normal flora.

Depending on the procedure to be undertaken and the documented care in the patient's care plan, use an aseptic technique, an aseptic non-touch technique or a clean technique. Always check the patient's care plan and/or with the practitioner in charge before carrying out the procedure. Not following the patient's plan of care could put the patient at risk of a wound infection, delayed wound healing or even **septicaemia**.

Key term

Septicaemia A severe bloodstream infection, which can be fatal.

Memory jogger

Can you remember the difference between aseptic technique, aseptic non-touch technique and clean technique? When should each be used? Look back at Topic 21 *Aseptic technique* on page 157.

The sterile field

To undertake the required wound care procedure, you must be proficient in setting up a sterile field and maintaining the sterility of the field during the procedure.

Asepsis and *sterility* are both defined as 'the state of being free from living pathogenic micro-organisms' (Hart 2007).

A sterile field is created by the use of sterile drapes or sterile towels that can be placed around the site of the procedure and/or on a dressing trolley, stand or dressing tray.

The following principles should be applied when setting up and maintaining a sterile field.

- Place only sterile equipment on the sterile field.
- Take care when opening packages to ensure that the sterile contents do not touch your exposed hands.
- Do not allow any other person to place any un-sterile objects on the sterile field.

- Do not allow any other person to touch the sterile equipment or lean across the sterile field.
- Once any piece of single-use equipment has become contaminated, make sure it is disposed of and then replaced, if needed.
- Keep contaminated reusable instruments separate from other sterile items until you can put them in the used medical instruments box, usually kept in the dirty utility room. Refer to your own organisation's policy on cleaning medical instruments before returning them to the Sterile Services Department.
- Ensure the procedure is undertaken in a clean area, e.g. a clinical treatment room or 30 minutes after any cleaning activity has taken place, to allow airborne particles to settle.
- Do not undertake a procedure by an open window: this will increase air movement and the potential for airborne contamination.
- The key principle of an aseptic non-touch technique is that, when handling any sterile equipment, you should not touch the key parts.

Evidence with a case study

Staff nurse Jo works in the Oral Health Clinic and is assisting the doctor to remove a lump from the mouth of a patient. Jo has washed her hands, has applied gloves and a disposable gown and is now in the process of setting up her sterile field ready for the procedure. Student nurse Emma is in her first year of nursing and it's her first day in the department. You are observing the procedure in the department. Emma is asked by Jo to open the sterile sutures for the procedure. Emma opens the sterile pack, takes out the inner suture pack with her bare hands and places it on the sterile field.

1 What mistake did Emma make?

2 Explain the implications of her mistake.

3 What should be your actions on witnessing the incident?

4 How could this mistake have been prevented?

Evidence may be gained for: CHS 12 K 1, 2, 5, 13, 15, 21

Patient observation during a procedure

(KS 1, 2, 3, 7, 8, 9, 26a, b, 27)

While carrying out the procedure, you must always observe the condition of your patient and listen out for cues that all may not be well.

Fainting

Patients can react very differently to the care they are given. If you have followed best practice and have discussed the procedure thoroughly with your patient, they may have informed you that they are prone to fainting at the sight of blood or an exposed wound. With this information, you can ensure that the patient is lying down for the procedure and ask a colleague to talk to the patient and keep them calm during the procedure.

However, not all patients will be aware of their potential to faint, so during the procedure you should be looking for:

- pale appearance
- rapid breathing
- sweating

and possibly the patient saying that they are suffering from:

- feeling warm
- light headedness
- blurred vision
- nausea
- rapid heart rate.

If the patient complains of any of the above, or if you are concerned about his or her condition, you must stop the procedure immediately and ask for assistance.

All that is usually required to prevent a patient from fainting is to lie them down or sit them with their head lowered but only if the patient's condition allows this. If the patient does faint, you need to call for assistance immediately by either using the emergency alarm or calling for help.

Memory jogger

How should you deal with a health emergency? Look back to page 66 to remind yourself.

First Aid: Fainting

Ensure that the environment is safe before you approach the patient, then check the patient for:

- **A**irway
- **B**reathing
- **C**irculation.

If no breathing or circulation, commence resuscitation. Refer back to page 68.

If the patient is unconscious, but breathing normally, lay them on their back and elevate their legs above heart level to help the blood supply to vital organs. Be aware of contraindications to this position such as pregnancy or respiratory disease. Loosen any restrictive clothing. Consciousness should be quickly regained.

If the patient vomits, or is bleeding from the mouth, if it is safe to do so, place them on their side in the recovery position.

If the patient was injured in the faint, then treat the injuries appropriately. Once help has arrived, explain exactly what has happened, giving any information regarding the patient's medical history, and assist the team as requested.

You will need to document your actions during the incident in the patient's nursing records (if your organisation allows this) or give a detailed report to the practitioner in charge so that they can document it. You may need to complete an incident form according to your organisation's policy. If so, write a simple, factual description of what happened and any care you provided.

An example of a completed incident form can be found on page 54.

Pain

It is good practice to offer analgesia before any wound care, particularly if you are aware that it could be painful for the patient. Analgesia could take the form of tablets, an injection or, in some departments, **Entonox**. You will need to liaise with the practitioner in charge of the patient's care in order to provide adequate analgesia for the procedure.

If the patient is able, ask them to rate their level of pain before, during and after the procedure using a pain assessment tool, such as a visual pain scale or numerical pain scale. This is an important aspect of the holistic wound assessment: it should be recorded on the appropriate documentation and communicated to the practitioner in charge of the patient's care.

During the procedure, you will still need to observe the patient for any signs that they may in pain. Even if they have been given analgesia before the procedure, this may not have been adequate and another form of analgesia may be required.

Observe for:

- verbal clues such as moaning, shouting or crying
- grimacing
- pulling away
- rapid pulse and breathing
- sweating.

If the patient complains of any of these, or you are concerned that they are still in pain, you must stop the procedure immediately and request the assistance of the practitioner in charge of the patient's care.

Evidence with a case study

Agnes is an 81-year-old lady who has come to your clinic to have her leg ulcer redressed. You have not undertaken her dressing in the past but have been passed as competent by your manager to carry out this procedure. Before the procedure, Agnes tells you that the last nurse really hurt her when removing the old dressing. She also tells you that it is still very painful.

What documentation would you access before undertaking the dressing?

What specific questions would you ask Agnes before commencing her dressing?

What could you do to reduce the level of pain Agnes experiences during the procedure?

How could you tell if Agnes was in pain during the procedure?

Who would you seek assistance from if you did not feel confident to undertake this dressing?

Evidence may be gained for: CHS 12, K 1, 2, 3, 6, 7, 8, 9, 10, 27

Discomfort

While you are undertaking the procedure, the patient should be made as comfortable as possible. If it is evident during the procedure that the patient is not comfortable (by patient comment or by visual cues), stop the procedure and reposition the patient. Check with the patient that they are happy to proceed.

Privacy, dignity and modesty

The patient's privacy, dignity and modesty should be maintained at all times. For some treatments and dressings, it will be necessary to expose areas of the body that may cause embarrassment to the patient. You need to manage this situation as sensitively as possible and expose only the minimum amount of the area. Only allow essential personnel in the treatment area and lock doors if this is possible. Consider offering a chaperone as per your organisation's policy.

If at any time the patient becomes distressed by the situation, you must stop the procedure immediately to maintain the patient's dignity and modesty. Gain the patient's consent before recommencing the procedure.

Evidence with a case study

Mrs Keith is an elderly lady who has recently had a hip replacement in hospital. She is booked into your GP's surgery for removal of her sutures. The procedure will take place in one of the consulting rooms.

What actions should you undertake to ensure that you maintain Mrs Keith's privacy, dignity and modesty?

What would be your actions if a student nurse asked to observe the procedure?

Evidence may be gained for: CHS 12, K 1, 2, 7

Documentation

Guidance on which parts of the patient's documentation you can complete will need to be agreed between you and your manager. The accurate and factual documentation of

0–10 Pain intensity scale

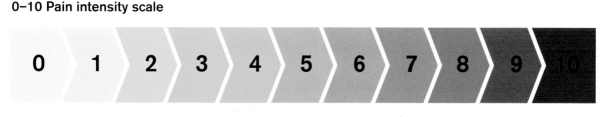

| 0 | 1 | 2 | 3 | 4 | 5 | 6 | 7 | 8 | 9 | 10 |

No pain   Moderate pain   Worst pain possible

People feel pain at different levels and will have their own pain threshold.

care provided, and the identification of future treatment plans, is vital for the continuity of patient care and communication between members of the multidisciplinary team.

Good record keeping is the mark of a skilled and safe practitioner; the quality of your record keeping is a reflection of the standard of your professional practice (NMC 2007).

Assessing wounds

In order to undertake a thorough wound assessment, you must take into consideration all factors affecting the patient and not just the wound itself. This is termed an 'holistic' assessment and includes aspects such as the patient's medical history, their psychological condition, their nutritional intake, their medication and their social history as well as the specific assessment of the wound itself.

While undertaking the wound assessment, you are looking for any improvement or deterioration in the wound. If noted, this needs to be conveyed to the practitioner in charge of the patient's care, so that they can decide if the patient's wound care needs revising.

Memory jogger

Look back at the section on factors affecting wound healing on page 259.

An initial wound assessment must be carried out to provide a baseline against which the effectiveness of future treatment choices can be evaluated.

There are various ways in which wounds can be assessed. Some organisations and departments use a wound assessment chart, kept in the patient's records so that it is available for review by all relevant healthcare personnel (see example on the next page). The chart provides a guideline as to which aspects of the wound need to be assessed and documented. Information may need to be collected from other assessment tools, such as

pain assessment tool. Other organisations may use care plans or care pathways or may simply write up care in the medical or nursing records. What is important is that the care and treatment given and any future plans are documented accurately at the time.

For more information on documentation, see CHS 4, page 239 on pressure sore assessment.

Types of wound

Wounds closed at the time of surgery
Information documented must include:

- the type of closure material used (e.g. staples, sutures and/or adhesive skin closure strips)
- **primary** and/or **secondary** dressings in place.

This information is generally found on the post-operative notes of patients returning from theatre, or in the patient's medical notes if the procedure took place in a department/ward area.

Wounds left open at time of surgery
Here information should include a description of:

- the wound bed, including its size, depth and colour
- any exudate present including consistency, colour and smell
- the condition of the wound margins
- primary and/or secondary dressings in place.

Key term

Primary dressing Dressing applied directly onto the wound.
Secondary dressing Dressing applied over the primary dressing.

Remember

With a secondary dressing, you will need to check that it is compatible with the primary dressing.

ASSESSMENT CRITERIA RELATING TO WOUND CARE

(Chart 2)

Patients Name: FRED   **Hospital Number:** 479268

Use a separate chart for each individual wound.

Wound number	①							
Wound site	RIGHT HIP.							
Date	22/1/08	23/1/08						
Wound size (Increasing, Decreasing, Stable)	D	S						
Wound depth (cm)	2 cm	2 cm	cm	cm	cm	cm	cm	cm
Grade of sore	4	4						
Wound Pain – (Worse, Less, Different)	L	L						
Wound Odour (None, Some, Offensive)	N	N						
Exudate – amount (Increasing / Decreasing)	D	D						
Exudate – Colour/type	YELLOW THIN	YELLOW THIN						
Base of wound bleeding (Yes / No)	N	N						
Swab (enter date sent & result)	22/1/08							
Wound -% Necrotic	0 %	0 %	%	%	%	%	%	%
Wound - % Sloughy	40 %	40 %	%	%	%	%	%	%
Wound - % Granulating	60 %	60 %	%	%	%	%	%	%
Wound - % Epithelialising	0 %	0 %	%	%	%	%	%	%
Surrounding Cellulitis (Yes / No)	N	N						
Wound margin – macerated (Yes / No)	N	N						
Objectives – Protection	✓	✓						
Objectives – Hydration								
Objectives – Absorption	✓	✓						
Objectives – Debridement	✓	✓						
Dressing – Primary (enter code)	4	4						
Dressing – Secondary (enter code)	2	2						
Dressing frequency	DAILY	DAILY						
Cleansing agent (enter code)	1	1						
Wound assessed by:								

Dressing codes:
1 – Bioclusive 2 – Allevyn 3 - Lyofoam 4 – Sorbasan 5 – Granuflex 6 – Aquaform 7 – Charcoal 8 – Other
Cleansing agents:
1 – Saline. 2 – Other (state)

Future dressings

The date and time of the next dressing may be indicated by the doctor on the operation notes or in the patient's medical notes. This information should be transferred to the wound assessment chart and/or written in the nursing notes by the practitioner in charge of the patient's care, so that all staff are aware of the patient's treatment plan.

If there is no documented information regarding the next dressing change, the practitioner in charge of the patient's care should make their decision regarding the next dressing change based on department protocols and an assessment of the wound type, ward bed and exudate if present.

What are you assessing?

When you assess a wound, you must consider a number of different factors:

- size and shape
- depth
- wound bed
- condition of surrounding skin
- exudate
- odour.

Size and shape

As you might expect, the bigger the wound, the longer it will take to heal. It is also easier for the wound to heal if it is boat-shaped rather than round or irregularly shaped.

To measure the wound accurately and to ensure standardisation of assessment, you should always measure the wound the same way. Measure the greatest length and greatest breadth, and record the measurement in centimetres.

Patient Label

B

Actual/potential nursing problem .... JOHN .... has undergone surgery under local / general* anaesthetic.   * delete as appropriate
Aim of nursing care: To reduce the potential for complications associated with post-operative recovery.

1. Explain to the patient that they are back on the ward	RTW @ 14.30 following incision + drainage of pilonidal sinus 22/1/08
2. Maintain airway.	Fully conscious on return 22/1/08
3. Observe and record temperature pulse, blood pressure and respiration and neuro-vascular checks as indicated.	Frequency of observations: 12 hours initially reducing as per policy if patient's condition dictates 22/1/08
4. Observe and record any pain and administer analgesia as required.	Morphine 10mg given in theatre + recovery. Further analgesia prescribed on drug chart 22/1/08
5. Observe for nausea and vomiting and administer anti-emetics as prescribed.	Ondansetron 4mg given in theatre. No nausea on return to ward. 22/1/08
6. Administer oxygen as prescribed.	...... LPM for ...... hours / until awake* — NOT REQUIRED. 22/1/08
7. Record fluid intake and output on appropriate charts.	Please chart Oral fluids ☐ Has passed urine @ IV fluids ☐ Urine Output ☐
8. Observe the wound site and take appropriate action as required.	Sorbsan pack insitu. Gauze to cover. Some minimal blood stained exudate 22/1/08
9. Offer and assist with post-operative wash and change of bed clothes/ night wear.	
10. Observe and record any specific post op instructions from doctor.	Redress wound in 24 hrs. Daily dressings by Practice / District Nurse 22/1/08

Evidence demonstrating research-based practice

Mitchell M (2004) *Pain management in day-case surgery.* Nursing Standard. 18, 25, 33-38.
Skilton M (2003) *Post-operative pain management in day surgery.* Nursing Standard.17, 38, 39-44
Wilkins I & Wheeler D (2003) *Preventing, recognizing and treating postoperative complications,* Surgery, 21:1 2003, 14-20.

Date for review 01/10/08

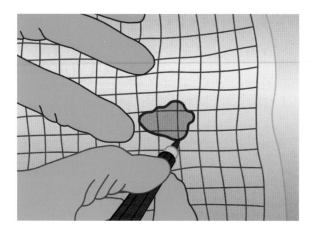

Ways to measure a wound

Acetate Place a sterile acetate over the wound and trace the margins of the wound. Then measure the wound's length and breadth and use these dimensions to calculate the surface area.

Two-layer acetates are also available. These are better than one-layer acetates because the layer in contact with the wound can be disposed of immediately, leaving the other to use as a guide.

Ruler Use a disposable ruler or tape measure. After use, dispose in the clinical waste.

Photography This can be a very good way to assess and evaluate wound care treatments, especially as it does not require any contact with the wound surface, but it does have its limitations. It can only be used where the entire wound can be photographed at once. Also, standardisation is extremely important when using photographs to assess wound progress: lighting, position and camera angle all need to be considered.

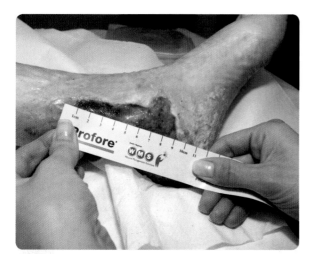

Each organisation will have its own policy on medical photography, which may cover:

- patient consent to have photograph taken
- concealing the identity of the patient
- what the photographs may be used for: evaluation of wound treatment, publication, teaching, etc.
- where the photographs may be taken: ward, department, clinic or patient's home
- where the photographs will be stored.

Moulds With a mould, a material is poured into a cavity and then removed when set, allowing the size and depth of a wound to be measured.

Other methods are available, but they require technical knowledge and skill to operate and can be very expensive to use.

Depth

Some of the above techniques can also be used to measure the depth of a wound. One simple method is to use a sterile foam-tipped probe to see how far down the wound goes: you insert the probe to its deepest point and then mark on the probe where it is level with the skin surface. This method is not reliable as it may miss any **sinus** or **undermining** present, and may not be standardised as each practitioner may probe a different area of the wound bed.

Care should be taken when probing the wound bed as the tip of the probe may damage any fragile granulating tissue present.

Key terms

Undermining wound An area of tissue destruction underneath intact skin.

Reflect

What methods do you use in your clinical area for measuring the size and depth of chronic wounds? How easy are these methods to use?

Is the information stored or documented anywhere? Is it easily accessible by all members of the health care team who need it?

Wound bed

Treatment options and wound dressings will depend largely on the condition of the wound bed. Here is an explanation of some of the key terms used to describe it.

Necrotic Recognised by the presence of dry, hard, black dead tissue. The black area can cover the wound completely, or be present in smaller areas in deeper wounds. The hard, black tissue may be covering an underlying abscess or cavity.

Necrotic tissue needs to be removed before wound healing can commence.

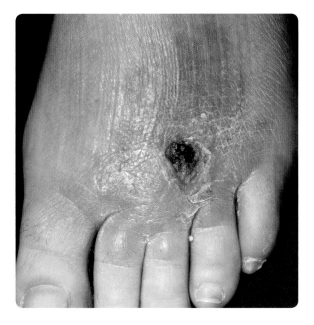

Sloughy This is dead tissue which is moist, stringy and yellow/cream in colour. Sloughy skin needs to be removed from the wound so that healing can take place.

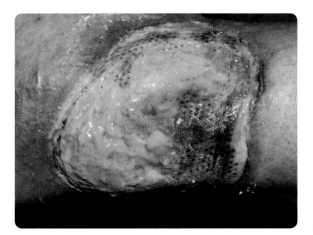

Granulating Appears bright red in colour and is very fragile. It is healthy tissue made up of delicate capillary loops, which can easily be damaged by inappropriate dry dressings.

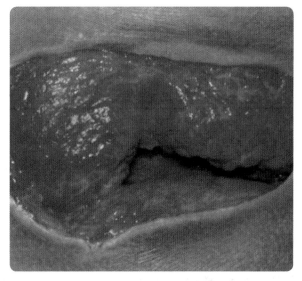

Epithelialising Once the wound is filled with granulation tissue, epithelialisation can begin. New epithelium begins to grow from the wound margins or from hair follicles. It is pale/dusky pink in colour.

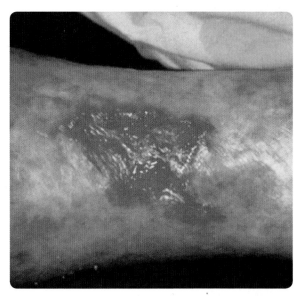

Condition of surrounding skin

The skin surrounding the wound needs to be observed during the wound assessment: future dressings may need to be changed in light of the findings.

You need to assess whether the surrounding skin is:

- healthy
- red – due to inflammation, infection or trauma
- dry and flaky
- macerated – soggy and white skin due to excessive moisture
- bruised, identified by purple/bluish skin.

Note your observations down on the wound assessment chart. If you are concerned about your findings, report them to the practitioner in charge of the patient's care.

Exudate

All wounds produce some form of exudate, which is most evident during the inflammatory phase of wound healing.

You need to make the following observations of wound exudate:

- amount – difficult to measure so scale may be based on '+', '++' and '+++'
- colour and consistency – What colour is it? Is it thin and watery or thick and opaque?
- dressing – Is the dressing containing the exudate, either at its edges or through the dressing?
- odour – Does the exudate have an odour?

Odour

This may be present due to necrotic tissue, infection, exudate or from the dressing itself. If noted during a dressing change, it should be documented and reported to the practitioner in charge so that further investigations and treatments can be started. Treatment will depend on the cause of the odour. Certain dressings and treatments can be used in the interim while the main cause of the odour is addressed. For the patient, having a wound that smells is very distressing and can lead to poor body image.

When re-assessing the wound, it is important to note if the odour has reduced. This is difficult to standardise as different practitioners undertaking the same dressing will each have a different sense of smell and may describe the odour differently.

Remember

Don't forget to document your findings on the appropriate records, e.g. wound assessment chart, patient's care plan

Also observe for signs that the patient may be allergic to the wound dressing or treatment applied. One such adverse reaction is contact dermatitis, which causes inflammation of the epidermis. There is normally a clear, defined reddened area which corresponds to the exact outline of the dressing. If you note this, remove the dressing and inform the practitioner in charge of the patient's care, as a different dressing will be needed. Sometimes patients are more allergic to the tape holding the dressing in place than they are to the dressing itself.

Evidence with a case study

Steve is a 27-year-old man who fractured his ankle while playing football. Yesterday morning, he went to theatre and had internal fixation of his ankle. Over the last 24 hours, he has developed a pyrexia. The practitioner in charge has asked you to undertake his dressing.

1 Before commencing the dressing, what information would you need to access – and where would you find this information?

2 On removal of Steve's dressing, what factors related to his wound would you assess?

3 What findings would you feel necessary to report back to the practitioner in charge of his care?

4 What further investigations or treatments might be required?

5 Discuss how and where you would document your findings and actions.

You may provide evidence for the following: CHS 12, K 3, 4, 12c, 19, 26b, 27

Nutritional assessment tool

As part of the holistic assessment of the patient, it is good practice to complete a nutritional assessment tool. However, you should refer to your organisation's policy on completing nutritional assessments, as not all patients with a wound will require one.

Identification of patients at risk of malnutrition (and hence of delayed wound healing) allows prompt referral to the appropriate healthcare professional.

Wound cleansing

Before a wound is cleaned, you should undertake a detailed wound assessment, as described above.

It is important to know that not all wounds need cleaning. Cleaning is not required where the wound bed is clean, there is little exudate and healthy granulation tissue is present. Removal of normal exudate present during the inflammatory phase will deplete essential growth factors and other vital components from the wound bed, leading to a delay in wound healing.

Reasons for cleaning include:

- removal of excessive exudate and/or slough
- removal of infected exudate or cell debris
- removal of foreign bodies in the wound
- removal of debris left from previous wound dressings.

Types of fluids used

In most hospitals, because sterile normal 0.9% saline is readily available, this is the preferred fluid of choice. Tap water which is suitable for drinking can be used for cleansing most chronic wounds such as leg ulcers or pressure sores.

Any fluid used should be warmed: cell production at the wound bed is reduced by cooling.

How to cleanse

Wounds should be cleaned by gentle irrigation using either a syringe or sterile saline pod. Do not use force to irrigate a wound: this may damage the delicate granulation tissue and could create a risk of splash back of the irrigation fluid, including the patient's bodily fluids.

After wound cleansing, make sure that the edges of the wound are clean and dry, but do not dry the wound itself.

Remember

Do not use cotton wool balls as they tend to shed fibres, which interfere in the wound healing process

Step by step: wound cleansing

1. With the sterile field already set up, open the cleaning fluid (usually sodium chloride 0.9 per cent at body temperature) and tip into sterile container.

2. Clean your hands with alcohol gel.

3. Put on sterile gloves.

4. Use moist gauze swabs to clean debris from round the wound edges only. Use one stroke, moving from centre out or down one side.

5. If the wound surface needs cleansing, use a syringe, spray can or pod (e.g. Steripod) to irrigate the wound and leave to dry naturally.

6. Dry the edges of the wound with sterile gauze.

Wound complications

(KS 3, 12b, c, 13c, 16, 17)

Haemorrhage

There is the possibility that the wound will continue to bleed when the patient returns from theatre or following a departmental procedure. If you are the first to notice the bleeding, you must get assistance immediately from a registered practitioner.

You will need to stay with the patient, remain calm and reassure them. If you have a thick dressing, a clean towel or something similar, then place this over the original dressing and apply pressure, but only if wearing gloves. When assistance arrives, a specific pressure dressing needs to be applied to the wound site and the site observed for further bleeding. Document your actions and any observations taken. Continue to monitor the patient's vital signs as requested by the practitioner in charge.

Dehiscence

This is the premature bursting open of a wound, which usually occurs 6–10 days post-operatively but can occur up to a month following surgery. The cause of dehiscence could be related to the patient's age, drug therapy, diabetes, nutritional intake or the presence of a localised infection.

If the complication also involves the protrusion of underlying **viscera**, it is termed **evisceration**.

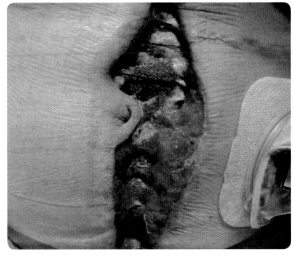

Abdominal wound dehiscene.

This is a medical emergency and you must seek assistance immediately. Use the emergency call bell to summon help, while you reassure the patient. If you have a clean, sterile towel or drape available, place this over the wound. If viscera are present, cover with a sterile, wet towel or pad. Keep the patient 'nil by mouth' until told otherwise, as the patient will most certainly need to return to theatre.

Once again, you must not forget to document your findings and actions. An incident form may be required, depending on your organisation's policy.

Wound infections

An infection in the wound will delay healing or could even lead to dehiscence (see above). Early identification of a potential wound infection is therefore vital.

As discussed in Topic 1 *Infection control*, the skin plays host to a number of micro-organisms called the 'normal flora'. These micro-organisms live happily on the skin's surface, but can become pathogenic if they invade deeper layers of the skin.

A wound provides the ideal opportunity for the pathogen to gain entry.

Types of wound infection

There are three categories of wound infection:

- contamination – the presence of bacteria that do not multiply and do not cause delayed wound healing
- colonisation – the bacteria can grow and multiply, but there is no damage to the individual or evidence of wound infection
- infection – there is multiplication of bacteria which overwhelms the host's defences, leading to an associated host response.

The host's ability to withstand the invasion of bacteria will depend on a number of factors such as their current medical condition, age, poor nutritional intake, smoking, certain medication, the presence of tissue ischaemia, wound haematoma or a foreign body in the wound.

Clinical signs

Cutting and Harding (1994) identify the following clinical signs of wound infection:

- abscess
- cellulitus
- discharge
- discoloration
- friable granulation tissue
- unexpected pain in a wound
- bridging of the soft tissue
- odour
- wound breakdown.

If there are signs of clinical infection, you may need to take a wound swab. Check with the practitioner in charge and, if one is required, follow your organisation's policy on taking a wound swab.

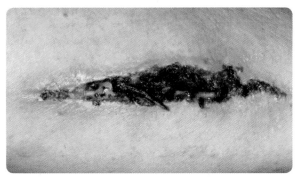

Clinically infected wound.

This table shows the pathogenic organisms specific to wounds and lesions.

Types of pathogens in wounds

Aerobic bacteria	Anaerobic bacteria
These bacteria thrive in the presence of oxygen but do not necessarily depend on it	These bacteria thrive in the absence of oxygen and so are suited to the conditions found in the bowel and the soil
Staphylococcus aureus	Bacteroides
Staphylococcus epidermidis	Clostridium welchii
Methicillin-resistant Staphylococcus aureus	Clostridium tetani
Beta-haemolytic streptococci	
Escherichia coli	
Klebsiella	
Pseudomonas	

Source: Bale and Jones, 2006

Evidence through reflection (CHS 12, KE 5, 12b, 13, 14, 16, 18c, 23, 24)

Identify an individual in your clinical area who has a wound infection.

What are the individual's signs and symptoms in relation to their wound infection?

What type of infection does the individual have?

List any other factors the patient has which will affect their wound healing.

When redressing this wound, what standard precautions will you take and why?

Make notes for your portfolio.

Dressing wounds

(KS 3, 5, 8, 18a, 19, 20, 22, 27)

The current dressing or treatment required by the patient should be documented on their care plan. It is important that you follow the plan exactly unless you notice any contra-indications, such as an allergy to the treatment. If noted, you must inform the practitioner in charge immediately, so that a different dressing or treatment can be started.

Your organisation may have a wound care formulary, used by practitioners to help them choose the appropriate dressing for a particular wound. These formularies are generally developed by the Tissues Viability/Wound Care Specialist and are based on current best evidence.

The ideal dressing should:

- maintain a high humidity at the wound/dressing interface
- remove excess exudate
- allow removal without causing trauma
- be impermeable to bacteria
- provide thermal insulation
- be free of particles and toxic contaminants
- allow gaseous exchange
- be acceptable to the patient
- be cost-effective.

Source: adapted from Turner (1985)

Types of dressing

The type of dressing required is based on the holistic assessment of the patient and their wound, taking into consideration the amount of exudate, the stage of wound healing, the surrounding tissue condition, any allergies the patient may have and any predisposing medical conditions.

Step by step: hydrocolloid dressing

1. Remove the old dressing, and clean wound if required according to the local protocol.

2. Assess the wound. If a hydrocolloid dressing is still appropriate, continue

3. The dressing should be big enough to extend beyond the wound edges by approximately 2 cm.

4. Remove part of the backing paper as per manufacturer's instructions and apply the adhesive side to the patient. Continue by smoothing down the dressing over the wound, removing the remainder of the backing paper as you go and firming it into place with your hand.

5. If you are applying the dressing to a difficult area, the dressing can be shaped with either sterile scissors or cuts made into the centre, so that it can be formed around a heel or finger, for example. Check first to see if your organisation has dressings specifically shaped for the site you are dressing.

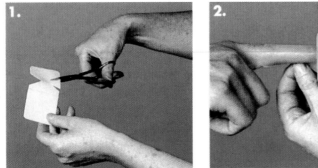
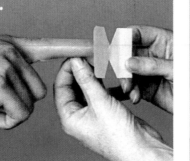
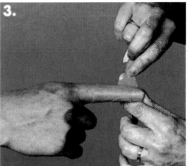

Applying dressing to a finger.

When applying the dressing, it is vital that you adhere to the manufacturer's instructions and guidelines regarding its use. Failure to do so will leave your organisation open to litigation should any harm come to the patient. Also, check the expiry date on the packaging and ensure that the package is not damaged or already open.

Type of wound	Aim of treatment	Treatment options	Examples of products available
Necrotic	To re-hydrate the eschar To debride wound	Hydrocolloid Hydrogel	Granuflex, Comfeel Intrasite gel, Purilon gel
Sloughy	To remove all debris, deslough and preserve healthy tissue	Hydrogel Hydrocolloid Alginate dressing Hydrocellular	Intrasite gel, Purilon gel Granuflex, Comfeel Sorbsan or Kaltostat Allevyn
Granulating	To keep moist and preserve delicate blood vessels	Hydrogel Hydrocolloid Alginate dressing Hydrocellular Non-adherent-silicone	Intrasite gel Granuflex Sorbsan or Kaltostat Allevyn Mepital – reserved for difficult-shaped areas
Epithelialising	To protect new tissue	Thin hydrocolloid Semi-permeable membranes	Duoderm thin Bioclusive, Opsite

Infected	To reduce bacterial numbers	Systemic antibiotic	See examples above
		Alginate sheet, rope or ribbon	
		Hydrocellular	
		Hydrogel with secondary dressing of either hydrocolloid, hydrocellular or polyurethane film	

Wound dressings.

The products in the table above are examples of those that can be used for specific wound types. You must however always refer to your own organisation's Wound Care Formulary or Wound Care Policy for the appropriate dressing choice for your Trust. It is equally important to follow the patient's wound care plan and/or instructions of the registered practitioner who delegated the task.

Wound care product choice will also vary depending on the depth of the wound and most primary dressings will also require a secondary dressing. Advice on an appropriate secondary dressing can usually be found in the manufacturer's literature for the primary dressing or your organisation's wound care formulary.

Evidence generator CHS 12 KE 20

Make a list of all the different dressings available in your department.

Against each dressing state:

- which group of dressings it belongs to, e.g. hydrocolloid
- its main purpose, e.g. maintains a moist environment

Give an example of what type of wound it might be used for, e.g. necrotic, odorous

Wound treatments

As well as applying a particular dressing, you may need to give the patient some other form of treatment.

Ointments and creams

Certain patients may require the application of topical ointments and creams during their dressing procedure. Before applying the ointment/cream you must ensure that:

- it is prescribed for the patient in question
- the product is in date
- the patient is not allergic to the product or any of its ingredients
- it is only applied to the relevant area of the wound or skin
- it is solely used for the patient for whom it is prescribed.

Step by step : applying a skin barrier treatment to a stoma site

Important: Follow your organisation's guidelines on procedure if available.

1. Following removal of the stoma appliance, ensure the stoma and surrounding skin is thoroughly cleaned and dried.

2. Assess the condition of the stoma site and the edges of the wound before applying any treatment or dressing.

3. Check the packaging of the barrier film for expiry date and sterility.

4. If using a foam applicator, apply a uniform amount of the barrier film around the stoma site.

5. If you miss an area, wait approximately 30 seconds and re-apply to that area only.

6. Apply the new stoma appliance to the manufacturer's instructions, ensuring that the patient is comfortable.

7. Follow your organisation's guidelines to complete the remainder of the procedure.

Some treatments or therapies may be carried out in specific departments where specialist practitioners are trained to deliver that treatment, e.g. laser therapy. Other treatments may be undertaken in your own department by appropriately trained staff, e.g. vacuum-assisted closure, use of sterile larvae. It is important that you have some understanding of these treatments, even though you will probably not be undertaking them yourself.

Larvae therapy

There has been an increased interest in the use of maggot larvae for wound debridement and the treatment of infected wounds. The maggots used are those of the green bottle fly, and are grown under sterile conditions. The larvae ingest necrotic tissue effectively, leaving healthy tissue in place. It has also been suggested that the secretions of the maggot have an antimicrobial effect, helping to heal infected wounds. The care of patients undergoing this treatment is an advanced role and should only be undertaken by knowledgeable, experienced wound care practitioners.

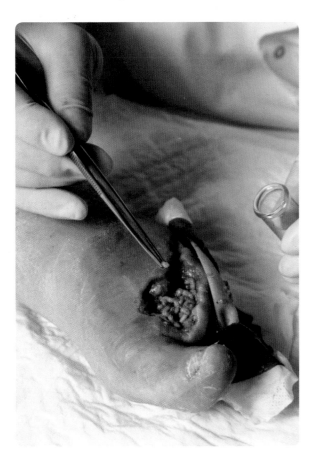

Activity

There are many journal articles on the subject of larvae therapy and vacuum-assisted closure. Carry out a literature search on the internet or speak to your librarian to find an article on each subject. Make some notes from each article and share your new knowledge with colleagues.

Evidence in action (CHS 12 KE 19, 22)

Make a list of all the different types of treatments that are undertaken in your department. Give a reason why each is carried out.

Why is it important to follow the dressing/treatment procedures exactly as specified – and what are the potential effects of not doing so?

Multidisciplinary approach to wound care

(KS 3, 10, 25)

Many different health care professionals can be involved in the treatment of a patient's wound or lesion:

* nurse
* doctor
* dietician
* prosthetist/orthotist
* podiatrist
* occupational therapist
* catering staff
* domestic staff
* specialist nurses.

In large organisations, there is generally a team of Tissue Viability/Wound Care Nurses employed to support staff in the clinical areas with wound care issues. Some of their roles are illustrated in the diagram on the next page.

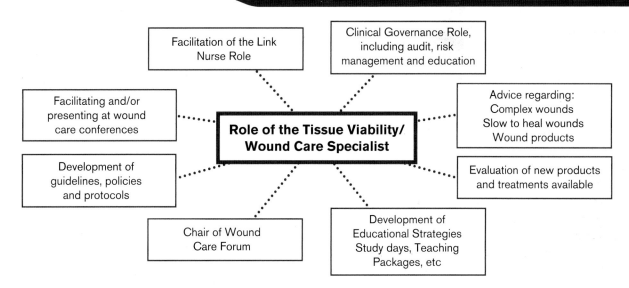

Roles of the Tissue Viability/Wound Care Specialist.

Evidence with a case study

As one of the department's link nurses for wound care, you have been asked by the department manager to tidy the cupboard containing all the wound care products and to make a list of their use and cost. You notice that, among the dressings you are familiar with, there are a couple you have never used before.

1 Who could you contact to give you information about these products?

2 What other possible activities could you arrange in order to develop the staff's knowledge of wound care products?

Evidence may be gained for: CHS 12 KE 10

References

Bale S. & Jones V. (2006) *Wound Care Nursing. A Patient-Centred Approach*, Mosby Elsevier, China.

Cutting K.F. & Harding K.G. (1994) Criteria for identifying wound infection, *Journal of Wound Care*, June, Vol. 3. No. 4, p198-201

Department of Health (2001) *Reference Guide to Consent for Examination or Treatment*, Department of Health, London.

Nursing & Midwifery Council (2007) *NMC Record Keeping Guidance*, A-Z Advice Sheet

Turner T.D. (1985) 'Which Dressing and Why?' In: Westaby S. (Ed) *Wound Care*. William Heinemann Medical Books, London.

Resources

Hampton. S (2004) Holistic Wound Care, JCN Online

Institute of Medical Illustrators National Guidelines – Clinical Photography in Wound Management http://www.imi.org.uk/guidelines/IMINatGuidelinesWoundManagement.pdf

Ramsey. C. (2001) *The Role of Sutures in Wound Healing*, Infection Control Today.

The Joanna Briggs Institute (2003) Solutions, Techniques and Pressure for Wound Cleansing, Best Practice – Volume 7, Issue 1, ISSN 1329 – 1874

World Wide Wounds – *Electronic Journal of Wound Management*

Undertake physiological measurements

Introduction

This unit will give you the required knowledge for taking physiological measurements of basic body systems. To ensure the body is working correctly and to identify underlying health problems, it is important to take appropriate physiological measurements as required. These measurements include blood pressure, pulse, pulse oximetry, temperature, respirations, peak flows, height, weight and Body Mass Index.

Through this unit, you will gain an understanding of how to prepare the environment for each of the measurements to be taken; this includes thinking about the individual and his or her comfort and rights. You will learn about and identify the different types of equipment used for each of the measurements, and how to follow correct procedures for their use. This will include developing an awareness of your limitations and of health and safety issues.

What you need to learn

- The importance of informed consent
- Legislation and organisational policies and procedures relating to your responsibilities
- Policies for safe use of equipment and techniques when taking the physiological measurements of an individual
- Job roles and responsibilities
- The importance of taking accurate body measurements
- Blood pressure
- Pulse
- Temperature
- Respirations
- Measuring height, weight and Body Mass Index
- Records and documentation

What evidence you need to generate for your portfolio

For this unit you will need to provide sufficient evidence to demonstrate your knowledge of and ability to undertake physiological measurements. You will need to plan with your assessor how you provide this evidence. The following is intended as a guideline as to the types of evidence you may wish to collect.

- ✔ Observation
- ✔ Witness testimonies
- ✔ Reflective accounts
- ✔ Written questioning
- ✔ Oral questioning

The importance of informed consent

(KS 5, 6, 27)

In this section, you will be looking at how to prepare the **individual** for taking physiological measurements. It is very important to put the individual first in this preparation period – he or she is just as important to prepare, if not more so.

> ### Key term
>
> **Individual** The person on whom the physiological measurement is being taken, whether an adult or a child.

What is consent?

(KS 6)

Consent can be defined as an individual's agreement to a prescribed therapy or treatment. Consent can be written, spoken or implied. If an individual rolls up her sleeve when informed of the need to take a sample of blood, this can be taken as the individual consenting. If the individual is not able to physically assist in his or her treatment but does not resist, this can also be taken as consent.

You do not always need the individual to say 'yes' for consent to be given.

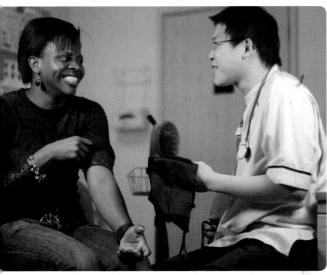

Regardless of the individual's physical or mental ability, you need to ensure that he or she is given the full correct information on the treatment to be given. This is known as informed consent. If an individual has no verbal or physical means of showing consent, treatment can be given if it is necessary to the individual's health.

Why you must obtain consent

(KS 5)

All individuals have the right to be informed about what is happening to them. Full information about the procedure needs to be given to the individual, as this will help him or her to feel more at ease when you take the measurements. Each individual has the right to information about his or her care or treatment, to ensure that any decision he or she makes is an informed one. Knowing what is happening, when and how, also **empowers** the individual to make choices around his or her individual beliefs, preferences, choice, needs and expectations. By ensuring the individual is fully informed, more accurate readings can be taken, as the individual will be less stressed and more cooperative.

> ### Key term
>
> **Empowers** Gives ability, skills or authority.

> ### Test yourself
>
> What is meant by the term 'informed consent' and why is this important? (KS 5, 6)

> ### Case study: Obtaining consent
>
> Harjinder is 87 years old. He lives at home with his wife and three children. He does not speak English, but is able to understand fairly well if you speak slowly. Harjinder has been admitted to your ward following a fall at home. You need to check his blood pressure.
>
> 1 How can you obtain consent from Harjinder before checking his blood pressure?
>
> 2 If Harjinder were not cooperative with you, pulling his arm away, what actions would you take?

Legislation and organisational policies and procedures relating to your responsibilities

(KS 1, 2)

Current European and national legislation

A range of legislation covers the rights of the individual. These are laws that must be adhered to, set by the national government and also the European Union. It is important to understand your own responsibilities related to the legislation to ensure good practice.

The table on the next page lists some of the European and national laws that affect both the rights of the individual and your responsibilities as a health care assistant.

Organisational policies and procedures

As well as current legislation, your workplace will have policies and procedures for you to follow when taking the physiological measurements of individuals. It is important to remember that these have been produced to ensure that your practices are safe and that the results you obtain are accurate.

How the law influences practice

When a law is passed, it then becomes necessary to ensure that the law is enforced in practice. This means that steps must be taken to ensure that those people to whom the law applies are informed of their new responsibilities under that law and act accordingly. For example, the Data Protection Act 1998 changed the law on how information is held about people: all people who store confidential information, such as contact details and medical records, need to be fully informed about how the law requires them to hold information on people (Freedom of Information Act 2000).

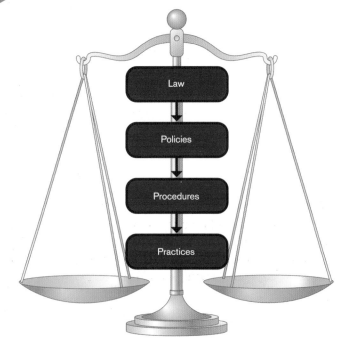

How the law influences practice.

Legislation	Rights of the individual	Responsibility of the health care assistant	Responsibility of the employer
The Human Rights Act 1998	The rights and freedoms of individuals are guaranteed by this Act. These include the right to privacy and the right to equal treatment.	To ensure that all care provided to the individual meets with his or her rights, beliefs and choice.	To ensure all staff are following the requirements by ensuring they are suitably trained and have the necessary resources to meet individuals' needs.
Equal Opportunities Act 2004	Individuals have a right to be given equal access to facilities, treatments, investigations and all other aspects of care.	To ensure individuals are given equal access to required facilities and that individual differences are respected.	To ensure all staff have full understanding of the policy, and that facilities, including access, meet with the varied needs of individuals.
Health and Safety at Work Act 1974	Individuals have a right to be kept safe and all practices should ensure that health, welfare and safety are maintained.	To ensure that all working procedures are adhered to and carried out safely, and that your acts or omissions do not put others at risk.	To ensure all staff have full training on health and safety practices, such as manual handling. To ensure equipment is regularly checked and maintained. To ensure the environment is fit for employees and individuals.
The Data Protection Act 1998	Information relating to the individual shall be processed fairly and lawfully. It will be kept safely and securely and used only for the purpose intended.	To ensure that all information is accurately recorded and stored in the appropriate place to prevent misuse or access by those who do not have permission. To ensure the confidentiality of an individual's details by sharing information with others on a 'need to know' basis only.	To provide suitable storage for records; to ensure staff are maintaining records appropriately; to ensure records are used only for the purpose intended and are kept no longer than required.
Control of Substances Hazardous to Health (COSHH) Regulations 2002	Individuals have a right to be protected from exposure to substances hazardous to their health.	To ensure that all chemical substances are stored, handled and disposed of appropriately, and used as per manufacturers' instructions.	To ensure a suitable, lockable storage area is provided and clearly marked and maintained.
Reporting of Injuries, Diseases and Dangerous Occurrences Regulations (RIDDOR) 1995	The individual has the right to expect any injury, disease or dangerous occurrence within the scope of this legislation to be reported.	To ensure that all injuries, diseases or dangerous occurrences are recorded and reported within the scope of this legislation as per procedures and job role.	To ensure all requirements under this legislation are met by those responsible.

It is your responsibility as a health care assistant to ensure that you are familiar with all your organisation's policies and procedures. Each health care environment will have its own policies and procedures clearly written and kept for all staff to access.

Evidence generator KS 1, 2

Identify the policy and procedure file where you work. Look at the policies and procedures for taking physical measurements and write a brief account on your responsibilities relating to these procedures.

Principles of good practice

Policies defined in health care are set around principles of good practice.

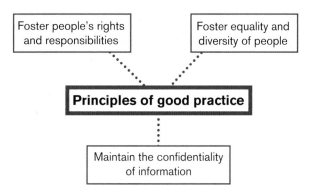

There are three main principles of good practice.

- *Foster people's rights and responsibilities*
  When working in a health care setting, tensions may arise between your values (what you see as being right) and those of other people (see page 77). We all have different values and there may be times when an individual wants to do something, which you do not agree with. This could be as simple as wanting to remain in the dining room while his or her blood pressure is taken. You need to separate your values from those of other people. You may not think it is appropriate for the individual to stay where everyone else can see him or her having blood pressure taken. However, you need to recognise the individual's rights and responsibilities and, providing the individual's request does not cause harm to him or herself or to others, you must respect the individual's right to choice.

- *Foster equality and diversity of people*
  Each individual has his or her own personality, likes and dislikes. This is what makes people different from each other. Within the principles of good practice, you need to ensure individuals are treated equally but differently. Everyone should be given the same opportunity but offered different means of meeting that opportunity according to their values, beliefs, preferences and choice. It is important as a health care assistant that you recognise an individual's diversity (difference). This could be in culture, religion, age, sex or ability. By meeting an individual's diverse needs you are promoting anti-discriminatory practice (see page 118). When preparing equipment or environments for individuals, you need to be mindful of their needs, ensuring that you take on each individual's rights to equality and diversity.

- *Maintain the confidentiality of information*
  You must have a clear knowledge and understanding of workplace policies, procedures and guidelines for storing and transmitting information (see page 36). This includes the recording systems and security arrangements for all information. When preparing records prior to taking physiological measurement, you must be aware of the possible consequences of leaving records unattended and prevent this from occurring.

Key term

Needs of the individual The characteristics of an individual that influence choice and set up of equipment and other resources, e.g. mobility, protection from radiation, etc.

Case study: Principles of good practice

Faharna is a young woman who is visiting the outpatients clinic of her local hospital for the first time. Faharna has lived in the UK most of her life and is a devout Muslim. On arriving in the department, she is informed by the male doctor that he needs to take her blood pressure. Faharna lowers her head and leaves the room immediately. The doctor follows her out into the corridor, asking what is wrong rather loudly.

1 What are Faharna's rights in this situation?

2 Was Faharna's equality and diversity met in preparation for taking physiological measurements?

3 What should Faharna do now?

4 What should the doctor do now?

Policies for safe use of equipment and techniques when taking the physiological measurements of an individual

(KS 4, 27)

Health and safety

Following health and safety policies and procedures keeps individuals, your colleagues, yourself and all visitors to the workplace safe. This is a particularly important part of your duties when preparing environments and resources for use.

When selecting and preparing environments and resources you must ensure they are correct for the task to be undertaken. The resource or equipment must be in full working order and clean. This is to reduce the risk to the individual or yourself from harm, injury or infection. It will also ensure accurate measurements are taken.

> ### Remember
> A **hazard** is something that can cause injury or harm to an individual or group, such as faulty equipment. A **risk** is the likelihood of the harm actually occurring, for example, the likelihood of faulty equipment causing harm or injury to an individual.

Environmental considerations should include:

- the room temperature: if the room is too hot or cold, this could provide inaccurate readings. For example, a person's body temperature may be recorded as very high if the environment is too hot.
- the room layout: Is it suitable to ensure privacy and dignity? Are there curtains at the windows? Can the door be closed securely?
- ventilation: poor ventilation or strong fragrances may possibly affect the individual's breathing, and this could give inaccurate readings when taking measurements relating to the individual's breathing.

Infection control

Infection control is important when taking any physiological measurement as it prevents cross-infection and ensures the accuracy of results. Infection control should be a **standard precaution in health and safety measures**. This means preventing infection and cross-infection by washing hands before, during and after preparation of environments and resources for taking physiological measurements, as well as wearing protective clothing such as gloves, aprons and masks where required.

> ### Memory jogger
> What are the six steps for good hand washing? Look back at page 143 to remind yourself.

> ### Remember
> When you put on any form of protective clothing, you must inform the individual why you are wearing it to prevent him or her becoming alarmed.

> ### Key term
> **Standard precautions and health and safety measures**
> A series of interventions that will minimise or prevent infection and cross-infection, including hand washing/cleansing before, during and after the activity, and the use of personal protective clothing and additional protective equipment where appropriate.

Check the Topics in this book on pages 244–45 for more in depth information about infection control.

Ensuring privacy is an important part of health care.

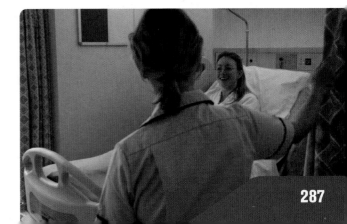

287

Have you remembered to:

- remove your jewellery before coming to work
- tie your hair back
- put on personal protective clothing – dress, tunic, trousers, plastic apron, theatre gown – both clean and sterile
- wash and dry your hands in the approved manner
- apply alcohol hand gel if necessary
- check and put on latex gloves – both clean and sterile.

Test yourself

Define the meaning of 'standard precautions' and explain its importance in relation to undertaking physiological measurements and the potential consequences of poor practice (KS 4).

Using a sterile field

In some circumstances, you may be required to undertake physiological measurements in a sterile field. A sterile field is an area that has been cleaned with chemicals to ensure that it contains no pathogens (bacteria or viruses). When commencing a procedure that requires a sterile field, you must use sterile gloves, wash your hands correctly, and ensure that equipment is sterilised to reduce the risk of cross-infection. More information on sterile fields can be found on page 265 of this book.

Wearing protective clothing

Employers have a legal duty to provide **personal protective clothing** to employees. Protective clothing reduces the risks of cross-**contamination** to both individuals and staff. It ensures that good hygiene is adhered to and protects **personal clothing** from damage. Some staff wear their work clothes outside the working environment. This can increase the risk of cross-contamination by transferring bacteria and viruses to other environments.

Key term

Contamination Something becoming unclean or non-sterile through contact with body fluids, chemicals or radionucleatides.

Did you know?

Any sterile pack/item which has been opened but not used should be treated as contaminated and be disposed of.

Wearing disposable aprons and gloves when working with body fluids and/or chemicals, and ensuring that they are changed after each task, ensures that you are meeting your health and safety responsibilities and keeping individuals safe.

Key terms

Personal protective clothing Items such as plastic aprons, gloves – both clean and sterile, footwear, dresses, trousers and shirts, and all-in-one trouser suits. These may be single-use disposable clothing or reusable clothing.

Personal clothing and fashion items Includes outer clothes worn from home to work, jewellery, acrylic nails, nail varnish and false eyelashes.

Case study: For whose protection?

Ahmed and Sheila work as health care assistants in a residential home for older people. They have had a very hectic day because a number of the individuals have stomach bugs. They decide to go to the local shopping centre for a coffee before going home. Both are still wearing their uniforms.

1 Do you feel this is acceptable practice?

2 Discuss this with your colleagues to identify their views.

Reflect

Is it easy for you to adhere to your organisation's policy on wearing work clothes outside of the working environment? Think about times when you've found it hard.

Storing and handling of equipment

These policies cover procedures for the appropriate storage and handling of equipment used for taking physiological measurements, such as portable blood pressure monitors.

Storing equipment

Storing equipment inappropriately increases the risks to both individuals and colleagues. Here are just some of the consequences of not putting equipment away correctly.

- Leaving a portable blood pressure monitor in the middle of the room could lead to an individual or colleague tripping over it and sustaining a serious injury.
- Leaving cleaning fluid on the work surface in the kitchen could lead to someone drinking it, resulting in poisoning. It could also contaminate food if spilt, again poisoning individuals.
- If an individual or colleague were to sustain an injury from equipment being stored incorrectly or not being stored at all, he or she could take legal action against whoever failed to follow the correct procedures.

Handling equipment

Equipment can be a potential hazard; when using any equipment you must always check that it is in full working order. The use of faulty equipment is unprofessional, shows poor practice and a lack of judgement, and could result in injury to yourself or the individual.

Electrical equipment should be checked to ensure there are no loose or exposed wires and that no electrical cable is frayed or split. You must also check that the electrical item has had a recent electrical test by a qualified electrician. Equipment that has been tested will have a sticker on it giving the date of the last test and who this was carried out by.

When you check equipment and find it is faulty, it is your legal responsibility to label it to ensure that no one else uses it, and to report the fault to the person in charge.

Evidence generator KS 4, 27

Discuss with your assessor the importance of applying standard precautions and the potential consequences of poor practice.

Job roles and responsibilities

(KS 3, 30)

Each job has its own role and responsibilities, which are set out in the job description. You should have your own job description and be aware of your role and responsibilities within your area of work. Following these roles and responsibilities ensures a safe and effective working environment. Knowing and understanding your role and responsibilities promotes good practice.

A safe practitioner is one who is aware of the limitations of his or her experience and job role and, as a result, never tries to do something outside of those limitations. If you are unsure of how to prepare the equipment or environment, it is safer for you and the individual to ask for help. This will not show you as being weak – quite the opposite. Asking for help is a strength: you will be demonstrating that you know what you are capable of and what you need support with.

Remember

Both you and your employer are accountable for your acts (what you do) and omissions (what you don't do) under the Health and Safety at Work Act 1974 (see page 49).

You need to be aware of your job description to be able to work within your area of responsibility.

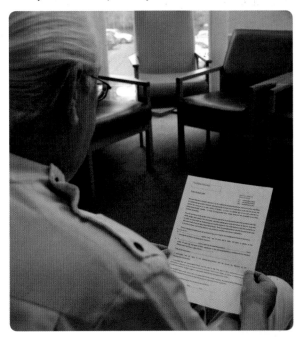

Accountability

Accountability can be defined as working responsibly within the limitations of your job role and taking responsibility for your actions. This includes your responsibilities to the individual and to your colleagues. It also covers whom you are 'accountable' to.

There is a line of accountability from the managers through to you. You are also accountable to the individual in respect of ensuring that he or she receives the treatment to which he or she is entitled, in the way in which he or she is entitled to receive it.

Remember

You are responsible for everything that you do and do not do in your work.

Accountability covers a range of issues when taking the physiological measurements of an individual. These include:

- awareness of your job role and your limitations within that role
- ensuring that you attend all training that is provided
- ensuring that the equipment is used safely – this includes ensuring that the equipment is in working order after use, storing it appropriately for others to use and reporting any equipment that is faulty
- awareness of the environment in which the equipment will be used
- awareness of the needs of the individual on whom the equipment is to be used.

Reflect

Read through your job description.

- Identify the daily tasks that you do in relation to your job role.
- Are there any things that you have been asked to do at work that have been outside your job role? If the answer is yes, what did you do?
- Is there anything you would do differently now that you have re-read your job description?
- How does knowing your job description help you to achieve good practice?

With your colleagues, discuss what you have learned from this activity. You do not have to give full details of actual examples; this activity is more concerned with your own reflections and learning.

Test yourself (KS 3)

Describe the importance of working within your own sphere of competence including why you should seek clinical advice when faced with situations outside your competence.

The importance of taking accurate body measurements

(KS 7, 8, 9)

Physiological body measurements are the signs of life in a person. They indicate the health and wellbeing of the individual, and monitoring them enables assessment of the level at which an individual functions physically. Accurate readings that are monitored, recorded and reported can ensure early interventions and treatment. This also helps individuals to make informed life choices regarding their health and lifestyle.

All of the physiological measurements can be observed, measured and monitored.

It is important to know how to take **accurate** body measurements as well as why they are being taken. This is a form of preventative health care designed to help and encourage us to live a healthier lifestyle, and is part of the Government White Paper *Choosing Health*.

Key term

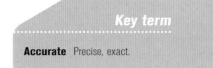

Accurate Precise, exact.

Baseline measurements

Baseline measurements are an essential part of planning appropriate care of the individual. A baseline measurement is one taken before any treatment or further measurements are taken. It is this first measurement on which all further measurements are compared; baseline measurements are essential in keeping track of any improvements. Gaining an understanding of the individual's 'normal' readings and the general physiological norms will ensure that appropriate care can be given. You will look at this in more detail further on in this section.

When taking physiological measurements it is essential to ensure that the individual receives the type of care that meets his or her full range of needs. Correct preparation of the environment promotes an image of competence and shows good working practice, which in turn can instil confidence and give reassurance to the individual. Discussing the tests with the individual also gives you the opportunity to assist him or her with repositioning of clothing in order to access the required parts of the body, if necessary.

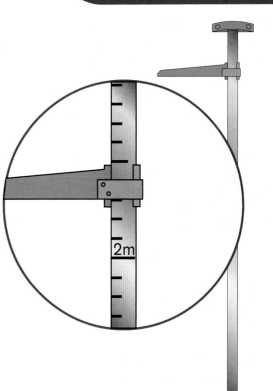

Case study: Under pressure

Sehlakubi is a student nurse on a busy admissions unit within a local hospital. A qualified nurse has shown her how to take patients' blood pressure. A new patient is admitted onto the unit and Sehlakubi is asked to check their blood pressure. Sehlakubi does not take the reading accurately, and notes it as being much lower than what it actually is. The doctor uses this reading to aid in his diagnosis of the patient.

1 What are the potential consequences of Sehlakubi's inaccuracy?

Reflect

Research the White Paper *Choosing Health* and identify the key targets set by the Government.

1 Pick one of the key areas and describe how you could change your practices to promote better health.

2 How do your current practices promote the key targets?

3 Do you feel you could promote the health issues in your current workplace?

Evidence generator KS 7, 8, 9

Describe the holistic reasons physiological measurements are taken and why it is important they are taken accurately.

Activity

Look at the illustration of the height stick and accurately state the measure it is pointing to.

Blood pressure

(KS 9, 10, 11, 12, 13, 14, 15, 27)

What is blood pressure?

Blood pressure is the pressure exerted by the blood on the walls of the blood vessels as it travels along. Every time the heart beats, the heart's natural pumping action pushes a volume of blood away from the heart into the arteries and around the body. This puts the blood under pressure and this is what is monitored when taking a blood pressure reading.

Understanding what blood pressure is will ensure that appropriate action is taken once the task has been completed. Communicating all of your findings ensures that an appropriate diagnosis can be made and that appropriate treatment can be given to the individual.

To fully understand what blood pressure (and pulse) is, you need to have a good understanding of the cardiovascular system.

The cardiovascular system

The cardiovascular system consists of the heart, lungs, blood vessels and blood. This system is also known as the circulatory system, because it circulates blood around the body within vessels (mainly veins and arteries) with the aid of a pump – the heart.

Arteries are the largest of the blood vessels. They connect to smaller arterioles, which connect to the tiniest of all the vessels – capillaries. Capillaries then connect to venules, which are smaller versions of veins. Arteries, arterioles, venules and veins all have the ability to dilate and constrict (open and close), which helps move blood along.

The main role of the cardiovascular system is to circulate blood around the body while carrying:

- vital substances that the body needs to keep its cells and tissues healthy – these include oxygen, food, water, hormones and enzymes
- waste products from the cells and tissues to the lungs and kidneys to be excreted – these include carbon dioxide and toxins
- heat around the body.

Did you know?

- The adult human body has on average 5.6 litres or nearly 10 pints of blood.
- In one day, your blood travels nearly 12,000 miles.
- Your heart beats around 35 million times per year.

How the cardiovascular system links to the respiratory system

Humans have what is known as a double circulatory system. This is because there are two loops - one from the heart to the lungs and back, and another from the heart to the rest of the body and back. The body needs a constant supply of oxygen to function properly. Oxygen is inhaled into the body via the lungs during breathing (inspiration), where it is absorbed into the blood supply. The oxygen-rich blood, known as oxygenated blood, then circulates from the lungs through the body, giving oxygen to the body's tissues, organs and cells. As oxygen is passed to the cells, it is exchanged for the waste product carbon dioxide. The blood containing carbon dioxide (deoxygenated blood) now returns to the lungs, where the carbon dioxide passes out and is exhaled from the body during breathing (expiration). With this, the process of passing oxygen to the blood and carbon dioxide from the blood starts again – this process is known as gaseous exchange. (For more on the respiratory system, see pages 213–17.)

The heart

The heart is a large muscular organ, which is divided into four chambers. The upper two chambers are called atria and the lower chambers are called ventricles; so the heart's four chambers are:

- the left atrium
- the right atrium
- the left ventricle
- the right ventricle.

Blood is pumped from the atrium to the ventricle through a one-way valve. The right side of the heart receives deoxygenated blood from the body through the veins. This blood is then pumped to the lungs where gaseous exchange occurs, i.e. carbon dioxide passes from the blood to the lungs

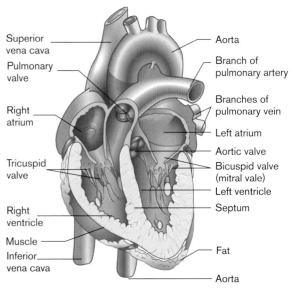

The structure of the heart.

Superior vena cava
Pulmonary valve
Right atrium
Tricuspid valve
Right ventricle
Muscle
Inferior vena cava

Aorta
Branch of pulmonary artery
Branches of pulmonary vein
Left atrium
Aortic valve
Bicuspid valve (mitral vale)
Left ventricle
Septum
Fat
Aorta

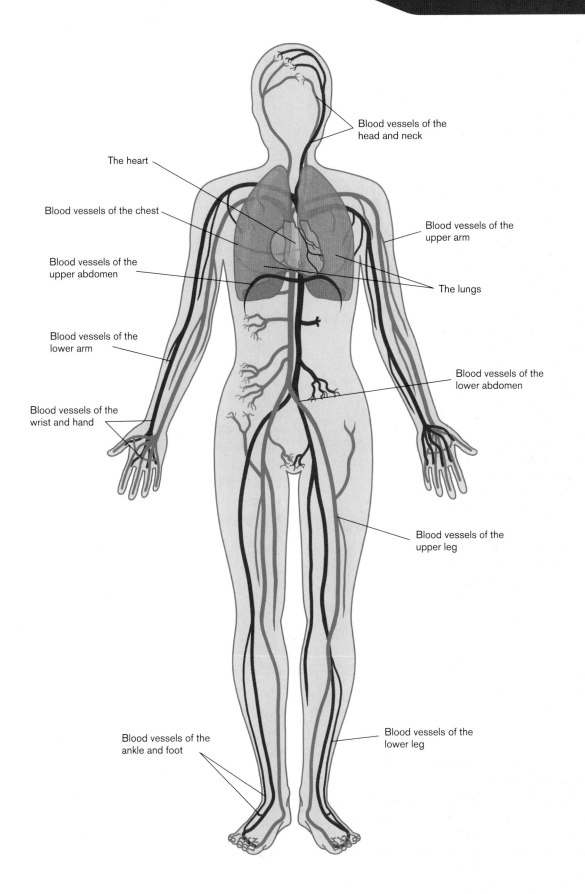

Blood vessels of the
head and neck

The heart

Blood vessels of the chest

Blood vessels of the
upper arm

Blood vessels of the
upper abdomen

The lungs

Blood vessels of the
lower arm

Blood vessels of the
lower abdomen

Blood vessels of the
wrist and hand

Blood vessels of the
upper leg

Blood vessels of the
ankle and foot

Blood vessels of the
lower leg

The cardiovascular system.

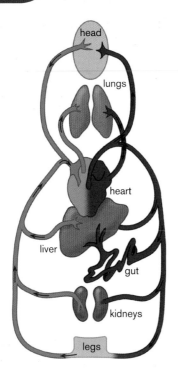
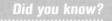

The double circulatory system.

and is exhaled during breathing, and the blood takes up oxygen, which has been inhaled during breathing. The oxygenated blood then returns to the right side of the heart where it is pumped out to the rest of the body. This process is then repeated.

> **Did you know?**
>
> On average, the heart pumps approximately 8,000 litres (14,085 pints) of blood around the body every 24 hours.

Blood pressure readings

Blood pressure is measured when it is at its highest and lowest, giving two figures.

- The highest pressure is the pressure within the artery when the heart contracts and blood is pumped out. This is known as systolic pressure.
- The lower pressure is the pressure within the arteries when the heart is being filled up with blood as the heart relaxes. This is known as diastolic pressure.

These two numbers are usually written with the systolic measurement over the diastolic measurement. On average, a healthy blood pressure reading in adults is 120/70 mmHg.

> **Did you know?**
>
> Blood pressure is measured in millimetres of mercury (mmHg).

The range of blood pressure	Measurement
Low	99/60 or less
Normal	100–129/61–80
Moderate	131–140/81–90
Severe	141–160/91–100
Crisis	161/110 or higher

This table should act as a guide only. An individual's blood pressure reading can mean a variety of things, depending on that individual. Low blood pressure could indicate either a good physical fitness or internal bleeding or a heart attack. You must ensure you record and report any recordings which:

- you are unsure of
- give you cause for concern
- are different from the individual's baseline measurement.

> **Test yourself KS 13**
>
> What is the difference between systolic and diastolic pressure?

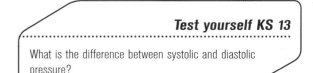

> **Did you know?**
>
> A person's blood pressure varies throughout the day, so this needs to be taken into consideration when taking a blood pressure reading. For example, when you wake up, your body is more relaxed and this can affect your blood pressure, giving it a lower reading. However, if you take morning medication and take a blood pressure reading before your medication, your measurement may be high. Evening blood pressure can be affected by the stress of the day and the fact that the heart has had to pump the blood around the body while it stands or sits – this can give a higher reading. Also, physical exertion raises the blood pressure and, in extreme heat, blood pressure will drop.

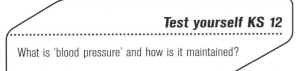

What is 'blood pressure' and how is it maintained?

Conditions where blood pressure may be high or low

KS 11

High blood pressure

High blood pressure is also known as **hyper**tension. It usually has recognisable symptoms, as shown in the diagram below. However, some individuals do not present any indications of having high blood pressure, which is why there is a need for regular monitoring.

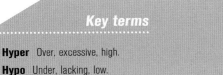

Key terms

Hyper Over, excessive, high.
Hypo Under, lacking, low.

There are two types of hypertension.

Primary hypertension, also known as essential hypertension. There is no clear cause for this type of hypertension; however, there are indications to suggest that it is hereditary. This means that you are more likely to get it if a close member of your family has it. Primary hypertension can also be linked to high salt and fat intake in food and excessive amounts of stress. Regular monitoring is essential for individuals who fit into either of these categories.

Did you know?

Statistics show that 95 per cent of hypertension is primary hypertension.

Secondary hypertension. The signs and symptoms of secondary hypertension are not always exhibited and often it is only during routine examination that it is picked up. This type of hypertension has a link to a recognised cause, which may be a symptom of another disease or illness, such as:

- kidney disease
- narrowing of the aorta
- pre-eclampsia in pregnancy
- adrenal gland disease.

Some forms of medication can also cause secondary hypertension, including steroids and some types of contraceptive pill.

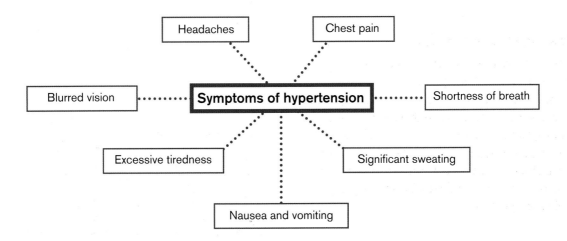

Diseases associated with hypertension

People with hypertension have a risk of major illnesses, as shown in this diagram.

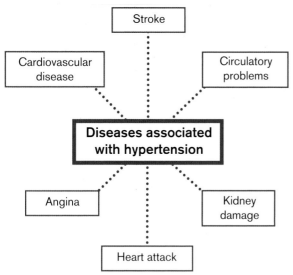

Treating hypertension

Hypertension treatment may include a range of medication. However, there are also lifestyle changes that can help to reduce high blood pressure, including:

- losing weight if overweight
- stopping smoking
- reducing alcohol intake
- reducing salt intake
- reducing fat intake
- eating at least five portions of fruit and vegetables a day
- taking regular exercise.

It is good practice to encourage individuals who have high blood pressure to consider these lifestyle changes and include all of them, if applicable, in their daily regime. Studies have shown that losing weight combined with a low salt and low fat diet significantly reduces hypertension, therefore avoiding the need for medication.

Low blood pressure

Low blood pressure is also known as **hypo**tension. Blood pressure that is too low results in an inadequate amount of blood circulating around the body to vital organs.

Low blood pressure is only a problem if it has adverse effects on the body. It is important to remember that different people have different blood pressures; some individuals will have a naturally low pressure in comparison to others, but are still healthy.

When taking an individual's blood pressure reading, it is important to ask questions about the person's medical history if his or her blood pressure is low. These questions may help other professionals to find a possible cause, and will help discover whether a low blood pressure reading is normal for the individual or not. It is important that you record the individual's responses to these questions in his or her notes and report any concerns immediately to the shift leader or nurse in charge.

Symptoms of hypotension

Sudden blood loss will reduce the blood pressure, leading to shock and, in the most serious of cases, unconsciousness. Others symptoms of hypotension that can build up over time include:

- fainting
- weakness
- dizziness
- tiredness
- light-headedness when standing from either sitting or lying – this is known as postural hypotension.

Causes of hypotension

There are many causes for low blood pressure, as you can see from the diagram. To accurately diagnose this condition, professional medical attention should be sought. If the individual's blood pressure is below 99/60 and he or she is experiencing the above symptoms, this would generally suggest hypotension and the individual should immediately be referred for further investigation.

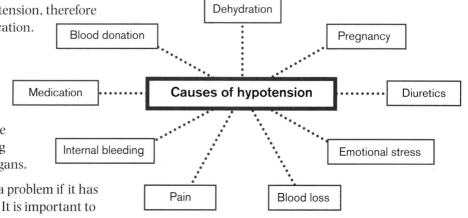

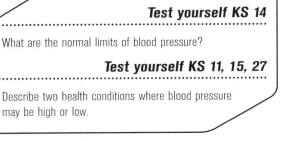

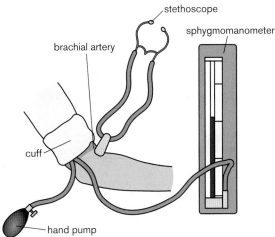

Taking a blood pressure reading with a manual sphygmomanometer and a stethoscope.

How to take a blood pressure reading KS 10

Blood pressure readings can be taken using:

- a manual sphygmomanometer
- a digital sphygmomanometer.

When using a manual sphygmomanometer, a stethoscope is also used. Manual sphygmomanometers used to be made with mercury, but are now being replaced with aneroid sphygmomanometers. This is because mercury creates health, safety and environmental risks.

Digital sphygmomanometers are modern and easy to operate. A stethoscope is not required (making them practical to use in a noisy environment) and they have become the preferred method within many health care settings. However, digital monitors can be affected by heat and moisture, and can be less effective if the individual's heartbeat is irregular. Some health care assistants therefore find a manual sphygmomanometer and stethoscope gives a more accurate blood pressure reading (if used correctly).

Using a manual sphygmomanometer KS 8, 9

A manual sphygmomanometer consists of an inflatable cuff, which wraps around the upper arm. It is important to use the right size of cuff for the individual to ensure that an accurate reading can be taken. Cuffs are available in small, medium, large and extra large, and the sizes are shown on the label of the cuff.

Encourage the individual to sit down and rest his or her arm on a table; alternatively, if lying down, the arm can be rested at the side on the bed. You should wrap the appropriate size of cuff around the individual's upper arm, just above the elbow.

Check the valve on the inflator bulb to make sure it is closed. By placing the head of the stethoscope over the brachial artery, on the inside of the elbow joint, you should be able to hear the 'thumping' of the pulse through the stethoscope. Inflate the cuff by squeezing the inflator bulb until the pulse can no longer be heard or felt. Inflating the cuff too much can cause the individual a great deal of discomfort.

Once the pulse sound has disappeared, release the valve on the inflator bulb slowly while you listen for the return of the pulse through the stethoscope. The first recording is taken at the point on the gauge when the pulsing can first be heard while deflating the cuff – this is the systolic pressure, the top number when recording. You must ensure you continue to deflate the cuff slowly until the pulsing sound disappears again. The bottom number – the diastolic pressure – is the recording taken at the point on the gauge when the pulsing can no longer be heard.

Remember

You only need to inflate the cuff on a manual sphygmomanometer until you can no longer hear or feel the brachial pulse. Inflating the cuff excessively can cause the individual a great deal of discomfort.

Checklist

Procedure for taking blood pressure using a manual sphygmomanometer

- Select the appropriate equipment and the correct cuff size.
- Explain the procedure to the individual and encourage him or her to sit with the arm extended on a table and to the front.
- Wrap the cuff snugly around the upper arm.
- Locate the brachial artery, placing the stethoscope over it so you can hear the pulse.
- Close the valve on the inflator bulb and ask the individual to be as quiet as possible.
- Pump up the cuff until you can no longer hear the brachial pulse.
- Deflate the cuff slowly and steadily.
- Listen for the pulsing of the systolic pressure to return and note the point on the gauge where this occurred.
- Continue deflating the cuff and listen carefully until you can no longer hear the pulsing (this is the diastolic pressure). Note the point on the gauge where this occurred.
- Deflate the cuff rapidly and completely.
- Remove the cuff from the individual.
- Record the blood pressure on the appropriate forms.
- Put the manual sphygmomanometer away in its appropriate storage place.
- Report any concerns or deviations to the baseline measurement to the shift leader nurse in charge.

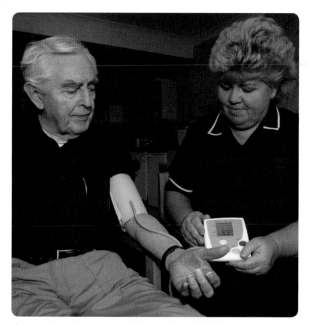

Taking a blood pressure reading using a digital sphygmomanometer.

sufficiently, it will begin deflating, taking digital recordings as it is does so. Once the machine has detected both the systolic and diastolic readings, it will give an audible sound to show it has finished. The cuff will then automatically completely deflate. The readings of the individual's blood pressure measurements will be displayed on the digital screen.

Remember

Always check the equipment is clean and in full working order before using.

If you put the cuff of a manual or digital sphygmomanometer over clothing, you will not be able to get a clear result. Remember to ask the individual to roll up his or her sleeve, or assist him or her to slip the arm out of a sleeve if it is too restrictive.

Memory jogger

What should you do to gain consent before undertaking any physiological measurements? Look back at page 283.

Using a digital sphygmomanometer

A digital sphygmomanometer has an inflatable cuff, which automatically inflates when the monitor is switched on. The cuff is fitted on to the individual's upper arm just like a manual sphygmomanometer. However, it is important that you position the tubing leading from the cuff to the monitor on the inner middle of the individual's arm. Once the machine has inflated the cuff

Procedure for taking blood pressure using a digital sphygmomanometer

- Select the appropriate equipment and the correct cuff size.
- Explain the procedure to the individual and encourage him or her to sit with the arm extended on a table and to the front.
- Wrap the cuff snugly around the upper arm, ensuring the tubing is running along the inner middle of the individual's arm.
- Switch the machine on, following manufacturer's instructions.
- Allow the machine to fully inflate the cuff and finish taking all of its readings.
- On hearing the audible signal indicating the measurements have been completed, remove the cuff from the individual's arm.
- Record the blood pressure on the appropriate charts.
- Put away the equipment in its appropriate storage place.
- Report any concerns or deviations to the baseline measurement to the shift leader or nurse in charge.

Evidence generator KS 10, 11

Show your assessor how you set up and use a manual or digital sphygmomanometer, according to your organisation's availability of equipment.

Test yourself (KS 10)

What equipment is used for taking blood pressure and how should it be prepared?

Pulse

(KS 10, 11, 21, 22, 23, 24, 25, 27)

The pulse is the wave of pressure from the heart. It is the force felt when blood is pushed from the left ventricle of the heart around the body (see page 208). An individual's heart rate may be very fast but his or her pulse may be slower if the individual is in heart failure or suffering from severe blood loss. This is because, although the heart is pumping quickly, the pressure and volume of blood within the arteries and veins is reduced, affecting the beats getting through to the pulse.

Pulse points

The pulse can be felt in various points in the body, which are known as pulse points. At each pulse point a steady beat can be felt. This beat is the expansion and constriction of the artery as the blood passes through it.

Here are the main points in the body for taking a pulse.

- Neck – the pulse point at the neck is called the carotid pulse. You can feel it by putting your forefinger and middle finger on the side of the neck, running them alongside the outer edge of the trachea.
- Wrist – the pulse point felt at the wrist is called the radial pulse. You can feel this by pressing your forefinger and middle finger approximately 1 cm from the wrist, with the tips of your fingers facing the thumb side of the wrist. This pulse point is possibly the one that is most familiar to you.
- Groin – the pulse point felt in the groin area is called the femoral pulse. You can feel this by pressing your forefinger and middle finger into the groin area. It can be found by imagining a line running from the hip to the groin, with the pulse being located approximately two-thirds of the way in from the hip.

You should always use the radial pulse when taking this body measurement as a general routine check-up. Pulses at the neck and groin are generally used in medical emergencies.

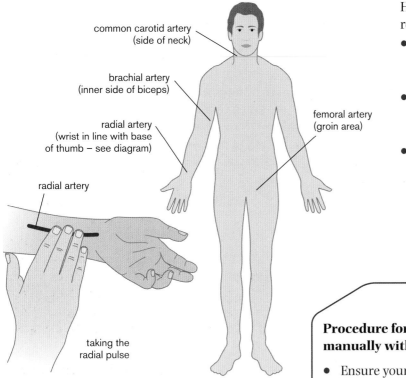

common carotid artery
(side of neck)

brachial artery
(inner side of biceps)

femoral artery
(groin area)

radial artery
(wrist in line with base
of thumb – see diagram)

radial artery

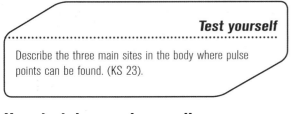

taking the
radial pulse

Common pulse points.

The average pulse is 72 heartbeats per minute, and the normal range of a resting adult pulse is between 60–90 beats per minute. A normal heartbeat is steady and rhythmical – it is so regular that the next beat can be predicted.

Test yourself

Describe the three main sites in the body where pulse points can be found. (KS 23).

How to take a pulse reading

You can take a pulse reading using one of two methods:

- manually with the aid of an accurate watch or clock with a second hand or stopwatch facility
- electronically with the aid of a pulse oximeter, which is a digital machine connected to a two-sided probe that is clipped to the fingertip or ear.

Test yourself

What are the normal limits of an adult's pulse? (KS 21)

Human error can affect the pulse reading.

- Moving about whilst taking a pulse will give an inaccurate reading.
- The thumb has a pulse of its own, so you should not use your thumb to take a pulse.
- Not using enough pressure on the site when taking a pulse can also give inaccurate readings, as beats may be missed or mistaken for being weak.

Checklist

Procedure for taking a pulse reading manually with the aid of a watch or clock

- Ensure your watch or clock has a second hand and is working correctly.
- Explain the procedure to the individual.
- Place your forefinger and middle finger gently on the artery at the base of the wrist.
- Locate the radial pulse, palm side up, just below the wrist.
- Count the beats for 1 minute.
- Take a note of the strength of the beats and how regular the beats are.
- Record the amount of beats on the appropriate recording form.
- Record the strength and regularity of beats on the recording form.
- Report results to shift leader or supervisor if you have any concerns or if there is a deviation from the baseline measurements.

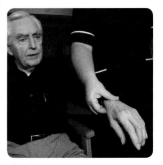

Taking a pulse from the wrist.

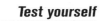

Reasons for different pulse rates

Variations in an individual's pulse, which could be a sign of illness include:

- irregular pulse
- weak pulse
- rapid pulse
- slow pulse.

Irregular pulse

An irregular pulse is one that is unsteady and not evenly spaced, with missing or skipped beats. An irregular pulse can indicate a range of illnesses including congestive heart failure, shock, internal bleeding, heart attack, stroke or cardiac arrest.

Weak pulse

A weak pulse is a pulse that is not strong or is hard to feel. It can be indicative of internal bleeding, shock or heart failure.

Rapid pulse

A rapid pulse is one that exceeds the average normal pulse rate of 60–90 beats per minute. Stimulants such as caffeine or cigarettes and medication such as amphetamines and some decongestants can increase the pulse rate. Stress, cardiac problems, infection and exercise all increase the pulse, as the body needs more oxygen at these times. The blood is pumped around the body quicker in the need to deliver oxygen where it is required.

Slow pulse rate

A slower pulse reading – one generally below 60 beats per minute – might be attributed to medication prescribed for hypertension, such as Beta blockers or digoxin, which is intended to reduce the pulse rate. However, if the individual is extremely physically fit, his or her pulse rate could be expected to be below 60 beats per minute.

Test yourself

What health conditions can affect the individual's pulse rate and how may the pulse be affected by the health condition? (KS 22, 27)

Taking a pulse using a pulse oximeter

When using a pulse oximeter, it is placed over the individual's index finger (see illustration) or ear. A two-sided probe transmits infrared lights through the body tissue, the majority of which

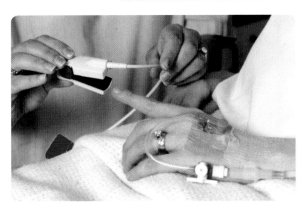

Taking a pulse reading from the finger using a pulse oximeter.

gets absorbed by the tissue. The probe on the other side of the fingertip detects the small amount of light that is not absorbed, and this measures the amount of haemoglobin saturation. The sensors in the pulse oximeter also recognise the pulse of the individual and these are displayed either in waveform or numerically.

When a pulse oximeter is switched on, it will start by going through a series of checks to ensure that it is in full working order. Some oximeters run on rechargeable batteries and the machine must be plugged in after each use to ensure that it is properly charged.

Checklist

Procedure for using a pulse oximeter

- Gather the equipment needed and ensure it is in full working order.
- Check the machine's battery power is sufficient or plug into an electrical socket if required.
- Turn the pulse oximeter on and wait for the machine to complete its checks.
- Select the correct size probe for the finger or ear that you are going to put it on.
- Put the probe on the finger or ear.
- Allow several seconds to pass to ensure pulse and oxygen saturation are detected.
- Check on the display for a waveform.
- Note the recordings on the display and record them appropriately.
- Report any concerns or deviations to the baseline measurement to the shift leader or supervisor.

More reasons to measure pulse oximetry

Pulse oximetry is a non-invasive process that measures the pulse and the amount of oxygen that is being taken up by the blood via the lungs (see also pages 205 and 215). Although a pulse oximeter measures the pulse, it is rarely used just for this. It can be used in the emergency department, during general anaesthetic, postoperatively and in intensive care. It can also be used to assess the viability of limbs after plastic and orthopaedic surgery. It is important to measure how much oxygen is taken up by the blood to ensure vital organs are given the oxygen they need. A monitor reading in the range of 96 per cent to 100 per cent is generally considered normal. Anything below 90 per cent could quickly lead to life-threatening complications including respiratory failure. A qualified medical practitioner should be alerted to identify any underlying causes of readings below 95 per cent.

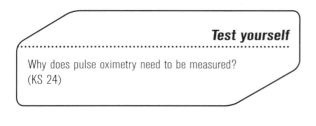

Test yourself

Why does pulse oximetry need to be measured? (KS 24)

Factors that can interfere with the use of a pulse oximeter

- Extreme bright lights – because the machine determines oxygen levels by reading light strengths.
- Very dark nail polish, such as blue, green or black – the infrared light is unable to penetrate the dark colour.
- The environment or individual being very cold.
- The individual shivering.
- The probe being placed on a finger where there is a reduced blood supply caused by serious injury, for example, a fractured wrist.

Test yourself

What are the normal readings of pulse oximetry and what are the implications of readings outside of this scale? (KS 25)

Evidence generator KS 24, 25

Show your assessor how you prepare and undertake an individual's pulse measurement using the manual method and, if available, using an oximeter.

Temperature

KS 10, 11 16, 17, 18, 27

What is body temperature?

An individual's body temperature is an indicator of the body's ability to generate and get rid of heat. The body is usually good at keeping its temperature within a very tight range, unless there is a problem with the individual's health.

Did you know?

Temperature is no longer measured in degrees Fahrenheit (°F). The preferred measurement is degrees Celsius (°C)

Normal body temperature, when taken orally, is 37°C, but anywhere between 36.5°C and 37.2°C may be normal. Maintaining the body's temperature as close to 37°C as possible is essential for the effective functioning of its cells.

Did you know?

Body temperature varies depending on where you measure it. Normal body temperature when measured orally (under the tongue) is 37°C; when measured in the ear (tympanic) is 38°C; and when measured axillary (under the arm) is 36.5°C.

How body temperature is maintained

Cooling the body down

When a person is too hot, the blood vessels in the skin dilate so that more blood circulates to the outer areas of the body. This allows more heat from the body to escape through the skin into the air. This is why the skin goes red when you are hot (for example, after running). The body also perspires or sweats when it is hot. This perspiration evaporates on the skin's surface, which cools the body down.

Warming the body up

When a person is cold, the blood vessels constrict, taking the blood supply into the body, away from the skin and extremities to supply heat to the vital organs such as the heart, lungs and kidneys. This conserves the heat in keeping the body warm. This explains why the fingers and toes are the first body parts to feel cold. Shivering also helps to warm the body up, as the extra muscle movement involved in the shivering process generates more heat within the body.

The role of the nervous system in temperature regulation

The nervous system provides a network of communication between different areas of the body, so that all the systems remain in contact with each other and the body maintains co-ordination. The nervous system also acts as a receiver for information from the external environment, so that the body knows what is happening in its surroundings and can respond in the appropriate way. These external stimuli are transmitted by sense organs in the form of sensations.

The nervous system consists of two main parts. The central part consists of the brain and spinal cord and is called the central nervous system (CNS). The part around the outside is called the peripheral nervous system (PNS) and is made up of nerves and receptors.

Body temperature is controlled by the central nervous system. The brain is the message centre of the body and all messages that go to and from the brain travel via the spinal cord. Receptors in the body register temperature and send messages to the brain, which then sends messages back, either getting the blood vessels to constrict or dilate in response.

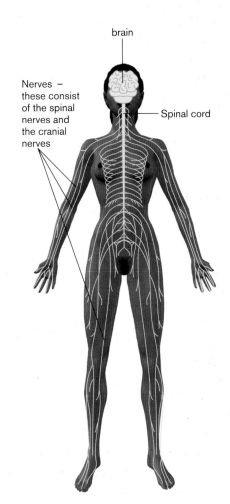

The nervous system.

Conditions where body temperature may be high or low

Hyperthermia

Hyperthermia is when body temperature goes above the 'normal' measurement due to environmental factors, such as time spent in hot weather: for example, sunstroke and heatstroke. The body can have difficulty in cooling down and so overheats, causing hyperthermia.

Pyrexia

Body temperatures between 37 and 38°C, when taken orally, are generally known as mild pyrexia. This is usually as a result of an internal imbalance, such as an infection or illness. In adults, a body temperature of over 38°C when taken orally is considered high and requires medical assistance to investigate the cause.

Causes of high temperature include:

- infection – for example, infected wounds on the body, meningitis
- illness – for example, influenza, shingles, chicken pox
- hormones – during the menstrual cycle and during menopause, the woman's body temperature can rise slightly
- dehydration.

A very high temperature (hyperpyrexia) can cause confusion, delirium, unconsciousness or even death. In these extreme cases, the body is unable to cool itself down because it stops sweating and is unable to transfer heat.

Hypothermia

Hypothermia is when the body temperature falls below the 'normal' measurement. A temperature below 36.1°C is classed as low. Older people and children are more susceptible to hypothermia as they have difficulty controlling body temperature. During cold weather they will therefore require closer monitoring due to the increased risks.

Test yourself

What are meant by the terms 'pyrexia', 'hyperpyrexia' and 'hypothermia'? (KS 18)

Causes of hypothermia include:

- exposure to the cold
- diabetes
- hypothyroidism
- alcohol or drug use
- shock.

The most common signs and symptoms include:

- shivering – this is the body's natural way of trying to warm up
- The 'umbles':
  - grumbles (the individual complains)
  - fumbles (the individual is unable to grasp small objects)
  - stumbles (the individual falls over frequently)
  - mumbles (the individual's spoken language is not very clear).

  These reflect the stages that someone with hypothermia goes through as his or her co-ordination and levels of consciousness change.

How to measure body temperature

Body temperature can be measured using a thermometer. There are several different types available:

- disposable thermometers
- digital thermometers
- tympanic (ear) thermometers.

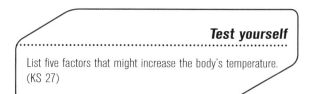

Test yourself

List five factors that might increase the body's temperature. (KS 27)

Did you know?

Glass thermometers, which contain mercury, are no longer recommended for use due to the risks associated with mercury poisoning. If you find a mercury thermometer in the workplace, inform your manager.

General procedure when taking a body temperature

When taking a body temperature you will need to ensure that:

- you have explained the full procedure to the individual;
- you have the appropriate equipment and it is in working order;
- the individual is comfortable and that he or she is not sitting in a draught or too near a heater, as this may affect the reading;
- the thermometer is left in place for the correct amount of time as per manufacturer's instructions. The amount of time required to take an accurate reading will vary depending on the method and equipment used;
- all readings are recorded;
- equipment is cleaned appropriately and put away in its correct storage place;
- you report any concerns or deviations to the baseline measurement to the shift leader or nurse in charge.

Checklist

Procedure for taking an axillary (armpit) temperature

1 When using a digital thermometer, ensure it is covered with a disposable cover to prevent cross-infection.

2 Place the thermometer under the individual's arm, with the bulb in the centre of the armpit.

3 Ensure the arm is held against the body and leave the thermometer in place for the stated time as per manufacturer's instructions. Time yourself if necessary, with a watch or clock.

4 Remove the thermometer and read it. On average, a normal axillary temperature reading will be approximately 36.5°C.

5 Remove the disposable cover before storing away correctly.

6 Record the measurement.

Checklist

Procedure for taking a tympanic temperature

1 Check that the probe is clean and in working order.

2 Turn the thermometer on.

3 Centre the probe tip in the ear and push gently inward toward the eardrum.

4 Press the 'ON' button to display the temperature reading. On average, a normal tympanic temperature reading will be approximately 38.0°C

5 Remove the thermometer and dispose of the used probe cover.

6 Record the measurement.

Possible causes and reasons for inaccurate body temperature readings include:

- temperature being taken within an hour of consuming hot or cold foods or drinks – the hot or cold food/drinks affect the oral temperature
- temperature being taken within an hour of exercise – exercise warms up the muscles and in turn the body's temperature can rise slightly
- temperature being taken within an hour of having a hot bath – as with exercise, the water can cause the body's temperature to rise slightly
- not leaving the thermometer in for the correct length of time – the thermometer is not able to register the correct body temperature
- not keeping mouth closed when taking oral temperature – the inside of the mouth is cooler when the mouth is open
- not following correct procedures
- faulty equipment.

Jacqueline is a health care assistant working on a medical ward. She has been asked to complete the hourly observations for four individuals in one of the bays. However, she is running late so she decides to save time by leaving the thermometer in for half the required time. She hurriedly completes the observations with no discussions or explanations with the individuals.

1 What implications will this have for the results?

2 What possible implications could this have for the care of the individual?

3 Why is it important to always follow set procedures?

4 Is this an example of good practice? Explain your answer.

5 Discuss with a colleague how you could improve on Jacqueline's practices.

Evidence generator KS 17, 18, 27

Show your assessor how you prepare the individual and environment for taking body temperatures. Using one of the above methods, show your assessor how you accurately take an individual's body temperature.

Respirations

(KS 10, 11, 19, 20, 27)

In order to understand respirations, it is first necessary to look at the respiratory system.

The respiratory system

The respiratory system comprises the lungs, trachea, bronchioles, bronchi and alveoli.

There are two lungs, which flank the heart in the thoracic cavity (the chest). The diaphragm is a sheet of muscle, which separates the chest from the abdominal cavity. When it moves up and down the lungs inflate and deflate, and this movement is known as breathing.

During inspiration (breathing in), oxygen enters the lungs via the air. The oxygenated air is taken in to the bronchi, bronchioles and alveoli. Alveoli are sacs inside the lungs, and here the oxygen is transferred into the blood through gaseous exchange (see page 215). There it oxygenates the blood by binding itself to haemoglobin in red blood cells, forming oxyhaemoglobin.

During expiration (breathing out), carbon dioxide, a waste product from the body's cells, is released from the haemoglobin and diffuses out of the blood through the walls of the alveoli to be breathed out.

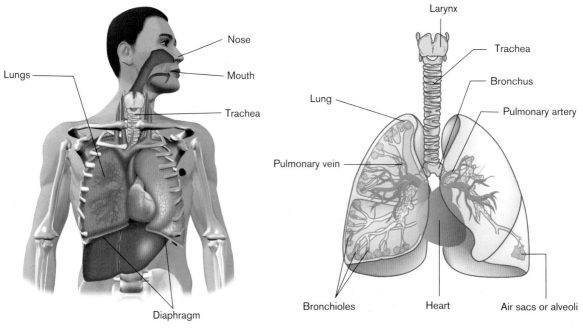

The respiratory system.

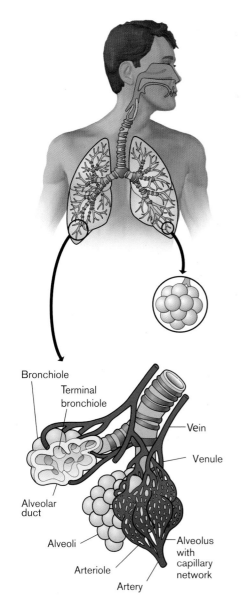

Gaseous exchange takes place in the alveoli.

So the purpose of breathing in and out is to keep the oxygen concentration high and the carbon dioxide concentration low in the alveoli, so that gaseous exchange can occur.

Measuring respirations

Respirations are counted by the amount of times the chest rises in one minute and are recorded as breaths per minute. You will need a watch or clock which has a second hand to be able to time a full minute. The amount of times that you breathe in and out in one minute is known as the respiratory rate.

The average respirations of an adult are 12–20 per minute; however, this will change throughout the day for a variety of reasons. You will breathe faster when you are doing physical exercise or when you are excited or scared. Breathing is slower when a person is calm and relaxed; it also slows down during sleep.

Why we measure respirations

The way a person breathes can be an indicator of possible lung conditions such as:

- bronchitis
- lung cancer
- tuberculosis
- emphysema.

Test yourself (KS 19)

What is the normal rate for respiration?

Reflect

Think about a time when you have been very short of breath – because of running for a bus or playing sport, for example. How did this make you feel?

Test yourself KS 20, 27

List three things that can increase and decrease respirations.

Did you know?

Tachypnea is rapid respirations (over 20 per minute) in an adult.

Checklist

Procedure for counting respirations

1 Gather together the equipment needed and ensure that it is in full working order.

2 On this occasion you should avoid explaining the procedure to the individual as this can affect the manner and speed of his or her breathing.

3 Ensure the individual is lying or sitting down.

4 Count the times the chest rises in one full minute.

5 Listen to the individual's breathing, noting if it is steady, shallow (fast), deep (slow) or wheezy. Always write down any noises that you notice about the individual's breathing. These noises could indicate a chest infection, fluid on the lungs or obstruction.

6 Record all of your observations and respirations on the appropriate chart.

7 Report any observations that cause concern to the shift leader or supervisor. Reasons to inform the shift leader include:
   - respiratory rate is higher or lower than the individual's 'normal' rate
   - you are concerned about any abnormal noises when monitoring respiration.

Measuring the oxygen saturation of haemoglobin using a pulse oximeter

It is important to measure the oxygen saturation of haemoglobin (how much oxygen the blood contains) in order to monitor the individual's health and promote recovery. As you read earlier (pages 292–94), the body requires oxygen to ensure effective maintenance and repair of its cells and organs.

The usual range of the total amount of haemoglobin (blood) that is filled with oxygen is 96–100 per cent. Generally, a reading of 90–95 per cent would require the individual to be given oxygen. However, if the individual has heart failure or chronic lung disease, a reading of 90–95 per cent may be seen as 'doing well' without oxygen. Below 90 per cent could indicate a life-threatening condition and the individual will need oxygen to be administered. Oxygen is classed as a drug and therefore has to be prescribed by a doctor or suitably qualified nurse.

Did you know?

Pulse oximetry readings can vary suddenly, going from the normal range to life-threatening very quickly. This can be due to the sudden movement of the individual or the probe being fitted incorrectly.

Remember

There are many factors that can affect the accuracy of the results when using a pulse oximeter. False low readings can be caused by anything that absorbs light, such as dried blood and dark nail polish, so it is essential to remove them and clean the skin thoroughly before putting the probe on.

Measuring lung capacity using a spirometer

Lung capacity is a medical term used to describe the amount of air an individual can hold within his or her lungs. A spirometer is used to measure lung capacity and lung function, and to monitor lung disease. The spirometer has a tube to blow into which is attached to a machine.

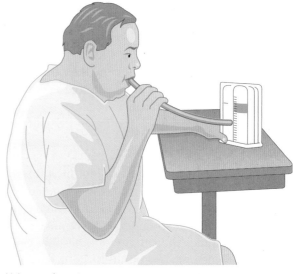

Using a spirometer.

A spirometer measures how much air is expelled from the lungs when the individual blows out and how quickly the air is expelled. This measurement is based on how much air can be expelled within the first second of expiration (known as Forced Expired Volume, or FEV1) and the maximum volume of air that can be forcibly expelled in total (Forced Vital Capacity, or FVC).

Checklist

Procedure for using a spirometer

1 Gather the appropriate equipment and ensure a disposable mouthpiece is fitted.

2 Explain the procedure to the individual.

3 Ensure the individual is sitting down.

4 Encourage the individual to take a deep breath.

5 Encourage the individual to close his or her mouth over the mouthpiece of the spirometer and blow out as forcibly as possible.

6 Read the recordings on the display.

7 Repeat the procedure two more times.

8 Record the highest reading from the three measurements on the appropriate forms.

9 Remove the disposable mouthpiece, clean and put the equipment away in its appropriate storage place.

10 Report any concerns or deviation to the baseline measurement to the shift leader or supervisor.

Measuring lung capacity using a peak flow meter

A peak flow meter is a portable tube with a reading gauge on the side, which is blown into very quickly. Peak flow readings indicate how open the airways are and this helps to determine any airway or lung changes. A peak flow meter measures how quickly and forcibly air is expelled from the lungs, and is another tool to help measure lung capacity. It gives a good picture of what is going on inside an individual's lungs.

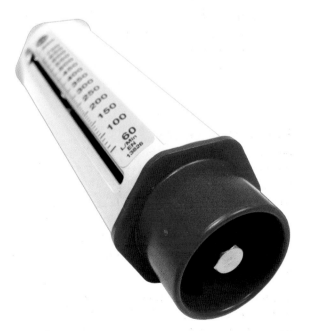

A peak flow meter.

Checklist

Procedure for using a peak flow meter

1 Gather all the appropriate equipment together.

2 Discuss the procedure with the individual.

3 Ensure the gauge is returned to the zero point.

4 Ensure the individual is standing up.

5 Ask the individual to take as deep a breath as possible.

6 Encourage the individual to place the meter in his or her mouth, closing the lips around the mouthpiece.

8 The individual should blow as hard and as fast as possible.

9 Write down the value on the gauge.

10 Repeat the process two more times and record the highest of the three recordings.

11 Put all the equipment away in its appropriate storage place.

12 Report any concerns or deviations to the baseline measurement to the shift leader or supervisor.

Remember

- Always reset the gauge before using to ensure accuracy of results.
- Ensure that you use the disposable inserts.
- Clean properly after each use to reduce the risk of cross-infection.

Clinical conditions requiring the use of a peak flow meter

Asthma

Asthma is a condition where the airways become irritated and inflamed. They become narrower and produce excessive mucus, which makes it more difficult for air to flow in and out of the lungs. In extreme cases, asthma can prove fatal.

There are three types of symptoms associated with asthma, and each varies depending on environmental conditions, physical health and time of day. These three types of symptom are:

- wheezing and coughing
- feelings of tightness in the chest
- shortness of breath.

The exact cause of asthma is not fully known, as it can sometimes flare up for no apparent reason. There are, however, some common triggers that appear to set off an asthma attack or make the symptoms worse. Allergies can narrow the airways, triggering an attack, as can some chemicals found in the workplace. Chest infections, colds and flu are possible causes of increased symptoms, and the weather can also affect people with asthma.

Did you know?

Hygiene hypothesis The developed world is no longer exposed to the range of infections that it used to be, so natural immunity is reduced. In some cases, the immune system overreacts to what used to be harmless substances, for example, house dust mites, medicine and animals, causing asthma.

There are other factors that can indicate a predisposition towards asthma. It tends to run in families so it has a hereditary link. Research indicates that boys are more likely to be asthmatic as children; however, this trend changes in adulthood with women becoming those more likely to develop asthma.

How peak flow meter readings can help in the management of asthma

Peak flow meter readings can be used to assess the severity of asthma and check responses to asthma treatments and monitor their effectiveness. Peak flow readings will drop before other signs and symptoms of asthma getting worse are detected. This is a very good preventative method, giving early warnings so that medication and other treatments can be altered whenever necessary. When monitoring peak flow, it is therefore important to constantly review the findings to ensure that the best values are maintained. This will also assist with ensuring effectiveness of treatment.

The 'traffic light' system is a recognised system to monitor peak flow and offers guidelines to help manage asthma.

Green zone	Peak expiratory flow rate (PEFR) is anywhere between 80 and 100 per cent of the individual's personal best. The individual's personal best is based on the highest that he or she, as an individual, is capable of achieving. This indicates relatively symptom-free asthma and the effectiveness of treatment.
Yellow zone	PEFR is anywhere between 50 and 80 per cent of personal best. This is the zone indicating the need for caution. A temporary increase in treatment may be required, so it is essential that the individual visit the asthma clinic or his or her GP.
Red zone	PEFR is below 50 per cent of personal best and is in the danger zone. Treatment is ineffective and urgent consultation is needed with the asthma clinic or GP to control the symptoms and treat any underlying cause such as a chest infection.

Did you know?

Stress affects the body in many ways:

- blood pressure rises and the pulse rate becomes faster
- breathing becomes shallow and quick
- the skin becomes clammy and sweaty.

It can also affect the physiological measurements you take, which can lead to false readings.

Evidence generator KS 27

Prepare the environment and individual for taking respiration measurements. Show your assessor how you undertake these measurements correctly using one or more of the methods described above.

Measuring height, weight and Body Mass Index

KS 10, 11, 26

A person's weight in relation to height can indicate the extent to which his or her health is being put at risk by being excessively underweight or overweight. There are ideal weights for height, which have been calculated to present the least risk to health. These can be identified by:

- a height/weight chart
- body mass index (BMI).

Using a height/weight chart

One way of checking height and weight is to plot them on a chart, which will give an indication of whether you are overweight, underweight, clinically obese or within the normal range. An example of a height/weight chart is shown here.

Reflect

What do you understand by the term 'clinically obese'? Write down your thoughts and assumptions, then do some research to see what the technical term means. How close were you?

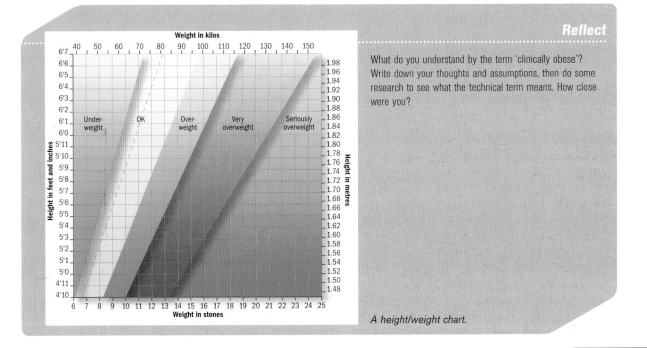

A height/weight chart.

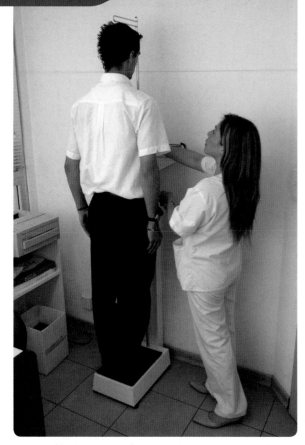

Using scales.

Measuring weight

Wherever possible when measuring weight, individuals should stand on a set of scales; any heavy items of clothing should be taken off before getting on the scales. The individual should stand still until the scales record the weight. Weight should be recorded in kilograms (kg) and then recorded in the individual's notes.

Measuring height

Height should be measured using a fixed ruler, which is attached to the wall. The individual should stand with his or her back to the wall in bare feet, with the heels touching the wall and their back as straight as possible. It is important that the individual does this in order to achieve an accurate recording.

You should move the measuring bar down the ruler until it sits gently on the individual's head. Then read the height from the ruler and record it in the individual's notes. Height should always be measured in meters (m) and centimetres (cm).

Measuring BMI

Body Mass Index (BMI) is a comparative measurement of a combination of the individual's height and weight. It is used to identify an individual's ideal weight and to check whether he or she is over or underweight and by how much (see the chart).

An individual's BMI is identified by dividing weight in kilograms by height in metres squared (height × height).

$$\text{Body Mass Index} = \frac{\text{weight (kg)}}{\text{height (m)}^2}$$

BMI < 20	Underweight
BMI 20–25	Normal
BMI 25–30	Overweight
BMI > 30	Obese
BMI > 40	Severely obese

Test yourself

How do you calculate individuals' BMI and how can it be used in weight/dietary control? (KS 26)

BMI readings and health

Body Mass Index can be used to monitor and encourage the individual to reach a healthy weight, which in turn reduces the risks to health. It is a useful guide when assessing health and can be used in conjunction with exercise and healthy eating.

Using the example of your own outcome from the activity above, you should have identified where on the scale you fall. To assist with your health needs and to reduce the associated risks, you can make lifestyle changes (see page 296). These changes can be monitored with regular weight checks and BMI calculations to see if they are working effectively. Plotting the results on a graph will give you a visual representation of your achievements and will show you clearly when you reach the ideal BMI range (a BMI of 20–25).

Health risks associated with being overweight or obese

There are many health risks associated with being overweight and obese. These include:

- gall stones
- diabetes
- coronary heart disease
- mobility difficulties.

Activity

Choose one of the above health risks that you have little knowledge about and identify how being overweight can cause the problem.

There are also some illnesses and treatments that can affect the weight of an individual.

These include:

- the use of steroids
- hyper- or hypothyroidism
- pituitary gland conditions
- hormone imbalances
- heart failure
- liver failure.

Activity

Choose two of the above illnesses or treatments you are unfamiliar with and identify how these can affect an individual's weight.

Records and documentation

(KS 28, 29, 30)

Recording the different body measurements is an important part of the overall process. There would be little point in taking the measurements if they were not recorded, since there wouldn't be anything to compare them with to see whether the individual's health was improved or had deteriorated. Diagnosis would be affected, as would the accuracy of treatment, and the needs of the individual would be less likely to be met.

How records are kept

Records are required to keep together with all information relating to the individual. Records are now kept in two ways:

- handwritten notes
- computerised records.

Access to records must be restricted to ensure confidentiality and to protect the individual's rights. Individuals now have a right to access their own files, under the Data Protection Act 1998 (see page 284). All records need to be **accurate**, **legible** and **complete** as they are legal documents; therefore the method of recording is essential.

- Accurate means 'containing the correct information of fact not opinion'.

- Legible means 'everyone is able to read it and obtain the same meaning without difficulty or misinterpretation.' Any mistakes should be crossed out with a single line and your initials inserted above. Correction fluid should not be used.
- Complete means 'the inclusion of date of entry and your signature, name and status'.

Test yourself KS 28

Describe why it is important to accurately and clearly record measurements.

Evidence generator KS 29

The Medical Records Act 1990 is a relevant piece of legislation for this area. Research it and explain to your assessor how it affects your working practices.

Recording physiological measurements

All measurements should be recorded on the appropriate forms and charts using the correct physiological measurement. These are shown in the chart below.

Measurement	Correct unit of measurement (with abbreviation)
Height	Centimetres (cm) and metres (m)
Weight	Kilograms (kg)
Blood pressure	Millimetres of mercury (mmHg)
Pulse	Beats per minute (bpm)
Respirations	Respirations per minute (rpm)
Temperature	Degrees Celsius (°C).

Other members of the care team require all recording forms; you need to ensure they are accurate, legible and complete for continuity of care to be given. Accurate and clear records ensure that correct information about the individual is collected. This is also a requirement of the Data Protection Act 1998. The Data Protection Act covers all records and individuals have the right to have their information kept confidential. All records must be accurate and fair, so it is important to ensure that correct training is received in how to complete paperwork.

Best practice

Record keeping and confidentiality of information

✔ Only pass on information to the people who have a right and a need to know.

✔ Keep records safe so that they cannot be seen or accessed by people who do not have a right to see or access them.

✔ Always write in black ink so that records are clear and are easy to photocopy.

✔ Always write what you see and hear, not what you assume. This keeps records accurate.

✔ Handwritten records must be legible.

✔ Records must only contain relevant information.

Activity

Each working environment will have its own charts and forms for each of the measurements described in this section. Collect one form for each measurement then practise filling them in. You could do this by practising some of the procedures on colleagues and then recording the measurements accurately.

Evidence generator KS 30

Show your assessor any recording documents you have completed when taking physiological measurements. Ensure they conform with the Data Protection Act 1998 in that they are accurate, legible and complete. Explain to your assessor why you have completed them the way you have.

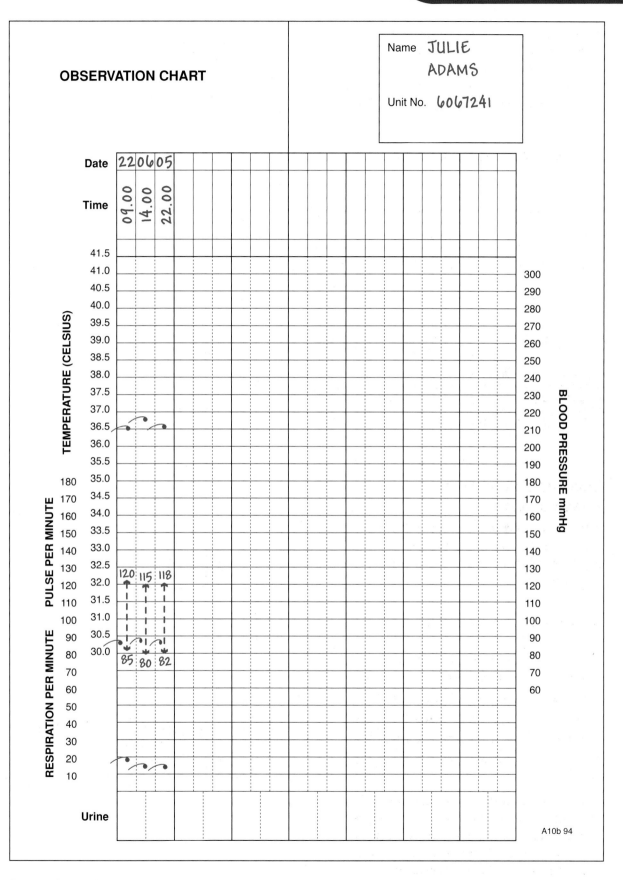

OBSERVATION CHART

Name   JULIE ADAMS

Unit No.   6067241

Example of a chart for taking body measurements.

A10b 94

Michelle works in a small nursing home for older people. Victor, one of the individuals, has not been well. He appears confused, looks sweaty and hot, and complains of headaches. He is also sleeping a lot and this has caused concerns regarding his health.

Michelle has accompanied Victor to the doctor, where Victor has had his temperature, blood pressure, pulse and respirations measured. All are raised above normal levels and, on listening to his chest, the doctor diagnosed that Victor has a chest infection, prescribing him antibiotics.

On returning to the nursing home, Michelle writes the following entry in Victor's case notes:

> 25/11 – Took V to the GP and was told he has an
> ~~infarction.~~ infection. MP

1 How do you think Michelle's entry into Victor's case notes will benefit his health?

2 What essential information do you think Michelle should have included in the case notes?

3 If you were working at the same home as Michelle, how do you think her actions would affect your own practice?

4 Who should Michelle have reported to with the information from the doctor?

Keeping good records is important in any health care setting as it not only ensures continuity of care but it also informs other health care assistants as to what has been done and what needs to be done.

When taking physiological measurements, clear records are a good indicator of whether treatment is working and they help with accurate diagnosis.

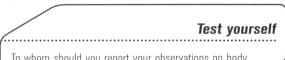

Test yourself

To whom should you report your observations on body measurements and why? (KS 29)

Prepare individuals for clinical/therapeutic activities; support individuals during and following clinical/therapeutic activities; prepare environments and resources for use during clinical/therapeutic activities

Introduction

These NVQ units are new workforce competencies developed by Skills for Health for the revised NVQ Health award.

Patients find themselves in different settings: for example, accident and emergency department, outpatients' department, labour wards, central treatment areas, day surgery and physiotherapy departments, in addition to clinics, health centres and GP surgeries. In any of these settings, patients can undergo procedures for both investigative and therapeutic reasons.

These units will give you the knowledge required for preparing the patient, the environment and the resources for such procedures. You will also learn how you can support the patient, both physically and emotionally, while they undergo the procedure or activity. It is essential too that you understand the limits of your job role and the actions to take if there are any problems during the preparation of the individual.

Specific procedures will be covered in this chapter but there are many more procedures that can be

covered by these units. The clinical or therapeutic activity will depend upon your work setting, but could include preparing individuals for procedures that may include:

- chest aspiration – withdrawing fluid from around the lungs
- lumbar puncture – withdrawing fluid from the spinal canal
- cardiac catheter test (coronary angiogram) – an X-ray examination of the coronary arteries
- examination of the colon and rectum (sigmoidoscopy)
- insertion of a urinary catheter, to remove urine from the bladder
- individual physiotherapy or occupational therapy activities
- group physiotherapy exercise sessions
- Caesarean section – delivery of a baby through an incision in the abdominal wall
- bronchoscopy – examination of the bronchi by means of a bronchoscope

What you need to learn

- Legislation and organisational policies and procedures
- Job roles and responsibilities
- Obtaining consent and confirming patient identity
- Infection control
- Checking documentation
- Resources and equipment needed
- Preparation of the patient: specific sites on the body
- Preparation of the patient: position, empty/full bladder
- Preparation of the patient: explaining, advising and supporting
- Actions to take in the event of adverse reaction or contra indication
- Follow-up procedures and post-procedural recovery
- Records and documentation

What evidence you need to generate for your portfolio

Your assessor must observe you as you prepare and support individuals undergoing clinical and therapeutic activities. You also need to provide evidence that you know and understand current legislation, policies and procedures, and that you understand the principles of best practice within your health care setting. If your assessor does not observe you dealing with problems, you could show that you can do so with a personal account of the actions you took on an occasion when problems did occur.

If you are completing more than one of these GEN units, some criteria can be cross-referenced between units. For example, knowledge question 5 in Unit GEN 4 asks you about the importance of standard precautions. This same knowledge question is included in GEN 5 (question 3) and in GEN 6 (question 3)

Legislation and organisational policies and procedures

All staff, including health care assistants and support workers, must ensure their working practices are not only in accordance with current legislation but also in line with their workplace's guidelines and procedures. It is your responsibility to ensure you are familiar with your care environment's policies and procedures and to know where these policies are kept in your workplace.

Individuals about to undergo a clinical procedure can expect to be kept safe from harm, to be fully informed about the clinical activity and to have their rights and choices respected as far as possible within the limits of the procedure. They can also expect that their personal details will be kept confidential.

Check the table on the next page in addition to the topics in this book for more in depth detail of legislation.

Evidence in action

Copy the table on the next page and add notes to it relating to your own work practice. This will help you to generate knowledge evidence for units GEN 4 and GEN 5.

Checklist: Referring to legislation

When you are preparing an individual, environment or resources for clinical activities, check that you have referred to:

- Human Rights Act 1998
- Health and Safety at Work Act 1974
- Manual Handling Regulations 1992
- Control of Substances Hazardous to Health (COSHH) 2002
- Reporting of Illnesses, Diseases and Dangerous Occurrences Regulations (RIDDOR) 1995
- Data Protection Act 1998
- Access to Medical Records Act 1990
- Mental Capacity Act 2005

Main legislation affecting the preparation of individuals and environments

Legislation	Relates to	Notes
Health and Safety at Work Act 1974	Ensuring the environment is safe and free from hazards Assessing risks Checking equipment before use Use of personal protective equipment Handling hazardous/contaminated waste Disposal of sharp implements Responsibilities – yours/employers	*Make sure the flex to the angle poise lamp is out of the way and won't cause anyone to trip* *Make sure you have a 'sharps box' to hand for disposal of used needles*
Manual Handling Regulations 1992	Safe moving and handling of patients Safe moving of equipment/loads Checking equipment before use Preparing the environment	
Control of Substances Hazardous to Health 2002	Storing cleansing materials Labelling of hazardous substances Bodily fluids – blood and urine Flammable liquids/gases Toxic/corrosive substances/liquids	*Store cleansing materials in locked cupboard.* *Used swabs to go into yellow bag – clinical waste*
RIDDOR 1995	Reporting accidents and injuries Reporting diseases Reporting dangerous occurrences Completion of relevant paperwork	
Data Protection Act 1998	Storing confidential information Paper-based information Information stored on computer Record keeping	*Ensure patients records are stored securely* *Ensure you log off and shut down computerised patient records*
Human Rights Act 1998	Involvement and informed consent Individual treatment and respect Patient need Rights and choices Privacy and dignity	*Ensure individual has given consent* *Maintain privacy and dignity throughout the procedure*
Mental Capacity Act 2005	Capacity to consent to/refuse treatment Best interests/advocacy Support individuals in the decision-making process	*Presume capacity to give consent unless it can be established that the individual lacks capacity*

Evidence in action
(GEN 4 K1; GEN 5 K1; GEN 6 K1)

Find out where the policy and procedure files are kept in your workplace and check the responsibilities these policies and procedures place on you. In some areas, these policies may be found on the individual organisation's intranet. Write an account of how your workplace's policies and procedures affect your work practice when you are preparing individuals, the environment and the resources for clinical activities.

Job roles and responsibilities

As a health care assistant, you need to be aware of the limitations of your experience and job role. It would be unsafe practice to undertake anything you have not been trained to do and are not competent to undertake. If you are unsure of how to prepare an individual for a clinical procedure or of the equipment and materials needed, you must ask for help from someone more qualified or experienced. It is essential that you understand your responsibilities when answering patients' questions: you need to know which questions you are able and qualified to answer, and when to refer questions to a more qualified member of staff.

Depending upon your workplace, a qualified member of staff could include a registered nurse, midwife, physiotherapist, occupational therapist, GP or medical practitioner. It is the role of the qualified staff member to both support and guide you in the development of your work practice.

Did you know?

The Nursing and Midwifery Council (NMC) code of professional conduct May 2008 states: 'You must be willing to share your skills and expertise for the benefit of your colleagues' and 'You must facilitate students and others to develop their confidence'.

Your employer's policies and procedure file will give you a framework for the development of your professional practice. The NHS Knowledge and Skills Framework (KSF) is the competency framework that provides the basis of the NHS Review and Development process. This has been introduced to provide you with the means to track and record your career development within the NHS.

Your job description will outline all the tasks that you are responsible for and will set out your line of accountability, by explaining who you are responsible to and what you are responsible for.

Here is a job description for a health care assistant working in an accident and emergency department.

JOB DESCRIPTION

Grade: Health Care Assistant
Role: Health Care Assistant A&E

Reports to: Shift Manager A&E
Responsible to: Matron A&E

Responsibilities

1 Assist trained staff to maintain high standards of patient care with regard to all policies and procedures laid down by the Trust and also attending to the Patients Charter.
2 Carry out assigned tasks involving direct patient care in support of and supervised by a Registered Nurse.
3 Assist in making the most efficient and economical use of available resources.
4 Help maintain department morale by presenting problems to the appropriate person.

Duties

a) Clean trolleys, mattresses and dressing trolleys.
b) Assist nurses in the moving and handling of patients.
c) Escort patients to and from specialised departments for treatment and investigations.
d) Collect X-rays and deliver specimens to the laboratory when necessary.
e) Apply synthetic and Plaster of Paris casts to fractured limbs.
f) Cleanse uncomplicated wounds and apply dressings using aseptic technique.
g) Apply a wide range of supportive bandages to limbs e.g. broad arm sling, tubigrip and crepe bandage.

h) Undertake NVQ Level 3 training in addition to mandatory training and updates.

Duties in conjunction with the nursing staff

a) Work on the department under the supervision of the nurse in charge.
b) Be aware of policies relevant to the department including:
   • Health and Safety
   • Moving and Handling
   • Resuscitation
   • Fire.
c) Record pulse, blood pressure, temperature and respiratory rate of suitable patients; pass on findings from the observations to the registered nurse.
d) Report defective equipment to the nurse in charge.
e) General cleanliness of the department considering the health and safety of all users.
f) Monitor and maintain stock levels under supervision of the manager.

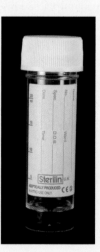

This job description outlines the main responsibilities. It is not a comprehensive list, but is intended as a guide for orientation and training. You should discuss your job description at your personal development review (PDR) and change it accordingly, in consultation with the Matron.

Evidence with a case study (GEN 4 K2, 7, 8; GEN 5 K2, 7, 8)

You are working in the accident and emergency department when a 40-year-old man is brought in with severe chest pain. The department is very busy, with all staff members engaged in caring for other patients. The doctor asks you to attach the electrodes and record an ECG (echocardiogram). Your job description doesn't include this in your responsibilities.

1 What would you say to the doctor?

2 Should you record the ECG?

3 What might be the consequences of undertaking this task when you are not qualified or trained to do so?

Reflection

If you are unsure of your job role and responsibilities and do not understand who you are accountable to, how might this affect the smooth running of your shift?

If you do not know the extent of your role, how might this make you feel?

How might the patients feel if staff members are not sure of their roles and responsibilities?

Evidence with a case study (GEN 4 K2, 7, 8, pc8; GEN 5 K2, 7, 8, pc8, pc9, pc12)

Mr B is a 72-year-old man who has recently had a stroke, which has left him with weakness in his left arm and leg. The physiotherapist has assessed Mr B and has provided him with a Zimmer frame to help him be more mobile. It is your role to support the patient to use this and to ensure that he is using the frame correctly before he is discharged. You notice Mr B is struggling to get used to his walking aid. He tells you that he has a walking stick at home and asks you to exchange his Zimmer frame for a walking stick.

1 What are your responsibilities to Mr B?

2 Who are you accountable to?

3 Who within the multidisciplinary team would you report this to?

4 What might be the consequences if you agree to Mr B using his walking stick rather than the Zimmer frame?

Reflection

Look at the case study again. Why do you think Mr B might have wanted to keep his walking stick rather than start using a Zimmer frame?

Imagine you are not a health care assistant, but a relative of Mr B's. Would you view this situation any differently?

Evidence in action (GEN 4 K2, 7, 8, pc7, pc8; GEN 5 K2, 7, 8, 9, pc8, pc9)

Check your job description and then write an explanation of your job role and your responsibilities when preparing patients for clinical procedures. Describe what action you would take if a patient asked you questions you were not qualified to answer. Explain the limits of your role and the roles of other team members. Include who you are accountable to and who you would seek advice from.

Obtaining consent and confirming patient identity

When preparing a patient for a clinical activity, it is important they are given full information about the procedure. Each person has a right to information about the clinical procedure they are to undergo, so that any decision they make is an informed one. Knowing what to expect also empowers the individual to make choices about their needs and expectations, and encourages the patient to make a rational decision based on the facts.

Consent can be defined as an individual's agreement to the procedure to be performed. This can be written (for example, when consenting to coronary angiography) or spoken (for example, when undergoing insertion of a urinary catheter).

As a health care assistant, it may not be your job role to obtain the patient's consent to the clinical procedure to be undertaken. However, it is your responsibility not only to obtain consent to prepare the individual for the procedure, but to also confirm you have the correct person. It is important that you check they are wearing a correctly completed identity wristband containing – as a minimum – name, date of birth and unique identification number. In addition, whenever possible, you must ask the individual to confirm their name and date of birth.

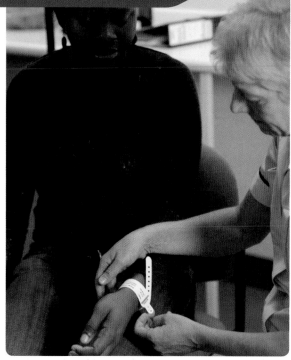

Confirming patient identity.

Infection control

Infection control is essential when preparing a patient for any clinical activity. It is important that you work within clinical guidelines to prevent cross-infection and that you understand these are standard precautions in health and safety measures. It may be your role to set up for the clinical activity and to prepare a sterile field for the practitioner to work in. Understanding how to handle equipment and materials safely is vital.

The Mental Capacity Act (2007) deals with the assessment of a person's capacity to consent to treatment. A person must be able to:

- understand the information relevant to the decision
- retain the information
- use the information as part of the decision making process
- communicate the decision.

Checklist

Before starting to prepare a patient, resource or environment, remember to:

- remove your jewellery before coming to work
- tie your hair back
- put on personal protective clothing – dress, tunic, trousers, plastic apron, theatre gown – all clean and sterile
- wash and dry your hands in the prescribed manner
- apply alcohol hand gel if necessary
- check and put on latex gloves – both clean and sterile.

Reflection

Imagine you are a patient being prepared for your dressing. How would you feel if you noticed that the health care assistant coming to help you had not washed their hands?

- Have you ever been busy and forgotten to wash your hands?
- Did anyone remind you and did you learn from this experience?
- Have you ever challenged a colleague about their bad practice?
- What was the outcome of this?

Memory jogger

Can you remember the correct procedures connected with infection control? Re-read Topic 1 to remind yourself.

Evidence in action (GEN 4 K5, 6, pc9, pc10; GEN 5 K3, 4, 5, pc5; GEN 6 K3, 4, pc7)

Explain what actions you must take to minimise or prevent infection and cross-infection when you are preparing patients for clinical procedures. Include the possible consequences if these hygienic precautions are not taken. What would be your response if a patient asked you why you were wearing an apron and gloves?

Checking documentation

Before preparing any patient for a clinical procedure, it is important to check all relevant documentation. This may include the care plan, case notes, doctor's letter or qualified practitioner's request for the procedure. It is essential to establish the exact clinical procedure the patient is about to undergo in order to undertake the correct preparation.

Evidence with a case study (GEN 4 K4, 7, 8, 10, 16, pc1, pc2, pc8; GEN 5 K7, 8, 13, 14, 15, pc3, pc8, pc9)

You are about to prepare Mrs Khan for urinary catheterisation. Here is her care plan.

Name	Mrs Khan	DoB 11/3/77	Ward	Gynaecology
Date	Problem	Action	Review date	Signature
6/11/07	Mrs Khan complained of abdominal discomfort. Unable to remember when she last passed urine. Seen and examined by Dr M who advised that a short term urinary catheter be inserted.	Urinary catheter to be inserted (continuous drainage via leg bag)	8/11/07	J Bloggs

Explain how you would check relevant documentation prior to preparing Mrs Khan. Include how you would confirm ID and how you would check that the patient understood and had consented to the procedure.

1 What concerns or worries might Mrs Khan have about having a catheter inserted?

2 How might you be able to support and reassure Mrs Khan?

3 Whose role would it be to insert the urinary catheter?

Preparing the environment, materials, equipment and resources

In order to correctly prepare the client and the resources for an activity, it is essential that you have a working understanding of the clinical activity to be undertaken. The resources you need will vary according to the activity. Before starting the activity, you must prepare all the resources and check all the materials and equipment, to ensure they are clean or sterile and in full working order. It would be unprofessional for a practitioner to have to wait because the resources are not there or are not sterile. Furthermore, having to wait could cause the patient unnecessary stress and anxiety.

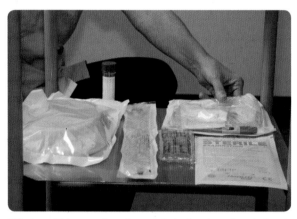

What would happen if a urinary catheter has been inserted and is draining urine, but the person preparing the resources has forgotten to put the catheter bag on to the trolley?

Preparation of the patient: specific sites on the body

It is important that you make the patient feel as physically and psychologically safe and comfortable as possible. The correct preparation of the patient, the environment and the resources demonstrate your competence in your work role and can give reassurance and confidence to the individual.

After you have confirmed the patient's identity, checked which procedure is to be undertaken, and ensured that the patient has given informed consent, you need to establish how much assistance the patient needs to prepare for the clinical activity.

It is important to encourage the individual to retain some ownership of what they have consented to, and to help them maintain as much independence as possible. If they are able to get onto an examination couch, get into a desired position or adjust their clothing, you should encourage this. It is your role to assist the patient as necessary to ensure that health and safety requirements are met. You also need to help maintain privacy by closing doors or pulling curtains around the bed: it is essential to respect the patient's dignity and keep them covered as far as possible within the limits of the procedure.

Having an understanding of the procedure to be performed will allow you to assist the individual into the desired position. For example, **chest aspiration** is usually performed with the patient sitting as upright as possible but, to undergo a

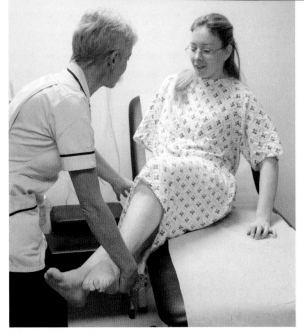

It is part of your role to encourage independence while also ensuring patient safety.

lumbar puncture, the patient will need to lie on their side, with their knees pulled up to their chin as far as they are able. It may be your role to physically support the patient to maintain this position or perhaps to hold their hand while the practitioner undertakes the procedure.

> ### Key terms
>
> **Chest aspiration** Withdrawing fluid from around the lungs.
> **Lumbar puncture** Withdrawing fluid from the spinal canal.

Urinary catheterisation and **sigmoidoscopy** can be very embarrassing procedures to undergo. It is essential to help the patient to maintain their privacy and dignity throughout the activity, and to only expose the necessary part of the body for as short a time as possible – hence the importance of good preparation.

> ### Key terms
>
> **Urinary catheterisation** Inserting a fine, hollow tube into the bladder to remove urine.
> **Sigmoidoscopy** An examination of the inside of the rectum.

> ### Reflection
>
> Consider how you would feel if you were to undergo a sigmoidoscopy. Imagine how you would feel if you are left lying on the couch partly exposed whilst the resources are prepared.

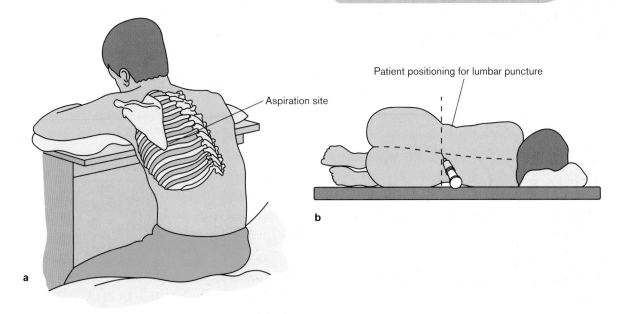

Aspiration site

Patient positioning for lumbar puncture

a

b

The correct positions for a) chest aspiration – sitting upright on the bed/examination couch, and b) lumbar puncture – lying on side, knees pulled up to chin.

Physical preparation

Some procedures, such as **cardiac catheter tests (coronary angiogram)**, require the patient to have nothing to eat or drink for a number of hours before the procedure. Some practitioners also request skin preparation for this procedure, and ask for the patient to be shaved three inches above and below the groins on both sides. This may be a task the patient is able to undertake or it may be within your job role: you will need to check this with your manager and medical practitioner performing the angiogram.

It is also important that you check that the patient has removed nail varnish and make-up, if this is a requirement of the procedure. For some procedures it is important the patient has an empty bladder, while others require the patient to have a full bladder to give the practitioner a better view of the bladder lining.

It is your role to check that the patient has complied with any prescribed pre-procedural instructions, and to inform the practitioner if these instructions have not been adhered to.

The table below offers a quick reference guide for you when you are preparing your patient for a procedure.

Key term

Cardiac catheter tests (coronary angiogram)
An X-ray examination of the coronary arteries.

Key term

Urethral meatus Where the urethra opens to the exterior.

Did you know?

Not all practitioners agree on the policy of shaving prior to a procedure. It can be argued that shaving may cause micro abrasions and encourages microbial growth causing infections.

Preparing patients for procedures

Typical procedure	Preparation	Why	Points to remember	Follow up
Cardiac catheter test (angiogram)	Shaving of groin and fasting Reassurance	Insertion of catheter into femoral artery in the groin	Fasting in case surgical intervention is needed	Check puncture site at regular intervals Monitor pulse and blood pressure
Sigmoidoscopy or colonoscopy	Prior to examination – low fibre diet, laxative and enema	Empty bowel needed to provide a good view of the inside of the bowel	Ensure toilet facilities are nearby	Outpatient appointment
Urinary catheterisation	Cleansing of **urethral meatus** Strict asepsis Reassurance	Infection control to prevent urinary tract infection	Use smallest catheter possible	Check/record urinary output Check documentation in care plan
Physiotherapy activities/mobility exercises	Correct clothing and footwear Explanation	Health and safety aspects	Ensure correct equipment used	Give patient constructive feedback Report to qualified member of staff
Exercise regimes	Prescribed medication close to hand e.g. GTN Explanation	In case of adverse effects to exercise	Observe clients for adverse effects during exercise routine	Give patient constructive feedback Report to qualified member of staff
Caesarean section	Pre-op shave Emotional support for patient and relative	Infection control	Ensure post-delivery resources are to hand	Check documentation

You are working in the endoscopy suite where it is your job role to prepare individuals for their procedure. Mr J arrives at 8.30 am for a sigmoidoscopy. You introduce yourself as a health care assistant and explain your role. You check Mr J's personal details and complete and place an ID bracelet on his wrist. You also check that the consent form has been signed and that Mr J has an understanding of what to expect. Mr J then tells you that he didn't take the laxative he had been given with his pre-admission guidelines because he had had his bowels opened and didn't think it was necessary. He asks you if this will make a difference to his test.

1 What might you say to Mr J?

2 What action would you take?

3 What records or documentation would you complete?

Look again at the case study. Imagine that you were sent to assist another patient, but had not recorded or informed anyone that Mr J had not complied with his pre-procedural instructions and you have not informed anyone. What might the consequences be?

Preparation of the patient: explaining, advising and supporting

It is understandable for the individual to be anxious when undergoing a clinical procedure. They will be in an unfamiliar and perhaps restrictive environment; they may be anxious about how much pain they will feel; and if they are undergoing a diagnostic procedure, they be worried about what the results may show. They may also be anxious about how long the procedure will take and whether they will be able to go home afterwards.

You may be able to allay some of the patient's worries by simple but important measures such as smiling, showing that you are listening to the individual and appearing calm and not rushed. It is important that you check the patient has understood what the practitioner has said to them. You will need to explain using language the individual is able to understand, avoiding technical terms and medical jargon.

No two patients are the same, and it is important that you demonstrate sensitivity in judging the amount of information individuals are able to manage. However, most individuals respond well to reassurance.

Individuals may have many questions – and if you are the staff member who is undertaking their preparation, you may be the person they will ask. It is essential that you answer any questions honestly while remembering you must not answer any questions that you are not trained or qualified to reply to.

During the clinical procedure, it may be your role to monitor the patient's condition: this could include observing facial expression, colour, breathing and pulse rate or perhaps recording blood pressure. If there are any changes in the patient's condition, you must inform the practitioner immediately.

For more information about physiological measurements, see CHS 19.

You are a health care assistant working on the cardiac catheter suite. It is your role to prepare Mrs K for her angiogram, help her maintain the correct position on the X-ray table and support and monitor her during the procedure. Mrs K is attached to the ECG monitor and has an inflatable cuff on her arm. During the procedure, you notice that Mrs K looks flushed, her blood pressure is elevated and her pulse rate has increased. Mrs K tells you her chest aches and asks you if this is normal for the procedure.

1 Explain how would you prepare Mrs K for her angiogram.

2 How might you physically support Mrs K during the procedure?

3 How can you emotionally support Mrs K during her angiogram?

4 What action would you take on noticing the changes to Mrs K's condition?

5 What might be your reply to Mrs K's question?

Reflection

Think of an occasion when you have been asked to remain with and support a patient undergoing a clinical procedure. Imagine no one had fully explained to the patient what to expect and the practitioner performing the activity was going to do so without speaking to the patient.

1 Would you speak to the patient?

2 How might you reassure them and check they are all right?

3 How do you think the above scenario might make the patient feel?

Problems

Occasionally there may be a change in the individual's condition or behaviour. This may indicate an adverse reaction or contra-indication in relation to the procedure. Such problems might include the patient feeling faint, dizzy and nauseous. In addition, the individual could become aggressive or may hyperventilate. If problems occur, it is important that you understand the action to take. This will usually involve stopping the preparation and informing the practitioner. However, it is possible you would need to activate the emergency alarm system and commence first aid, providing this is in line with your workplace's policies and procedures.

Reflection

Think of a time when you felt ill – perhaps you felt nauseous or dizzy. Did it help if someone took notice and listened to your explanations of how you felt? How might you feel if no one noticed you were not feeling well?

Did you know?

A patient may complain of light-headedness during the insertion of an enema. This is due to vagal nerve stimulation, which can slow the heart rate and alter its rhythm.

This table provides a quick reference guide to the problems that may occur during clinical or therapeutic activities.

Problems that can occur during clinical or therapeutic procedures

Activity	Problem	Action
Angiogram	Chest pain/ dizziness, discomfort/ nausea or vomiting	Inform the practitioner/ administer GTN spray
Physiotherapy exercises	Chest pain, breathlessness or muscle strain	Inform the practitioner/ administer GTN spray or prescribed inhaler
Chest aspiration/ insertion of chest drain	Pain/ breathlessness	Inform the practitioner
Urinary catheterisation	Patient discomfort	Inform the practitioner
Sigmoidoscopy/ colonoscopy	Patient needs the toilet while undergoing the procedure	Inform the practitioner
Lumbar puncture	Patient complains of pain	Inform the practitioner
Caesarean section	Haemorrhage	Assist the practitioner as necessary

Test yourself (GEN4 K14, 16, 17, 18, 21, 22, 23; GEN 5 K17, 18, 19, 22)

1 Before either a clinical or therapeutic activity, what type of physical and emotional support might an individual need?

2 What concerns, anxiety and discomfort might the individual have?

3 Why might you have to adjust or help the individual to remove clothing in preparation for certain activities?

4 When might the client's rights and choices have to be restricted due to the nature of certain activities?

5 Why is it important to keep the individual informed about what you are doing and the nature of the activity?

6 Why is it important to consider the individual's level of understanding when answering their questions? How might you communicate with an individual who has a communication difficulty?

7 How would you monitor the individual's condition during and following the procedure? What physiological measurements might you record?

Evidence in action (GEN4 K27, pc15)

Explain the action you would take if you were preparing a patient
for coronary angiography and they told you they had central
chest pain.

Records and documentation

It is important that, when you have prepared
your patient for the clinical procedure, you
document all the activities you have undertaken.
The practitioner undertaking the procedure and
other members of the care team will refer to these
records, so it is essential they are accurate, legible
and complete. It is also important to record your
activities as soon as possible after the episode of
care. Good record keeping not only informs other
members of staff of what has been done, but also
ensures continuity of care. Records may be kept
by handwritten notes or stored on a computer, but
you must remember that access to documentation
must be restricted to ensure confidentiality and
protect the patients' rights.

Memory jogger

What are your duties under the Data Protection Act? Look back
at pages 313–14.

Sigmoidoscopy preparation checklist

Have you checked?		Confirmed with patient	Staff signature
Date	30/5/08		
Time	10.15am		
Name	John Smith	✓	S White
Date of birth	11/3/37	✓	S White
Hospital number	AC 2349	✓	S White
ID bracelet in place	Yes	✓	S White
Consent obtained	Yes	✓	S White
Low fibre diet adhered to	Yes	✓	S White
Laxative/enema given	Yes	✓	S White
Result	Very good result	✓	S White
Clear fluids only taken orally	Yes	✓	S White

An example of a patient's case notes. These are for a patient due to have a sigmoidoscopy.

Evidence in action
(GEN 4 K28, 29, 30, pc16; GEN 5 K31, 33, 34, pc 11; GEN 6 K23)

Explain the records you would complete when preparing the patient, the environment and the resources for a clinical activity. Include information you would record in relation to your activities, the procedure and any follow-up instructions.

Evidence with a case study
(GEN 4 K28, 29, 30, pc1, pc3, pc16; GEN 5 K32, 33, 34, pc11)

Your colleague has just been sent home ill and you have been asked to take over managing her group of patients, who have started their physiotherapy exercise session. Your colleague left in a rush and has not completed any documentation, nor has she passed on to you the fact that Mrs S has asthma and needs to have her inhaler to hand.

1 What might be the consequences of you not being aware of this?

2 What documentation might you need to check before continuing with this exercise session?

Reflection

Look at the case study above. Think of the possible consequences of the above situation. Who might be accountable? What could you learn from this scenario?

Follow-up procedures and post-procedural recovery

Following the clinical or therapeutic activity, the individual may need a period of rest before they are ready for discharge either home or back to a ward or department.

If the individual was asked to have nothing to eat or drink prior to the procedure, then they might be offered a cup of tea and a biscuit, a slice of toast or perhaps a sandwich.

Lumbar puncture

Following a lumbar puncture, the patient may be asked to remain in a horizontal position for up to twelve hours. This may help to prevent the adverse effects of headache caused by the reduced pressure of the cerebro-spinal fluid.

Coronary angiogram

After a coronary angiogram, the patient will be kept lying flat for approximately an hour and it may be your role to check the individual's blood pressure and pulse at regular intervals. It is important you also check the puncture site to ensure it is not bleeding. The patient will gradually be allowed to sit out of bed and mobilise.

Chest aspiration

Following a chest aspiration or insertion of a chest drain the practitioner may request the patient undergoes a chest X-ray to determine the lungs are inflated and the position of the drain.

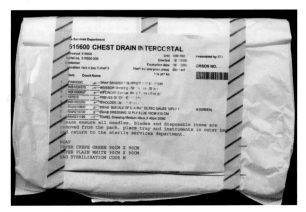

A Chest Aspiration Pack.

Sigmoidoscopy or colonoscopy

Following a bowel examination, the patient may need to use the toilet before going home. Air may have been introduced to dilate the bowel wall and this may cause the patient to have the desire to go to the toilet.

Physiotherapy exercises

During any exercise session, it is important that the individual is advised to do both 'warm up' and 'cool down' exercises. It is essential the individual has fully recovered from the exercise session prior to discharge.

Caesarean section

Prior to a Caesarean section, the patient may have had an epidural anaesthetic. Until the effects of the anaesthetic wear off, it is important the patient is monitored and remains in bed.

It is important the patient is made aware of any post-procedural instructions. While it may be the role of the qualified practitioner to explain any instructions to the individual, it could be your role to reinforce what has been explained. Following some clinical procedures, you may need to apply a dressing to the individual and it is important you inform them of how to care for this and when the dressing needs to be changed. On occasions, you may need to give the some quite detailed instructions. If this is the case then, in addition to a full explanation, it may also be helpful to provide an information and advice sheet for them to refer to. Following coronary angiography, the patient is discharged with an instruction sheet advising them to continue to check the puncture site and to contact the angio suite on their direct telephone number if there is persistent bleeding. They are also advised to take two days off work, to avoid any heavy lifting or exercise for two days and to refrain from driving for four days.

Once the individual has recovered and the practitioner has said they can be discharged, it may be your role to arrange this and book transport either to their home address or back to a ward. It may be that an outpatient appointment is needed and you should inform the individual when they need to return. If the individual is returning to a ward, it is essential that you give staff all the relevant information.

Evidence in action (GEN 5 K31, pc10)

Explain how you arrange a follow-up appointment and how you arrange for the patient to be returned to the ward.

OR

Explain how an outpatient appointment would be made and how transport home would be arranged.

Reflection

Consider the consequence if a patient is told that they need to return to see the doctor in the outpatients' department but no one makes them an appointment.

- What might your reaction be if the patient was a relative of yours?
- What confusion might this cause for the patient?

Test yourself (GEN 5 K10, 21, 29, 30, 31)

1 Explain when an individual might need a recovery period and refreshment after a procedure.
2 What is your workplace policy for discharging individuals following either a clinical or a therapeutic procedure?
3 What instructions might the individual be given following either a clinical or a therapeutic procedure/activity?
4 What could be the outcome if these instructions are not followed?
5 Explain how you would arrange transport and escort services for the individual, this could be return to a ward or discharge home.

Memory jogger

Can you remember all the issues surrounding communicating detailed and complex information? Look back at see HSC 31 page 13 to remind yourself.

The following examples of procedures might help you to see an overview of how units GEN 4, GEN 5 and GEN 6 interlink.

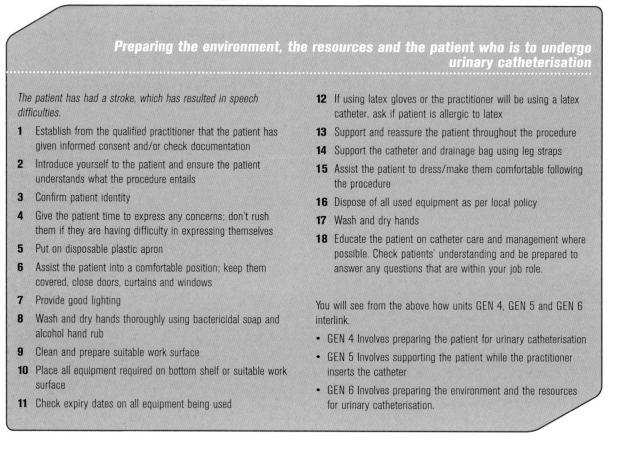

Preparing the environment, the resources and the patient who is to undergo urinary catheterisation

The patient has had a stroke, which has resulted in speech difficulties.

1 Establish from the qualified practitioner that the patient has given informed consent and/or check documentation

2 Introduce yourself to the patient and ensure the patient understands what the procedure entails

3 Confirm patient identity

4 Give the patient time to express any concerns; don't rush them if they are having difficulty in expressing themselves

5 Put on disposable plastic apron

6 Assist the patient into a comfortable position; keep them covered, close doors, curtains and windows

7 Provide good lighting

8 Wash and dry hands thoroughly using bactericidal soap and alcohol hand rub

9 Clean and prepare suitable work surface

10 Place all equipment required on bottom shelf or suitable work surface

11 Check expiry dates on all equipment being used

12 If using latex gloves or the practitioner will be using a latex catheter, ask if patient is allergic to latex

13 Support and reassure the patient throughout the procedure

14 Support the catheter and drainage bag using leg straps

15 Assist the patient to dress/make them comfortable following the procedure

16 Dispose of all used equipment as per local policy

17 Wash and dry hands

18 Educate the patient on catheter care and management where possible. Check patients' understanding and be prepared to answer any questions that are within your job role.

You will see from the above how units GEN 4, GEN 5 and GEN 6 interlink.

- GEN 4 Involves preparing the patient for urinary catheterisation
- GEN 5 Involves supporting the patient while the practitioner inserts the catheter
- GEN 6 Involves preparing the environment and the resources for urinary catheterisation.

References

Nursing and Midwifery Council (2004) *NMC Code of Professional Conduct*

Further reading

Baxter A, Lloyd PA (2004) *The Royal Marsden Hospital Manual of Clinical Nursing Procedures Sixth edition.* Blackwell Publishing, London

Storey, L (2005) *Delegation to Healthcare Assistants.* Practice Nursing 16(6):4

Nursing and Midwifery Council (2007) *NMC Advice for delegation to Non-regulated Healthcare staff.* NMC London

Prepare environments and resources for use during clinical/therapeutic activities

Introduction

This NVQ unit is a new workforce competence developed by Skills for Health for the revised NVQ Health award.

Unit GEN 6 links with Dimension HWB7: Interventions and treatments in the Knowledge and Skills Framework, Level 1. HWB is the Health and Well Being Dimension. This dimension relates to intervening and treating individuals' physiological and/or psychological needs.

Patients find themselves in different settings: for example, accident and emergency department, outpatients' department, labour wards, central treatment areas, day surgery and physiotherapy departments, in addition to clinics, health centres and GP surgeries. In any of these settings, patients can undergo procedures for both investigative and therapeutic reasons.

This unit focuses on your role in preparing both the environment and the resources so that they are ready for the designated clinical or therapeutic activity to take place. You will also learn how to set up and prepare resources in an appropriate manner and time for the activity to be carried out, while at the same time meeting the needs of the individual. You will look at what actions you should

take if items of equipment are damaged, faulty or contaminated or if the environment is too hot or too cold.

Specific procedures will be covered in this chapter but there are many more procedures that can be covered by these units. The clinical or therapeutic activity you may need to prepare the environment and resources for could include:

- chest aspiration – withdrawing fluid from around the lungs
- lumbar puncture – withdrawing fluid from the spinal canal
- cardiac catheter test (coronary angiogram) – an X-ray examination of the coronary arteries
- examination of the colon and rectum (sigmoidoscopy)
- insertion of a urinary catheter, to remove urine from the bladder
- individual physiotherapy or occupational therapy activities
- group physiotherapy exercise sessions
- Caesarean section – delivery of a baby through an incision in the abdominal wall
- bronchoscopy – examination of the bronchi by means of a bronchoscope.

What you need to learn

- Legislation and organisational policies and procedures
- Job roles and responsibilities
- Safety checks that must be made on equipment prior to use
- Reporting problems with equipment and resources
- Infection control
- Preparing the environment
- Preparing the equipment, materials and resources
- Storing resources
- Records and documentation

What evidence you need to generate for your portfolio

Your assessor must observe you as you prepare the environment and the resources for clinical/therapeutic activities. You also need to provide evidence that you know and understand current legislation, policies and procedures and that you understand the principles of best practice within your health care setting. If your assessor does not observe you dealing with problems, you could show that you can do so with a personal account of the actions you took on an occasion when problems did occur.

If you are also completing unit GEN 4 and/or unit GEN 5, then some criteria will also be covered in these units and can be cross-referenced between units.

Legislation and organisational policies and procedures

Before you start to prepare the environment and resources, you need to be aware of your organisation's policies and procedures in addition to health and safety legislation. The Health and Safety at Work Act 1974 places certain responsibilities on both employers and employees.

When you are preparing the environment and the resources for both clinical and therapeutic activities, it is important that the environment is safe not only from environmental hazards such

as wet floors but also from infection – especially when dealing with bodily fluids or soiled dressings. The workplace must also be safe from hazardous fumes and gases and flammable liquids you could be dealing with.

Patients undergoing certain procedures may require oxygen therapy and it is essential you are aware of the precautions needed at such times.

Further information can be found in the previous chapters – GEN 4 and GEN 5 in addition to the topic section in this book.

Check the table opposite in addition to the Topics in this book for more in-depth detail of legislation.

> ### Key term
>
> **Vicarious liability** Being liable for something you did not actually do yourself. For example, an employer is vicariously liable for negligent acts or omissions by his employee in the course of employment, whether or not such act or omission was specifically authorised by the employer.

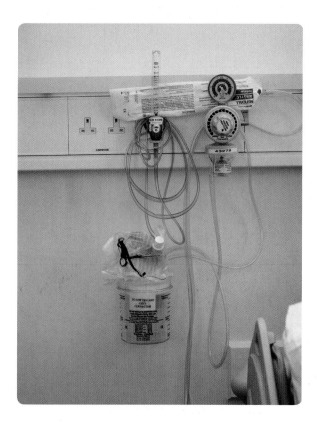

Special precautions are required for oxygen therapy.

Main legislation affecting preparing environments and resources

Legislation	Relates to	Notes
Health and Safety at Work Act 1974	Ensuring the environment is safe and free from hazards Ensuring work areas are well lit Assessing risks Checking equipment before use Infection control Use of personal protective equipment Contaminated items Responsibilities – yours/employer's **Vicarious liability**	*Check resources are fit for use.* *Dispose of damaged or out-of-date items*
Manual Handling Regulations 1992	Safe moving and handling of patients Safe moving of equipment/loads Checking equipment before use Preparing the environment	*Check the hoist has been serviced* *Ensure the correct sling is available and is fit for use* *Ensure there is enough room to undertake the manoeuvre*
Control of Substances Hazardous to Health 2002	Storing cleansing materials Labelling of hazardous substances Flammable liquids/gases Toxic/corrosive substances/liquids	
RIDDOR 1995	Reporting accidents and injuries Reporting diseases Reporting dangerous occurrences Completion of relevant paperwork	
Data Protection and Access to Records 1998	Storing confidential information Paper based information Information stored on computer Record keeping	*Keep patient case notes confidential* *Use password to access computerised data*

Evidence in action

Copy this table and add notes to it relating to your own work practice. This will help you to generate knowledge evidence for GEN 4.

Checklist

Have you referred to:

- The Health and Safety at Work Act 1974?
- Manual Handling Regulations 1992?
- Control of Substances Hazardous to Health (COSHH) 2002?
- Reporting of Illnesses, Diseases and Dangerous Occurrences Regulations (RIDDOR) 1995?
- Data Protection Act 1998?

Job roles and responsibilities

As a health care assistant, you need to be aware of the limitations of your experience and job role. It would be unsafe practice to undertake anything you have not been trained to do and are not competent to undertake. Your job description will set out your line of accountability by stating what you are responsible for and who you are responsible to.

It is also essential that you understand your responsibilities for checking the safety of the equipment and the environmental conditions you will be working under, and that you know which adjustments you are able and qualified to undertake and when to refer problems to another member of staff or perhaps to another department.

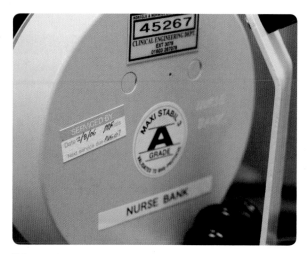

Who would check equipment and attach such stickers? Find out for your workplace.

may be your workplace practice to report faulty equipment directly to the estates department with a telephone call, or it may be your role to complete a requisition slip and send this to the relevant department. It is essential that you make a record of what action you have taken and that you include the date and time you reported the problem.

Electrical equipment must always be checked to ensure it is safe and fit for use. It is your role to check that electrical items have had a recent electrical test by a qualified electrician.

Your employer's policies and procedures file will give you a framework for the development of your professional practice. The NHS Knowledge and Skills Framework (KSF) is the competency framework that provides the basis of the NHS Review and Development process. This has been introduced to provide you with the means to track and record your career development within the NHS.

Did you know?

The qualified practitioner is responsible for delegating work appropriately, providing feedback and supervising the health care assistant (HCA). However, if the HCA has received training and does not carry out the task competently, it is the HCA who is responsible.

Reporting problems

As well as understanding when to refer problems, it is essential that you know who to report problems to and how to do this.

Depending upon the fault or the adjustment needed, you may have to report this to your manager or qualified practitioner. However, it

Test yourself
(GEN 6 K6, 7, 8, 9, 10, 11, 14)

1 Why is it important that you do not undertake tasks you are not trained or qualified to undertake?

2 When preparing the environment and the resources for a clinical or a therapeutic procedure, what is your role? What are the roles of other staff members?

3 Explain all the resources you would need to prepare for one procedure.

4 How do you ensure you handle equipment safely?

5 Why is it important to prepare all resources before the start of the activity?

Department	Date	Time	Equipment	Reported by	Signature
Physio and OT department	10/12/07	10.15am	Electric fan not working	J Bloggs	J Bloggs

Here is an example of a job description for a health care assistant supporting a qualified physiotherapist.

JOB DESCRIPTION

Grade: Support Worker

Role: Physiotherapy Support worker

Reports to: Physiotherapist in charge

Responsible to: Senior Physiotherapist in charge of the department

Responsibilities

1 Assist the physiotherapist in maintaining high standards of patient care with regards to all policies and procedures laid down by the Trust and also attending to the Patients Charter.

2 Carry out assigned tasks involving direct patient care in support of and supervised by a qualified physiotherapist.

3 Assist in making the most efficient and economical use of resources.

4 Ensure there are adequate supplies of resources and equipment.

Duties

1 Implement physiotherapy programmes and treatments under direction.

2 Undertake mobility and movement programmes – with and without gym equipment – under direction.

3 Ensure all equipment is safe and fit for purpose.

4 Provide and fit assistive devices to meet individual needs.

5 Support individuals to develop skills to manage their lives.

6 Undertake NVQ Level 3 qualification in additional to mandatory training and updates.

This job description outlines the main responsibilities of a support worker in the physiotherapy department. It is not a comprehensive list, but is intended as a guide for orientation and training.

Evidence in action (GEN 6 K2, pc 2)

Find and read your job description, then, explain what it says about your responsibilities and your accountability within the health care environment when you are preparing the environment and the resources for an activity.

Include what you are responsible for and who you are accountable to when resources are found to be damaged, faulty or contaminated. The table on the next page may help you.

Equipment and resources	Employer responsibility	Your responsibility
Suction	Electrician to check	Check it is working and has an adequate supply of suction catheters
Oxygen	Oxygen supply working	Ensure adequate supply of oxygen masks and nasal catheters
Fixed lighting	Electrician to check	
Angle poise lamp	Electrician to check	Check it is working Check it has correct size bulb
Moving and handling equipment	Manufacturer to service regularly	
CSSD packs	Quality checks	Check pack is sterile and unopened – check seal is unbroken
Foley catheters	Manufacturer to monitor	
Sterile water	Manufacturer to monitor	Check date of manufacture and use-by date Ensure it has been stored correctly
Sterile gloves	Ensure sufficient supplies	
Exercise equipment	Manufacturer to service	Ensure equipment has been serviced Ensure it is in good working order and fit for use
Portable fan	Electrician to check	
Laboratory forms	Adequate supplies	Ensure sufficient stocks are available for histology, cytology, microbiology and haematology
Specimen containers	Adequate supplies	
Syringes and needles	Manufacturer to monitor	Ensure they are sterile, have adequate supplies and different sizes of both syringes and needles. 'Sharps box' needed for disposal
Local anaesthetic	Qualified practitioner to check	

Evidence with a case study (GEN 6 K6, 15, 16, 20, pc2, pc10)

You are working in the physiotherapy department and are assisting clients to exercise to improve their mobility. Part way through the session, Mr N complains that it is too hot in the room. There are no windows you can open so you decide to put on the electric fan to cool the room down. When you check the fan, the plug is loose and the fan does not work.

Which of the following actions would you take?

1 You rewire the plug – you have done this before at home with no problems.

OR

2 You inform someone else – if so, who would you inform?

Explain the reasons for your actions in the above situation.

Reflection

You are competent to rewire a plug – you have done it at home, what might be the consequences if you did rewire the plug on the fan?

Infection control

Infection control is essential when preparing resources for any clinical procedure and should be standard precautions in health and safety measures. Infection and cross-infection can be minimised by washing hands before, during and after preparing environments and resources for clinical or therapeutic activities. For some procedures, you may also need to wear protective clothing such as apron and gloves; for other procedures, you may need to use **additional protective clothing and equipment**.

It may be your role to clean and prepare trolleys and also to prepare a sterile field for the practitioner to work in. You need to have a good understanding of the cleaning materials needed to disinfect or to sterilise the environment. It is also essential that you understand how to check that instruments packaged and prepared in the central sterilising supply department (CSSD) are in fact sterile and fit for use. It is important that you handle both equipment and resources in a way that prevents cross-infection.

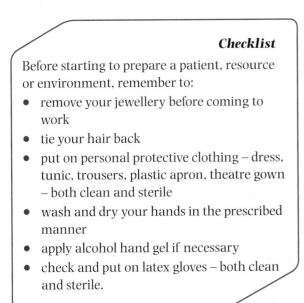

Key term

Additional protective clothing and equipment
Items such as protective eyewear, visors and radiation protective equipment.

See Topic 1 Infection control *for more detail about infection control and sterile field.*

Checklist

Before starting to prepare a patient, resource or environment, remember to:

- remove your jewellery before coming to work
- tie your hair back
- put on personal protective clothing – dress, tunic, trousers, plastic apron, theatre gown – both clean and sterile
- wash and dry your hands in the prescribed manner
- apply alcohol hand gel if necessary
- check and put on latex gloves – both clean and sterile.

Memory jogger

See pages 160–64 for a reminder of how to set up a sterile field and how to put on sterile gloves.

Evidence in action (GEN 6 K3, pc 7)

Explain how you prevent infection and cross-infection when preparing the environment and the resources for an activity.

Preparing the environment

It is essential you have a working understanding of the clinical or therapeutic activity to be undertaken in order to prepare the environment and the resources correctly. The environment could be a treatment or clinical room where the window would need to be closed in order to provide a dust-free environment, or an operating theatre with its own air circulation system. However, the environment could also be a gym or physiotherapy department where individuals might undergo an exercise session. While it is important that the room is not too cold for the individuals, it would not be helpful if it were uncomfortably hot during the exercise session. You will need to check your workplace policies and procedures file to determine the optimum temperature, humidity and air conditioning requirements.

Most procedures and activities need good light, so it is essential that both general and any directional lighting needed are checked before starting the activity. For example, in an operating theatre, it may be your role to ensure that the theatre light is in working order; in a treatment room, it could be essential that the angle poise lamp is functioning.

Evidence with a case study (GEN 6 K4, 5, 9, pc1, pc5)

You are working in the central treatment room where the majority of patients undergo clinical procedures. You are short staffed and have a busy list including routine dressing changes, removal of sutures and, just after lunch, a patient has been booked in to have a lumbar puncture. In an attempt to keep the department running smoothly, you decide to prepare for the lumbar puncture before you go to your lunch.

You prepare the trolley, open the basic pack to save time and leave the room with the door closed.

1 Is this acceptable practice?

2 What problems could arise?

Preparing and storing equipment, materials and resources

Once the environmental temperature, humidity, ventilation and lighting have been prepared, you need to collect together and check the resources that will be needed. These will vary depending on the activity to be performed, and may include both fixed and portable items. All resources must be prepared and materials and equipment checked to ensure that they are not only clean or sterile, but also safe and in full working before starting the activity.

Evidence in action (GEN 4 K11, 12, 13; GEN 6 K8, 9, 10, pc1, pc4, pc5)

Give an example from your work practice of the resources you need when preparing an individual for a clinical procedure. Include how you handle equipment and materials safely, and explain why you prepare all resources before the start of the activity.

Reflection

Think of the time you first prepared all the necessary resources for a urinary catheterisation.

1 Who explained what would be needed?

2 Did you 'get it right' first time?

3 If you forgot something, what did you learn from this?

Examples of the resources needed for common procedures

Here you will see the resources needed for three common procedures: urinary catheterisation, lumbar puncture and chest aspiration.

Depending on your workplace, your central sterilising supply department (CSSD) may supply packs containing all of the sterile resources you will need for many different procedures.

Resources for the insertion of urinary catheter

- Trolley – cleaned and disinfected
  - Top shelf – autoclaved catheterisation pack
  - Bottom shelf – sterile water for cleansing purposes
- Waste disposal bag attached to the trolley
- Foley catheters – more than one in case of wastage
- Syringe and sterile water to inflate the balloon if not included with the Foley catheter
- Latex gloves
- Leg bag with straps or night bag with stand
- Lubricating anaesthetic gel, if required
- Urine specimen bottles, if sample requested
- Laboratory forms, if sample requested
- Intake and output chart or other documentation

Did you know?

Autoclaving is a very effective way of destroying organisms and spores. It is the method of choice for sterilising gauze and cotton wool, cotton gowns and some types of plastic kidney bowls and gallipots.

Key term

Autoclaving Sterilising by steam under pressure.

Resources for chest aspiration and lumbar puncture

As above but in, place of the catheterisation pack, you will need a large basic pack or lumbar puncture pack.

In addition you will need:

- skin sterilisation solution or hibitane swabs
- local anaesthetic, which usually only the qualified practitioner has access to
- syringe and needles to administer the local anaesthetic
- laboratory specimen bottles
- laboratory forms.

If a chest drain is inserted, you will need to include an underwater drainage system and appropriate dressings to cover the puncture site.

In addition to any specialised equipment you might need, such as catheters, sigmoidoscope, chest drain and exercise equipment, you may also need some of the following:

- anglepoise lamp – make sure it works
- dressing pack and other sterile equipment – make sure the pack/seal is intact, not damaged, sterile and in date.
- sterile gloves
- skin cleansing solution
- syringes and needles – check they are of the correct size/gauge and ensure you have spares
- local anaesthetic – it may not be your job role to have access to this but you need to check it is to hand before the practitioner starts the procedure
- laboratory forms
- containers or bottles for the collection of samples or specimens.

Reflection

Look at the case study. If this happened to you in your workplace, how do you think you would feel? How you would feel if you were the patient and this happened to you?

Storing resources

(GEN 6 K12)

It is essential that you know where the required equipment, materials and resources are stored in your workplace. Failure to do so might mean the procedure has to be delayed, which in turn could cause the patient unnecessary anxiety and would not help the smooth running and efficiency of the department. It is also important to understand which resources are sensitive to environmental changes and how this affects their storage. For example, sterile dressing packs are usually stored in a cool, dry place while skin cleansing solutions may need to be stored in a cool, dark and locked cupboard.

Evidence with a case study (GEN 6 K1, 2, 4, 9, 19, 21, pc1, pc2, pc3, pc10)

You are a health care assistant in a busy GP practice and it is your role to set up for and assist the doctor with his minor operations clinic. Mrs H arrives. She is to undergo the removal of a small skin lesion from her back. You have made sure the room is warm enough and have a blanket to cover Mrs H when she has removed her jumper and blouse. You have prepared all the resources including a specimen jar and laboratory forms in case the doctor wishes to send the skin sample off to the laboratory. You only have one sterile basic pack left but this appears to be damaged and some of the contents appear to be missing.

1 What would your first action be?
2 Who would you inform?
3 Would the doctor still be able to go ahead with the procedure?
4 How could this situation could be prevented in the future?

Test yourself (GEN 6 K12, 13, 15, 16, 18, 19, 20, 21, 22)

1 For one activity, explain where all the resources you need are stored.
2 Which resources must be stored in a cool, dry place?
3 Do any resources have to be protected from light and heat?
4 What could the consequences be if resources were stored incorrectly?
5 Explain how you check environmental conditions: for example, light and heating.
6 Explain how you ensure that equipment is working before use.
7 If equipment is found to be faulty, what would you do?
8 To whom would you report problems with equipment or materials?
9 What might the consequences be if the sterile field were contaminated?

Records and documentation

When you are preparing the environment and the resources for clinical or therapeutic activities, it is important to include the correct documentation. This may include laboratory forms, patient's case notes, theatre list or department diary. All procedures require some form of documentation so that either you or the practitioner can document what activity has taken place, describe any treatment given or type of specimen taken.

Effective record keeping is essential in health care settings. If all care given, and any problems or progress are documented, it enables staff to communicate effectively and deliver the best possible care.

Did you know?

If you have received training and do not carry out record keeping competently, then you are responsible.

(Source: *British Journal of Healthcare Assistants* (2007))

Test yourself (GEN 6 K23, 24)

1 When preparing the resources for a procedure, what paperwork might you need to get ready?

2 Why is it important to report problems immediately?

The following examples of procedures might help you to see an overview of how units GEN 4, GEN 5 and GEN 6 interlink

Preparing the environment and the resources and undertaking a supervised exercise session

1 Establish from the qualified practitioner the nature of the exercise session. Check documentation.

2 Introduce yourself to the patients and ensure they understand what is expected of them.

3 Give time for any of the patients to express any concerns.

4 Ensure patients who need to have taken any prescribed medication have done so.

5 Ensure all patients are wearing well fitting footwear and appropriate clothing.

6 Ensure the environment is well ventilated and not too hot.

7 Ensure all equipment to be used has been safety checked and is fit for use.

8 Introduce 'warm up' exercises.

9 Observe individuals for signs of adverse reaction to the exercise session.

10 Support and reassure patients throughout the exercise session.

11 Ensure you encourage appropriate 'cool down' exercises.

12 Offer refreshments and ensure all are comfortable following the exercise session.

13 Arrange discharge or return back to the ward or department.

You will see from the above how units GEN 4, GEN 5 and GEN 6 interlink.

- GEN 4 involves preparing individuals for the exercise session
- GEN 5 involves supporting individuals during the exercise session
- GEN 6 involves preparing the environment and the resources prior to an exercise session.

References

Nazarko, L Record keeping: the role of the healthcare assistant. *British Journal of Healthcare Assistants* 2007 Vol 1

Further reading

Baxter A, Lloyd PA (2004) *The Royal Marsden Hospital Manual of Clinical Nursing Procedures* Sixth edition. Blackwell Publishing, London

Storey, L (2005) Delegation to Healthcare Assistants. *Practice Nursing* 16(6):4

Nursing and Midwifery Council (2007) *NMC Advice for delegation to Non-regulated Healthcare staff*. NMC London

The following grid is an example of where evidence generated for specific units/topics in this book may support the requirements of your KSF outline and the dimensions therein. The dimensions are addressed on and following the page numbers shown.

Unit/topic	Page	Knowledge specification framework dimension	Level
HSC 31 Promote effective communication for and about individuals	2–43	Core 1	2
		Core 6	2
		HWB 2	2
		HWB 3	1
		HWB 5	2
		HWB 7	1
HSC 32 Promote, monitor and maintain health, safety and security in the working environment	44–75	Core 3	1
		Core 4	1
		Core 5	1
		Core 6	2
		HWB 3	1
		HWB 7	1
HSC 33 Reflect on and develop your practice	76–100	Core 1	2
		Core 2	2
		Core 4	1
		Core 5	1
HSC 35 Promote choice, well-being and the protection of all individuals	101–133	Core 1	2
		Core 3	1
		Core 5	1
		Core 5	1
		Core 6	2
		HWB 2	2
		HWB 3	1
		HWB 5	2
		HWB7	1
Topic 1: Infection control	134–155	Core 3	1
		Core 4	1
		Core 5	1
		HWB 2	2
		HWB 5	2
		HWB 7	1
Topic 2: Aseptic technique	156–165	Core 3	1
		HWB 2	2
		HWB 5	2
		HWB 7	1

Unit/topic	Page	Knowledge specification framework dimension	Level
CHS 4, CHS 5, CHS 6 Identify the individual at risk from skin breakdown; undertake risk assessment and pressure area care, move, and position individuals	222–247	Core 1	2
		Core 3	1
		Core 6	2
		HWB 2	2
		HWB 5	2
		HWB 7	1
CHS 12 Undertake treatments and dressings related to the care of lesions and wounds	256–281	Core 1	2
		Core 3	1
		Core 6	2
		HWB 2	2
		HWB 5	2
		HWB 7	1
CHS 19 Undertake physiological measurements.	282–316	Core 1	2
		Core 3	1
		Core 6	2
		HWB 2	2
		HWB 3	1
		HWB 7	1
GEN 4, GEN 5, GEN 6 Prepare individuals for clinical/therapeutic activities; support individuals during and following clinical/therapeutic activities; prepare environments and resources for use during clinical/therapeutic activities	317–343	Core 1	2
		Core 3	1
		Core 6	2
		HWB 7	1

Core 1 – Communication
Core 2 – Personal and people development
Core 3 – Health, safety and security
Core 4 – Service improvement
Core 5 – Quality
Core 6 – Equality and diversity
HWB 2 – Assessment and care planning to meet health and well-being needs
HWB 3 – Protection of health and well-being
HWB 5 – Provision of care to meet health and well-being needs
HWB 7 – Interventions and treatments

Abuse Physical, psychological or sexual maltreatment of a person.

Accurate Precise, exact.

Active support Support that encourages individuals to maintain their independence and to achieve their potential.

Additional protective clothing and equipment Items such as protective eyewear, visors and radiation protective equipment.

Additional protective equipment Types of personal protective equipment such as visors, protective eyewear and radiation protective equipment.

Advocate A person who is responsible for acting and speaking on behalf of an individual when he or she is unable to do so.

Anaemia A condition when there is lack of red cells or haemoglobin, the substance that carries oxygen round the body.

Antibiotics Chemicals that attach to particular parts of bacteria and either destroy them or prevent them multiplying.

Antibodies Particular proteins that can lock on to foreign or diseased molecules and make them harmless or enable them to be destroyed by white cells in the body.

Antigen A molecule, or part of a molecule, that is detected by the body immune system as 'foreign'. An antibody is produced in response, which will react with that antigen.

Aphasia A condition where someone has difficulty understanding and expressing meaning through words.

Assessment tool In relation to skin breakdown, a process of assessment using a variety of risk factors, including continence, weight and nutritional status, against which a score is identified, clarifying the degree of risk that an individual's skin will break down. Assessment tools have various names according to their authors or developers.

Assumptions Something believed to be true without proof.

ATP Adenosine Triphosphate, the chemical that provides energy for all cellular material.

Aura A sensation that precedes the onset of certain disorders.

Autoclaving Sterilising by steam under pressure.

Bacteriocidal Killing bacteria.

Bacteriostatic Preventing the growth or multiplication of bacteria.

Beliefs Mental acceptance of something as being true or real.

Blood-borne Carried in the blood.

Bronchoscopy Examination of the bronchi, the two branches into which the trachea divides.

Cardiac catheter tests (coronary angiogram) An X-ray examination of the coronary arteries.

Carrier Someone who has their body colonised by a pathogen, yet does not show the signs of infection.

Chest aspiration Withdrawing fluid from around the lungs.

Cognitive Intellectual ability.

Colonisation When a micro-organism establishes itself on a body without causing any disease.

Commensal Living in harmony with another without harming or benefiting it.

Confidentiality Treating patient's information with discretion according to the law.

Conflict Clash or difference of viewpoints.

Consent Freely given, specific and informed indication of wishes.

Constructive feedback Helpful response.

Contaminated Infected or polluted.

Contamination Something becoming unclean or non-sterile through contact with body fluids, chemicals or radionucleatides.

Cytoskeleton Filaments forming the supportive scaffolding of the cell.

Debrief Go through what happened after an event.

Dehiscence Bursting open of a wound.

Desquamation The natural process where surface dead cells rub off as they are replaced by new cells from the germinative layer.

Development at work Developing the qualities and skills necessary for the workforce.

Discrimination Unfair treatment of a person or a group of people.

Distress Suffering resulting from anxiety, grief or unhappiness.

DNA Deoxyribonucleic Acid, the genetic material that provides the blueprint for all cell types.

Electron microscope A microscope that uses small particles – electrons – and electromagnets to magnify up to half a million times.

Empathy The ability to identify someone else's feelings.

Empowerment Helping people make choices, promoting self-esteem and confidence, and encouraging individuals to take action for themselves when possible.

Empowers Gives ability, skills or authority.

Endogenous infection Caused by micro-organisms already present on the body.

Entonox A gas made up of 50 per cent oxygen and 50 per cent nitrous oxide. It is an excellent analgesic for short procedures and wound dressings as it has a very rapid onset of action and is quickly eliminated from the body.

Enzymes Complex chemicals that control reactions in living cells and speed up changes.

Evaluation Considering something to judge its quality, condition or importance.

Evisceration When the viscera protrude through the wound.

Exogenous infection Caused by micro-organisms transferred from another person or object.

Extrinsic Originating from the outside.

Hazard Something which could possibly cause harm.

Holistic Looking at a person or situation as a whole.

Humidity The amount of water vapour in the air.

Hyper Over, excessive, high.

Hypo Under, lacking, low.

In utero In the womb.

Individual The person on whom the physiological measurement is being taken, whether an adult or a child.

Individuals at risk People whose health is particularly vulnerable, because they are: unconscious; very elderly; people with reduced mobility or immobility due to surgery, stroke, etc.; suffering from malnutrition, dehydration, skin conditions, sensory impairment, acute illness, vascular disease, severe chronic or terminal illness; people with a previous history of pressure damage or incontinence; people with diabetes; those with an altered mental state.

Induction Being taught about general principles at the beginning of a new job.

Infection The multiplication of harmful micro-organisms within the tissues, leading to damage

Intellectual Acquiring knowledge.

Intercostal Between the ribs.

Interstitial [definition to follow]

Intrinsic Within, on the inside.

Invasive Relating to a technique in which the body is entered by puncture or incision.

Joints Where two bones meet.

Knowledge and Skills Framework (KSF) Part of the NHS Agenda for Change pay system. It is an organisational tool for describing the knowledge and skills health care staff need to apply at work in order to deliver high quality services.

Labelling Describing someone in a way that treats them as one of a category, rather than as an individual.

Language Communication with words.

Ligaments Fibrous tissue that connects muscle to bones.

Limb An arm or leg.

Lumbar puncture Withdrawing fluid from the spinal canal.

Malpractice Immoral, unethical or illegal behaviour.

Mandatory Required by law.

Matrix Base material forming a framework for other cells or substances.

Mental state The mental condition of an individual. This can include the individual being withdrawn, depressed, agitated or confused.

Metabolism The processing of nutrients by cells to produce energy, with the production of waste products.

Micro-organism An organism that can only be seen through a microscope, including bacteria, protozoa, fungi, some algae and viruses.

Milestones Indicators for short-term objectives.

Molecule Tiny particle made up of one or more small units called atoms.

Motility How well something can move and be active.

Muscles Strong fibrous tissues, which shorten to give the body strength.

Needs of the individual The characteristics of an individual that influence choice and set-up of equipment and other resources, e.g. mobility, protection from radiation, etc.

Non-verbal communication or **body language** Ways of communicating without words, through positioning and posture, gestures, facial expression and eye contact.

Normal flora The community of micro-organisms that normally live on the surface of the body.

Objective Not influenced by emotions or personal prejudices.

Organelle A minute structure within a eukaryotic cell that has a particular function. Examples of organelles include the nucleus, mitochondria and lysosomes.

Orifice An opening, mouth of a cavity.

Pathogens Micro-organisms that cause disease.

Peritoneum A serous membrane which covers the digestive organs and the upper surface of the female uterus and is reflected back to line the wall of the abdominal cavity. This forms a double layer with a small amount of fluid between the layers allowing easy movement.

Personal clothing and fashion items Includes outer clothes worn from home to work, jewellery, acrylic nails, nail varnish and false eyelashes.

Personal development Developing the personal qualities and skills needed to live and work with others.

Personal development plan (PDP) Document used to summarise work activities and identify aims and goals over a defined period.

Personal protective clothing Items such as plastic aprons, gloves – both clean and sterile, footwear, dresses, trousers and shirts, and all-in-one trouser suits. These may be single-use disposable clothing or reusable clothing.

Personal protective clothing Items such as plastic aprons, gloves (both clean and sterile), footwear, dresses, trousers and shirts, and all-in-one trouser suits. These may be single use disposable clothing or reusable clothing.

pH The percentage of hydrogen ions in a substance, which is a measure of the acidity or alkalinity of a solution.

Physical Relating to the body.

Prejudice A belief which is not grounded with any knowledge of what is true or real.

Primary dressing Dressing applied directly onto the wound.

Reflection Deep and careful thought.

Reflective practitioner Someone who evaluates the work they do.

Register Degree of formality or informality in language.

Risk The likelihood of a hazard causing harm.

Risk assessment A formal evaluation of a particular risk.

Secondary dressing Dressing applied over the primary dressing.

Self-confidence Belief in your own abilities.

Self-esteem An individual's sense of their own worth.

Septicaemia A severe bloodstream infection, which can be fatal.

Serous fluid Thin, watery fluid produced by serous membranes which serves as a lubricant. It reduces friction where organs might rub together.

Sigmoidoscopy An examination of the inside of the rectum.

Sinus A blind-ended channel that permits the drainage of wound exudate. It extends from the surface of the wound to a cavity.

Social How people in groups behave.

Speech community A group of people who have particular ways of speaking.

Standard precautions and health and safety measures A series of interventions that minimise or prevent infection and cross-infection, including: hand washing/cleansing before during and after the activity, and the use of personal protective clothing and additional protective equipment when appropriate.

Standard precautions and health and safety measures A series of interventions that will minimise or prevent infection and cross-infection, including hand washing/cleansing before, during and after the activity, and the use of personal protective clothing and additional protective equipment where appropriate.

Stereotype Oversimplified opinion of a person.

Stimuli Physical event causing a change we are able to detect, for example, heat, cold, etc.

Synapse The minute gap between neurones, across which impulses pass.

Synovial fluid A thick, clear lubricant made mostly of carbon dioxide and some nitrogen.

Systematic Orderly.

Transient micro-organisms Micro-organisms that lie on the surface of the skin and which can easily be transferred to another person or object by touching it. They can easily be removed by proper hand washing.

Ultraviolet (UV) light Energy from sunlight, which can burn the skin if over exposed.

Undermining wound An area of tissue destruction underneath intact skin.

Universal precautions Standard infection control practices used universally in health care settings to minimise the risk of exposure to pathogens. Also known as standard precautions.

Urethral meatus Where the urethra opens to the exterior.

Urinary catheterisation Inserting a fine, hollow tube into the bladder to remove urine.

Values Principles or standards which underpin the way individuals behave.

Vicarious liability Being liable for something you did not actually do yourself. For example, an employer is vicariously liable for negligent acts or omissions by his employee in the course of employment, whether or not such act or omission was specifically authorised by the employer.

Viscera Internal organs, particularly those of the abdomen.

Vital capacity The largest amount of air we can breathe out in one expiration.

Index

Pages in *italics* indicate figures and diagrams. For definitions of terminology see the Glossary.

Index